THE MEXICAN
SALT-FREE DIET
COOKBOOK

Merle Schell

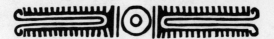

THE MEXICAN SALT-FREE DIET COOKBOOK

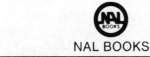

NAL BOOKS

NEW AMERICAN LIBRARY

NEW YORK AND SCARBOROUGH, ONTARIO

NAL BOOKS TRADEMARK REG. U.S. PAT. OFF. AND FOREIGN COUNTRIES
REGISTERED TRADEMARK—MARCA REGISTRADA
HECHO EN HARRISONBURG, VA., U.S.A.

SIGNET, SIGNET CLASSIC, MENTOR, ONYX, PLUME,
MERIDIAN and NAL BOOKS are published *in the United States* by
New American Library, 1633 Broadway, New York, New York 10019,
in Canada by The New American Library of Canada Limited,
81 Mack Avenue, Scarborough, Ontario M1L 1M8.

Designed by Julian Hamer

Library of Congress Cataloging-in-Publication Data

Schell, Merle.
  The Mexican salt-free diet cookbook.

  Includes index.
  1. Salt-free diet—Recipes.   2. Reducing diets—
Recipes.   3. Cookery, Mexican.   I. Title.
RM237.8.S29   1986   641.5′632   86-5326
ISBN 0-453-00509-8

First Printing, August, 1986
1 2 3 4 5 6 7 8 9
PRINTED IN THE UNITED STATES OF AMERICA

For Thelma and Jules Smolker,
my very dear parents,
for their constant love and support

Acknowledgments

Once again, I have the pleasure of publicly thanking some very caring and special people:

My good friend Amy Shouse, who dedicated days, nights, weekends and gave me untold support in assembling this book; Jennifer Maguire, who cheerfully handled countless details; my parents, Thelma and Jules Smolker, who continually provide me with valuable information and understanding; my editors, Irene Pink and Molly Allen, who worked so hard to help me realize the concept for this book.

And last, but never least, my readers. My efforts are for you, and your expressions of pleasure and thanks I gratefully and joyously acknowledge.

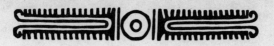

Contents

Foreword by Carl Franzblau, Ph.D.   xi
Foreword by Roman Chapa   xiii
Author's Note   xv

The Evolution of Mexican Cooking   1

History of a Civilization   1
Culture and the Arts   3
The Terrain   4
The Development of Mexican Cuisine   6

The Ingredients and Where to Find Them   9

A Mexican Pantry   10
A Low-Sodium Pantry   19

For Ease of Preparation   23

Utensils   23
Preparation and Assembly   24

**How to Adapt Your Favorite
Mexican Recipes**   25

Other Diet Tips   27

Food Watching   27
Travel and Other Pleasures   29

RECIPES 31

  Appetizers and Snacks 33

  Tortillas, Tacos, and the Like 47

  Breads 65

  Soups 75

  Salads 97

  Fish and Shellfish 109

  Poultry 131

  Meat 149

  Beans, Potatoes, Pasta, and Rice 173

  Vegetables 191

  Sauces 209

  Eggs 231

  Desserts 243

A Mexican Menu for Entertaining 255

A Mexican Diet 285

Tables of Nutritional Values 319

Bibliography 331

Index 337

Foreword

Sodium chloride, or table salt as it is commonly known, is truly an enemy of the people. It is a substance, for which we, as humans, have an absolute requirement. Yet, taken in excess, it causes all sorts of problems, including the development of hypertension. We don't think of salt in the same way we think of other food substances, such as cholesterol or sugar. It is not fattening. It doesn't give you that rush of energy. However, when used on food, it has a profound, addictive effect on taste and, consequently, there are very few cultures in the world that don't abuse the use of salt.

I can remember when my family would sit down to dinner, several of us added salt to our food even before we tasted it. Therefore, I cannot help but admire Merle Schell's efforts. Not only does she bring to the public an awareness of the salt problem, she has created a series of books that clearly are designed *not* to take the fun out of eating. On the contrary, she has chosen to focus on ethnic foods, which we all have learned to love, and has created an astonishing variety of dishes so tasty, even "salty," they do not require the overwhelming salt content usually present. This book—*The Mexican Salt-Free Diet Cookbook*—is the second in her series of salt-free ethnic cookbooks. It is not a run-of-the-mill low-salt diet book. It is unique, imaginative, and truly a labor of love.

For anyone interested in the nutritional value of food, it is extremely helpful to have the data one sees in Ms. Schell's book. Not only is the sodium content given but the calorie, carbohydrate, and fat content per serving for each recipe has been calculated. For those of us who not only want to restrict sodium intake but are also mindful of calorie, fat, and carbohydrate intake, these data are invaluable.

In summary, this book, and Ms. Schell's other efforts, serve to reintroduce us all to the art of healthy, tasty cooking. For these reasons we urge the author to continue her quest for more unusual low-salt ethnic recipes. We all need them!

—CARL FRANZBLAU, PH.D.
Professor and Chairman
of the Biochemistry Department
Boston University School of Medicine

Foreword

I am most pleased to write an introduction to Merle Schell's new book, *The Mexican Salt-Free Diet Cookbook*. I was impressed by her thorough research and knowledge of Mexican cuisine and its multi-national origins, and by her ability to translate that knowledge into recipes which everyone, including those people with special dietary requirements, will enjoy.

Most people think of Mexican food as synonymous with tacos, tortillas, guacamole, refried beans, and chile, and so endorse the myth that—while it is delicious and great fun to eat—Mexican food is also heavy, greasy, fattening, and unhealthy.

But true Mexican food is peasant food in the best sense . . . honest, basic, and simple, more often simmered than fried. Its rich flavor comes from the natural good taste of its sauces made with fresh herbs, spices, corn, tomatoes, and other vegetables.

Ms. Schell knows this and does a wonderful job of capturing the versatility, charm, and authentic eating pleasure of Mexican cuisine in recipe after recipe of this very fine book.

—ROMAN CHAPA
Owner, Pancho Villa's
restaurant chain in
New York City

Author's Note

Writing this book was a special challenge and joy! A challenge because so many thought it could not be done. And, I confess, the task of replicating, faithfully, but without salt, the mouthwateringly delicious and numerous sauces which are intrinsic to almost every Mexican dish was awesome.

But a joy, too, because after many visits to Mexico, I have grown to love the people, the country, the cuisine which so wonderfully embodies both—and I was excited and determined to do justice to them all.

So, for a variety of reasons—both personal and professional—I approached this project with great enthusiasm.

Some of my work was done for me. First, I knew I would not have to explain the merits of salt-free living. I would have been happy to do so, and did in my first two books (*Tasting Good* and *The Chinese Salt-Free Diet Cookbook*). But today, so many of us are watching the salt that it has passed the point of being a trend. It has become a fact and a way of life.

Indeed, salt is not the only target. Today, we are health conscious. Period. Physical fitness is the rule, not the exception. That is why fat, sugar, cholesterol, as well as calories, are all under attack in our determination—tantamount to a crusade—to realize our twin objectives: slimmer and healthier bodies.

In pursuit of these goals, we have witnessed many changes in the American diet over the last five years. Liquor consumption is way down. The martini lunch and before-dinner cocktail have all but disappeared, replaced, to a great extent, with seltzer water and other low-calorie, low-sodium soft drinks. Quick-trim fad diets have been rejected in favor of the old-fashioned, common sense approach to weight loss: namely, nutritional balance coupled with exercise.

This winning combination is being pursued with relentless, and typically American, enthusiasm. Health club memberships are soaring; sales of diet foods, booming. Yet despite our devotion to the healthy body beautiful, a 1986 *Time* magazine study documents that more Americans are overweight than ever before.

xv

The reason can be summed up in one word. Life-style. Think of your own jam-packed day. When it is all over, including a vigorous workout, how often do you have the time, energy, or opportunity to fix a tasty and nutritious meal to accompany that diet drink? You are not alone. Not only do we travel more, eat out and order in more, but we also like to experience more new tastes and new foods.

The explosive popularity of Mexican food is just one example. Once enjoyed primarily in the Southwest and on the West Coast, Mexican cuisine has captured the imagination and the taste buds of the entire country. Restaurants are opening everywhere. More telling are the local supermarkets where Mexican food staples and specialty items are no longer tucked away on an out-of-reach shelf, but are prominently and substantially displayed within easy vision and access of the shopper.

The trick, then, is to reconcile these seemingly contradictory needs and desires: our on-the-go, active life-styles with the control and stability most diets require to assure success; our new passion, Mexican food (well-known for its high oil, high calorie, very salty content) with our sincere desire to slim down and shape up.

It is really an easy trick to master. All it takes is a little know-how, a little compromise, and you can have your enchilada, eat it, and never pay the price.

The Mexican Salt-Free Diet Cookbook is designed to show you how. For all the popularity of Mexican cuisine, there is not one cookbook on the market especially created and taste-tested for the special- or health-conscious dieter. It is truly a shame because, in addition to providing a spectacular variety of flavors, Mexican food is basically very nutritious and can be admirably and easily adapted to suit the most rigorous dietary needs.

For example, fried foods can be simmered, flash-fried, or roasted in a very hot oven, thereby minimizing the amount of oil required. Tuna and Apricots (page 124) and Festival Chicken in Wine (page 142) deliciously demonstrate the point. Moreover, the cuisine tantalizes and sparkles with an astonishing array of herbs, spices, and condiments so pungent and distinctive that they need no other accent. When you sample the classic Beef Chile (page 150) and the exotic Chicken and Bananas (page 134), I am sure you will agree.

Knowing what to leave out, where to cut back, how to use the flavor enhancers generic to the cuisine and still produce authentic-tasting dishes—these are some of the puzzles I am happy to solve for you in *The Mexican Salt-Free Diet Cookbook*.

Once you discover the secrets and the joys of cooking delicious and healthy Mexican food, it is a very small step to apply what you learn outside the home. Let me reassure you that Mexican people are both gracious and tireless in their efforts to bring pleasure to their guests. The Mexican chef is no exception. How to help him help you get the meal you want will be explained in detail.

So, let us not waste another minute. Mexican food, and its south-of-the border charm, is something I am most eager to share. From the Pacific Ocean to the Gulf Coast, from Tijuana to the Yucatan, together we have thousands and thousands of years of glorious food to feast upon.

Note: Before using this or any other diet book and its tips, you should check with your own doctor to be sure it is compatible with your needs.

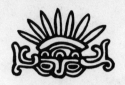

THE MEXICAN
SALT-FREE DIET
COOKBOOK

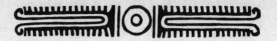

The Evolution of Mexican Cuisine

Mexican food is a spectacular blend of many cuisines and cultures. Its origins date back more than 3,000 years when the nomadic Asiatic Indian settlers first began experimenting with the strange foods of their new country.

But it is the Spanish Conquest of August 13, 1521 that must be credited for initiating modern Mexican cuisine and the diversity of tastes and foods with which we are now so familiar. The staples and delicacies from Europe, Asia, and Arabia, which were assimilated at that time, set the culinary tone for more than 300 years. The foods and cooking methods of France, Italy, and Austria arrived later, during the nineteenth-century reign of the Emperor Maximilian and Empress Carlota. Thus, modern Mexican cooking is a fusion of the finest the world's kitchens had to offer.

To better understand and appreciate the remarkable route Mexican cuisine has taken in its development, we want to take you on a brief tour back through time so that you can marvel for yourself at the emergence and growth of one of the most historically rich and exotic cultures of the world.

History of a Civilization

Archaeologists discovered that between 50,000 and 10,000 years ago, Asian Indians crossed what is now the Bering Strait in pursuit of mammoths and mastodons. They traveled on foot over a land bridge connecting Siberia and Alaska, formed during the Ice Age. Years later, when a warming trend melted that same bridge, the Indians were stranded in the New World, and the civilization of the Americas was born.

Ancient Mexico, called Mesoamerica, was comprised of 10,000 cities which reached as far south as Honduras. Trade routes were painstakingly carved through the mountains and wilderness and were, indeed, the genesis of an elaborate and highly developed exchange system through which the rituals, beliefs, and foods of one tribe permeated and became part of the culture of every other. So it was that the fundamentals of Mexican cuisine took hold.

Unfortunately, little survives of the civilizations predating 1200 B.C. But around this time, a tribe known as the Olmec established themselves in the tropical lowlands along the west coast. Power then shifted to the mountain valleys of central Mexico which produced the next great civilizations: the Tlatilco; who dominated the country from 1000 to 550 B.C.; the Cuicuilco, whose society lasted 400 years, from 500 to 100 B.C., and who were famous for building the first stone pyramid on the continent; and the mighty Teotihuacan, the most powerful of these early cultures, who reigned supreme from 150 B.C. to 700 A.D.

All the Mesoamerican civilizations lived in constant fear that the wrath of the gods would bring drought, famine, pestilence, and even annihilation to the world. And there were so many gods before whom to tremble: gods of rain, fire, sun, moon, and the most dreadful of all, Quetzalcoatl, god of wind and air. To appease these terrible beings, the ancients held nightly ceremonies during which many people were sacrificed in the midst of grotesque rituals.

Paradoxically, although savage on the one hand, these early people, particularly the Mayans, were scientifically brilliant on the other. When we consider that their magnificent cities, temples, and pyramids were built with rudimentary Stone Age technology, their architectural and engineering feats become all the more awesome. Moreover, their Calendar Round system enabled them to plot the solar and agricultural cycles so necessary to insure abundant harvests with almost as much precision as we do today.

In the 3,000 years of continuous civilization, which began with the Olmec, it is the Mayan and Aztec cultures in which modern Mexico has its deepest roots. Indeed, the marvelous Great Temple, Sacred Precinct, and other spectacular ruins of the Aztec capital, Tenochtitlan, lie beneath the busy thoroughfares of today's capital, Mexico City. Symbolically, the palace of the great Aztec leader Montezuma II is entombed directly below Mexico's seat of government, the National Palace.

The Mayans, who brought major cultural and scientific advances to the Indian civilization, were also masters of war. But their ferocity paled beside the force and sheer numbers of the warlike Aztecs who slaughtered and plundered their way to power in the 200 years before the Spanish Conquest. Ironically, they fell victim to the same fate when, with even greater dispatch, the Spanish ravaged and laid bare city after city in the first years after their victory. Almost nothing remains of this proud nation, which was obliterated in Cortes's quest for jewels, silver, gold, and other precious metals.

The treasure he sought for the Spanish Crown and for himself was displayed in the breathtaking splendor which greeted the Spanish army as it marched into Tenochtitlan and the kingdom of Montezuma II. Borne aloft on a litter bedecked with blindingly beautiful gems, the Aztec king came to meet his visitors. His mantle blazed with jewels; his feet were shod in gold. Dazzling opulence was everywhere. And Montezuma, by nature a peaceable man, lavished these riches on the strangers in his midst, choosing to treat them like gods rather than enemies. By the time he realized his mistake, it was too late.

Aided by Montezuma's Aztec foes, Cortes's meager band of 550 men vanquished a city of 100,000 people. With the defeat of this mightiest of Indian nations, the fall of all Mesoamerica was virtually assured.

In the 400 years following the Spanish Conquest, the country was repeatedly scarred by uprisings, warfare, and cultural clashes. But as in all things, the pain of the past forged the future. Mexico has emerged a unique and colorful new nation which, happily, continues to reflect the richness of its remarkable legacy.

Culture and the Arts

Mexicans have a saying: North Americans live to work, but Mexicans work to live. That is because family, friends, religion, and hospitality are the center of their lives. Thus, if work must be delayed to accommodate love, duty, and honor, so be it.

Every birthday, every baptism, every personal occasion is cause to celebrate, with an extended family of immediate and distant relatives, godparents and their relatives, co-workers and passersby. This effusive warmth and goodwill are bestowed on strangers as well.

Several years ago, on my first trip to Mexico, I got lost on my way to Chapultepec Park and the National Museum of Anthropology. Observing my distress, an elegant Mexican gentleman offered to be my guide. Thanks to this charming escort, I enjoyed a delightful, informative, and memorable day. All of which proves that a little Mexican spontaneity is good for the soul.

Mexicans pour the same unbridled exuberance into every aspect of their lives. Homes, buses, office buildings are splashed with rich, vibrant reds, purples, pinks, oranges, and yellows. The rainbows of flowers which sprout untamed throughout the countryside are also whimsically displayed in every nook and cranny, lending a heartwarming gaiety to even the most impoverished locale.

On a higher artistic plane, Mexican handicrafts—rugs, jewelry, pottery, and clothing, including rebozos (shawls) and huipils (long blouses)—strikingly exhibit the bold, geometric patterns of their Indian heritage.

But the full force of Mexico's artistic passion is experienced in her architecture and art. Soaring Mayan pyramids and Aztec temples, which rival the spectacular structures of ancient Egypt, stand in breathtaking contrast to the ornate baroque edifices of European design. The same sweeping intensity is captured, on a smaller scale, in the art of Mexico's finest painters. The works of Diego, Orozco, Siqueiros, and Rivera are almost painful in their beauty and emotional force. To see them is to understand why Mexicans elevate their artists to heroic heights.

If artists are her heroes, music is Mexico's soul. Every major religious and personal celebration is accompanied by the strains of mariachi music —Mexico's version of the blues. Costumed caballeros strum their guitars on December 12, as pilgrims make their way to the Basilica in Mexico City to honor the Virgin of Guadalupe. They join in the raucous parade on November 2, marking the Day of the Dead, each one sporting a marigold, which the Aztecs believed was the flower of the dead. And every January 6, they help celebrate the third of Mexico's national fiestas, the Day of the Three Kings. At once rhythmic, undulating, and driving, this music captures the essence of the sensual Mexican personality.

The wonderfully rich heritage of their culture forms a bond uniting the fifty-four ethnic groups which co-exist in modern Mexico. Predominant among them are the mestizos, who account for more than 90 percent of the country's 74 million people. Descendants of the Spanish conquistadores and Indian women, mestizos were once despised as half-breeds. However, then and now, the mestizos were and are Indian in their cultural habits and philosophy. They cling to their centuries-old bloodlines and revere the glory of ancestral accomplishments with as much fervor as do their pure Indian cousins.

Sadly, of the remaining 10 percent little more than 3 percent of the population can trace their roots directly to the early Mesoamericans. The remainder are the criollas—Mexicans of pure Spanish blood.

Although 13 percent of the populace still speaks Indian, Spanish is the national language, and Catholicism the universal religion. These are major accomplishments of the conquistadores. So, too, is their helping to shape one of the world's greatest cuisines. It is significant, however, that despite the slavery, persecution, and vilification, which they inflicted on their captives, the Spanish could not destroy the deeply rooted culture of these Indian people. Indeed, the National Museum of Anthropology is Mexico's greatest national treasure. It proudly and beautifully displays the relics and history of its splendid past.

The last Aztec king, Cuauhtemoc, surrendered to the Spanish in 1521. He would be pleased if he knew how much of his world lives on in the hearts and traditions of the Mexican people.

The Terrain

The Mexican terrain is as much a study in contrasts as is the mosaic character of its people. Lush, primeval forests stop abruptly at the edge of desolate desert, untouched and uninhabited since the beginning of civilization. Cool green valleys wander lazily through the tropical jungle lowlands, ending at the glittering blaze of golden sand that stretches along the coast. Craggy, bleak mountain ranges split the country north to south, and even they hide a world of extremes.

For example, the western Sierra Madres, located in the state of Jalisco, cut through the north central plains, and are as treacherous as they are beautiful. Their pristine, snow-capped peaks conceal volcanoes—like the dangerous El Paricutin—threateningly poised for eruption. Yet cradled within their midst are tranquil highland forests, resplendent with vegetables, herbs, spices, and fish-filled lakes.

These apparent contradictions echo throughout Mexico's almost two million square miles. But it is because the terrain is so filled with extremes that it can produce the extraordinary assortment of foodstuffs which makes Mexican cuisine unfailingly interesting and impressive.

The Central Valley is the heartland of Mexico. The area spans 3,000 square miles and is nestled 7,000 feet above sea level among three mountain ranges: the Sierra Las Cruces on the west, the Sierra Ajusco on the south, and the Sierra Nevada on the east.

Cattle graze on the plains, wheat flourishes in the northern region, and the Mexican staples—maize and beans—grow here as they do in every part of the country. Yet, more important than its crops is the Central Valley's function as a passageway. Since prehistoric times, trade routes have snaked through its mountains connecting key cities, which today include Acapulco on the Pacific Coast, Oaxaca to the south, and Veracruz on the Gulf Coast.

The Central Gulf Coast is one of the country's most fertile provinces. Thanks to a hot, tropical climate and abundant rainfall, it is an agricultural bonanza. Citrus and tropical fruits, corn, sugarcane, and coffee thrive, and there is ample grazing for cattle. Numerous rivers and the Gulf Stream provide a lavish and almost infinite supply of fresh seafood. What is more, via Veracruz, these rich harvests are easily and quickly transported to the rest of the country.

Although the Central Valley is extraordinarily productive, virtually every Mexican region, except the desert, is a horn of plenty. Even the Yucatan, with its poor limestone soil, is able to harvest crops.

There are three reasons for this happy state of affairs. First, three of Mexico's borders are bounded by water, which is a source of both food and irrigation. Second, even at its highest altitudes, Mexico is spring-like all year, rarely dipping below 60° Fahrenheit in the mountains, and averaging 85° Fahrenheit in the interior and coastal lowlands. Third, the many mountain ranges which zigzag across the country create myriad plateaus and valleys where animals and foods flourish.

From the days of the Mayans and Aztecs, agriculture and fishing have been the livelihood of Mexico's people. That they remain so today is natural and good. That they spring from the majesty of the mountains and the mystery of the seas seems allegorical, and so, the birthright of the Mexican people.

The Development
of Mexican Cuisine

Of all the cuisines of the world, Mexican is among the most brilliantly diverse, the product of an exquisite and fascinating commingling of many cultures.

Thousands of years ago, in early Mesoamerica, the nucleus of Mexican cuisine was formed. Chiles, tomatoes, beans, and corn were its cornerstones. Corn, in particular, was deified by the Mayans and Aztecs in this pre-Christian era. Interestingly, the ancient corn specialties—tortillas, tacos, tamales, and quesadillas—have emerged intact from that ancient time, the same now as they were then.

The foods of these primitive cultures were unknown outside the Americas, and were precious booty for Cortes. Today they are still very much part of the cuisine, as are chocolate, vanilla, peanuts, avocados, squash, sweet potatoes, pineapples, bananas, papaya and other tropical fruits.

In the post-Hispanic period European foods and cooking styles gradually became part of the Mexican kitchen. The tender chickens, which Spain introduced, quickly replaced the tough, gamey wild turkeys. Spain was also responsible for bringing in many of the foods now synonymous with Mexican cuisine—namely, pork, cheese, onions, and garlic. A veritable avalanche streamed from the larders of Spanish ships, including oil, wine, cinnamon, cloves, rice, wheat, sugar, almonds, beef, dairy products, and citrus fruits.

It is important to note that this bounty was not endemic to Spain alone. Honey, sausage, and beer were German in origin; other foods, Asian. The Arab countries—which had dominated Spain for centuries just prior to Spain's own conquest of Mexico—contributed many more.

Of course, recipes and cooking styles emigrated along with the foods. For example, the classic dish ceviche could not have existed without the lemons and limes of Spain. Marinating foods in succulent wine sauces and simmering them to tender perfection are cooking methods used in many of Mexico's most famous dishes. Both techniques are Spanish as well as French in origin.

Moreover, the most basic condiment on the Mexican table, salsa, is based on Italian tomato sauce. It is hard to believe that this important staple did not appear in Mexico's food repertoire until the brief French-dominated reign (1864–1867) of Archduke Maximilian of Austria. He and his Belgian wife Carlota introduced the ingredients, recipes, and cooking styles of France, Austria, and Italy, and so put the finishing touches on Mexican cuisine.

Over the last 150 years, since Mexico became an independent country totally free of foreign rule, Mexican cooking has truly come into its own. Regional specialties have emerged. The Gulf Coast city of Veracruz established its artistry in the preparation of the seafood which flourish off its shores. On the western boundary, the seafood dishes of Acapulco, Puerto Vallarta, and, especially, Mazatlan are almost as well known. Yucatan, at the country's southern tip, is noted for its suckling pig. Inland, Oaxaca is justifiably acclaimed for its many delicious moles, and Puebla is honored for originating Mexico's national dish, Chicken Mole (page 140).

The evolution of hundreds of centuries is complete. Mexican cuisine is no longer an exciting, colorful, ever-changing patchwork quilt, but a tapestry, extraordinarily rich, of lustrous depths, recalling the past and preserving for the future an excitingly singular cuisine.

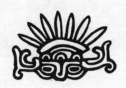

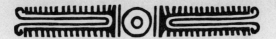

The Ingredients and Where to Find Them

The experience of shopping in a Mexican open-air market is an innocent joy like no other. You will not know where to look first as your eyes are dazzled by the colorful, riotous clutter and splendid array. Tropical-size zucchinis, tomatoes, avocados, platanos, hundreds of chiles, and more, peak in precarious pyramids high over the tops of baskets, stalls, wagons, and trucks.

Dogs, cats, babies, donkeys, chickens seem to be everywhere you turn, heightening the festive confusion, their mingled chorus a counterpoint to the good-natured bantering and arguing of the vendors and their customers. And flowers—shimmering blues and whites, brilliant yellows, pinks, and reds—dance in every available sliver of space. The air is ripe with scents and sounds, while overhead a technicolor-blue sky embraces the mountains which arch and stretch to meet it.

Mexican (and Spanish) food stores cannot duplicate this spectacular opulence. But they can and do offer an equally prodigious display of foodstuffs, herbs, and spices, along with the same warmth and easy charm of the Mexican market. Of course, you can buy almost all the Mexican ingredients you will need in your own supermarkets, but it will not be as much fun.

Many ingredients generic to Mexican cuisine are not to be found in this book. That is because some of the more exotic items are only available in Spanish or Mexican markets, which do not exist in every part of this country, and because some of the ingredients are usually available only in canned, salted form.

But this book neither pretends nor intends to be an authentic replication of Mexican cuisine. What it does promise is authentic taste, true to the style and flavor of the Mexican kitchen and its heritage.

The ingredients list which follows itemizes not only those Mexican foods used throughout this book but those forbidden to us low-sodium dieters as well. For the latter, substitutions and low-sodium options are noted where appropriate.

In addition, you will find a list of low-sodium "musts." Once you stock your pantry with the foods described on the following pages, you will be fully equipped to embark on your Mexican culinary excursion.

A Mexican Pantry

ACHIOTE
Used for coloring as much as for flavoring, achiote are the dark red seeds produced by the annatto tree. Because it is not readily available here—unless you are lucky enough to have a Spanish market nearby—we have substituted cayenne pepper or dried chiles where achiote would normally be called for.

ALCOHOL (See also individual listings.)
Except for sherry and wine, alcohol is used sparingly in Mexican cuisine, but when called for, it adds a distinctive and important flavor. Although alcohol is low in sodium, its sugar content may be unacceptable for diabetics, who may either substitute orange juice or eliminate it altogether.

ALLSPICE
Although so named because its rich scent hints of a clove, cinnamon, and nutmeg combination, allspice is actually a berry of the evergreen family. Native to Mexico and other Caribbean countries, allspice is available whole or ground in supermarkets everywhere and is most often used in baked goods or with sweet vegetables. Stored in jars in a cool, dry place, it will keep indefinitely.

ANISEED (FENNEL SEED)
Originally from the eastern Mediterranean and used as a medicine in ancient Syria, the small, grayish aniseed is a member of the parsley family. Its licorice flavor is a common presence in Mexican food, where it is used to accent meats and vegetables, and baked goods as well. Aniseed and its taste-alike, fennel seed, are readily available in Mexican food stores and in most supermarkets. Stored in jars or plastic bags and kept on a cool, dry shelf, both aniseed and fennel seed will keep indefinitely.

AVOCADO
The base for one of Mexico's most famous dishes, Guacamole (page 34), ripe avocados are a delicious and healthy treat—low in sodium, high in potassium. Ripen hard avocados at room temperature. When ready for eating, they should be tender but not soft to the touch, and the flesh should be firm and creamy. Cut avocados turn slightly brown in the air, but putting lemon juice on the exposed surface should prevent this occurrence. This lovely, nutty-flavored fruit is available at food stores everywhere.

BANANAS
Known as platanos, the Mexican variety of this popular fruit is more fibrous and generally larger than its United States counterpart and comes in a variety of colors. Platanos are always available in Mexican and Spanish markets, but our domestic fruit is a more than acceptable replacement. Both platanos and bananas should be allowed to ripen at room temperature, and then refrigerated to retard spoilage. They should be used within 2 to 3 days of ripening.

BAY LEAF
The dried leaf of the laurel tree, native to the Mediterranean, bay leaf probably came via Turkey or Portugal to Spain and from there to Mexico, where it became an important part of the cuisine. Its slightly sharp taste is an essential flavoring for many of the soups, sauces, and stews that are featured at the Mexican table. Stored in a tightly closed plastic bag or jar and kept in a cool, dry place, bay leaf will keep its delightful pungency indefinitely.

BEANS
Black, pink, pinto, green, brown, yellow—beans of every variety are an integral part of Mexican cuisine, predating the Spanish Conquest. Happily, they are available everywhere and will keep indefinitely on the shelf in a tightly closed plastic container.

CAYENNE PEPPER
The dried and powdered form of the moderately hot cayenne chile, cayenne pepper adds a zesty bite to the cuisine of Mexico as well as to that of China and India. Because of its increasing popularity, cayenne pepper is readily available in food stores everywhere. Kept in a tightly closed jar and stored in a cool, dry place, it will keep its rich, full flavor indefinitely.

CHEESE
Now an integral and important part of the cuisine, cheese was unheard of in Mexico until the Spanish brought dairy cattle to the country about 1530. Today, Mexicans have developed a marvelous variety of cheeses, which admirably complement their corn- and chile-based diet.

Because these cheeses contain salt, we have, of course, substituted low-sodium varieties. For example, for the stringy, slightly acidic *quesillo de Oaxaca*, we use low-sodium mozzarella with spices or low-sodium Muenster. For the slightly sharp *queso Chihuahua*, also known as *queso asado*, we substitute low-sodium Cheddar or Swiss. For the very salty *queso añejo*, we again use low-sodium Cheddar or Swiss sparked with sharp spices. And for the Mexican cream cheese with its mildly sour taste, we choose low-sodium cream cheese, usually blended with a wine or vinegar.

Available in health food stores and many supermarkets, most low-sodium cheeses will keep up to one month in the refrigerator if tightly sealed in plastic or aluminum foil. If a white or green mold does form, simply cut it off (the cheese is still good).

There are a few exceptions: cartoned cheeses, such as cottage cheese and ricotta, will stay fresh only 1 week after opening. Mozzarella will start to soften and form a brownish mold 2 to 3 weeks after opening, but wonderfully, in this state, mozzarella tastes very much like Brie or Camembert.

Note: For the nutritional content of low-sodium cheeses, consult the Tables of Nutritional Values (page 320).

CHILES

Chiles are synonymous with Mexican cuisine. One or more of over 100 varieties, in fresh or dried form, is found in the majority of dishes. The misconception is that all chiles are fiery hot. Indeed, some are, including the popular jalapeño and serrano and the less familiar morita, chipotle, and pequín (or tepín). But many more are merely spicy (picante) or mild, ranging from the long, dark pasilla, the large ancho, the tapering mulato, the well-known poblano, and the sweet valenciano and güero.

Mexican dishes often call for specific chiles. However, not all chiles are available everywhere, so part of the fun of Mexican cooking is substituting one chile for another to suit your own tastes and creative whims, just as the Mexicans do. In fact, it is this experimentation that partially distinguishes one region's cuisine from another's.

The innovative use of chiles underlies the charm and versatility of Mexican cooking. Not only are fresh varieties exchanged on a whim, but dried chiles, chili powder, cayenne pepper, and paprika are often used as substitutes.

Dried chiles will keep indefinitely when stored in a plastic bag on a cool, dry shelf. They are available in Mexican and Spanish markets, at most vegetable stands, and in some supermarkets, particularly those in the southern and western United States.

As for fresh chiles, traditionalists always peel them before use by broiling, grilling, or frying the chiles until the skin blisters. Once cooled, the skin is then easily removed.

Although we are not going to be as exacting in this book, we do caution you to always remove the veins, as well as the seeds, for it is in the veins that the heat-producing ingredient capsaicin is found.

Fresh chiles may be bought wherever dried are sold. They will stay fresh about one week in the vegetable bin of your refrigerator.

Note: Canned chiles can be found everywhere, but avoid them because they are packed in a salt solution.

CHILI POWDER

A finely ground powder made of dried chile peppers, cumin, oregano, garlic powder, cayenne or black pepper, and, sometimes, paprika. Available bottled in the spice section of food stores everywhere, most commercial varieties contain salt. Therefore, we have supplied our favorite salt-free blend in the Sauces and Seasonings section of this book. Like its salty counterparts, our Chili Powder (page 210) will keep its potency indefinitely if stored in a tightly closed container on a cool, dark shelf.

CHOCOLATE
Mexican chocolate is a blend of ground cacao beans, almond, and sugar which dates back to pre-Columbian days. Its bittersweet flavor is most closely duplicated by our own semisweet or bittersweet varieties. For our purposes, we have gone one step further and substituted low-sodium bittersweet chocolate (which is also sugar-free). Low-sodium chocolates are widely distributed in health food stores and many supermarkets by a number of manufacturers. If refrigerated, they will keep indefinitely wrapped in plastic or aluminum foil.

CHORIZO
A spicy sausage, sometimes made with beef, but most often with pork. The store-bought chorizo found in Mexican and Spanish markets always contains salt, but a delicious replacement is provided in the Meat section of this book. Once prepared, our Chorizo (page 158) should be tightly wrapped in plastic or aluminum foil. It may be refrigerated up to 1 week, or frozen indefinitely. *Note*: If you freeze our Chorizo, divide it into small, serving-size packets.

CILANTRO
See Coriander.

CINNAMON
More than 2,000 years ago, cinnamon was prized in Egypt for its magical effect on the body and on the emotions. It is held in much the same esteem today in Mexico—although no longer as a medicine or perfume, but rather as a sweet, intoxicating flavor for a great variety of dishes. Mexican cinnamon, both the stick and ground form, comes from the soft cinnamon bark imported from Ceylon. Although slightly more pungent, the Indian cinnamon imported for the United States is an acceptable substitute. Cinnamon will keep indefinitely if stored in a tightly sealed container on a dark, cool shelf.

CLOVES
Cloves are seeds from tropical evergreens and were first discovered in the Moluccas of Indonesia. In ancient times, cloves were rare and so precious that those parents who could secure them planted the seeds to bless and honor the birth of a child. Today, although cloves are readily available, ground or whole, in supermarkets everywhere, they are as wonderful as ever, lending their aroma and flavor to any number of Mexican dishes. Stored in a tightly closed container and kept in a cool, dry place, they will keep indefinitely.

CORIANDER

This fresh, green, slightly sharp-tasting herb is known as cilantro in Mexico, but is most commonly known here as Chinese parsley. It is easily found in Chinese markets everywhere. Fresh coriander will keep up to one week if refrigerated in a tightly closed plastic bag. When dried, it is very perishable. Thus, the more readily available, though milder, parsley, to which coriander is related, is the substitute used throughout this book in both fresh and dried forms. Like coriander, fresh parsley will keep about one week if refrigerated. In dried form, it will keep indefinitely if stored in a tightly sealed container in a cool, dark place.

CORN (See also Masa Harina.)

Corn can be traced in Mexico to 5,000 B.C. This vegetable is one of the cornerstones of Mexican culture and cuisine. Indeed, corn is as much the Mexican staff of life today as it was long ago. Every part of the plant is used: young ears for tamales, dried corn for flour called masa, corn husk for tamale wrappings, and corn silk for a tea believed to have medicinal properties. In this book, we use the already prepared corn flour called masa harina, which is described later in this section.

CORN HUSKS

Used for enclosing tamales, corn husks (or *hojas*) are dried until they are wafer-thin and papery. To prevent cracking, they must be softened in hot water, then drained before use. Available in Mexican and Spanish food stores everywhere, corn husks should be purchased as needed, for they tend to become brittle. Aluminum foil, though unorthodox, is a more accessible container, however, and is, therefore, used throughout this book.

CREAM

Mexican cream is similar in taste and texture to the tart French *crème fraîche*. It is made by adding 4 to 6 tablespoons of buttermilk to 1 pint of heavy cream. This mixture should be covered and set in a warm place to "sour" for 4 to 6 hours, then refrigerated, where it will keep for about 1 week. Because buttermilk contains salt, we have opted for heavy cream in the recipes in this book. But if your restrictions are not severe, by all means use this puckery treat whenever heavy cream is called for.

CUMIN SEED

Cumin seed, along with aniseed and mint, predates biblical times and is, indeed, mentioned in the Bible as a precious offering. Superstition and romance mark its history, for cumin was said to bring luck to newlyweds and guarantee a bountiful harvest. Originally found in Egypt, today cumin is an integral part of many international cuisines, including that of Germany, whence it entered Spain and then Mexico. It is hard to conceive of Mexican food without the pungency of cumin in ground or seed form, and it is one of the primary ingredients in our Chili Powder (page 210). Available everywhere, cumin will keep indefinitely if stored in a tightly closed container in a dark, dry place.

DRIED CHILES (HOT PEPPER FLAKES)
Dried chiles are used as often as fresh in Mexican cuisine. Small bursts of fire, dried chiles are available whole or crushed in most markets. Cayenne pepper is a reasonable substitute. Dried chiles should be stored in a tightly closed plastic bag and will keep indefinitely on the shelf. In this book, crushed dried chiles are referred to as hot pepper flakes.

EPAZOTE
This pungent herb is worthy of mention because no Mexican cook would prepare black beans without it. Its sharp odor is as distinct as its somewhat medicinal flavor, making epazote an acquired taste. For these reasons, as well as because it is not easy to come by, we beg the purists' pardon for not having used it in this book.

GARLIC
An ancient herb, this bulb plant, which grows best in warm climates, can be traced to Egypt 5,000 to 6,000 years ago. Although garlic is available in many forms, including powder, flakes, and juice, the fresh is so easily found in supermarkets that we prefer to use it most often. Fresh garlic will keep several weeks if refrigerated. The various dried forms will keep indefinitely if stored in tightly closed containers; likewise, the juice, if refrigerated.

GREEN TOMATOES or TOMATILLOS
The green tomato is actually not a tomato at all, but a tiny, puckery fruit related to the gooseberry. They grow wild in papery husks which remind one of Japanese lanterns, and are so delicate they can only be exported canned. Unfortunately, canned green tomatoes contain salt, so we have had to forego their lovely taste and color in this book and have adapted our recipes for the red tomato.

JICAMA
This white root vegetable, which resembles a turnip, is covered with a hard brown skin and should be peeled and sliced or chopped before eating. Its crisp, crunchy, and refreshingly sweet taste is especially delightful in salads. Although plentiful in California, jicama is not widely available in the rest of the country. An adequate substitute is the Jerusalem artichoke, which is more commonly found in food store produce sections. Unpeeled, both jicama and Jerusalem artichokes will keep up to 3 weeks in the vegetable bin of your refrigerator.

KAHLUA
A coffee-flavored liqueur of which Mexico is justly proud.

MASA HARINA
The corn flour used for making tortillas, masa harina is sold in bulk in Spanish and Mexican markets everywhere. Stored in a tightly closed container, it will keep indefinitely on the shelf.

MINT
Once known as a symbol of hospitality, mint adds a welcome and refreshing flavor to food. In Mexican cooking, spearmint, known as *yerba buena*, is the most widely used variety of this sweet-tasting herb. Although easy to grow, spearmint is not easily found in the more convenient dried form. However, since the somewhat stronger-tasting plain mint is readily available both fresh and dried in supermarkets, we use it throughout this book. Fresh mint will only keep about one week in the crisper section of your refrigerator. However, dried mint will keep indefinitely if stored in jars or plastic bags in a cool, dark place.

MOLE
This highly flavored sauce of chocolate, chiles, and numerous other spices is a Mexican delicacy. It is available in canned form in Mexican food stores, but since this commercial blend is heavily salted, it is not for our consumption. We do not offer a specific unsalted recipe in this book because mole is an acquired taste. But it may very well be to your taste and, if so, by all means savor its unique pungency in Chicken Mole (page 140). If you choose, you can then make your own mole sauce from this recipe; it will keep up to 2 weeks in the refrigerator or 1 month in the freezer if stored in a tightly closed plastic container.

NUTMEG
Nutmeg, yet another product of the evergreen family, originated in the Moluccas. It was probably first discovered on an Arabian foray into the West Indies. The nutmeg spice is actually the pit of the nutmeg fruit, sold whole or ground. It is available in all food stores and will keep indefinitely if stored in a tightly closed container in a cool, dark place.

NUTS
Nuts of every kind play an important role in Mexican cuisine. Not only are they used to add their particular subtle flavors to every conceivable type of dish, but when crushed to a fine powder, they also serve as a delicious thickening agent in sauces and stews, replacing cream, eggs, or flour.

Interestingly, the only nuts indigenous to Mexico are pecans, peanuts, and pumpkin and squash seeds. One debt Mexicans owe their Spanish conquerors is the latter's introduction of walnuts, filberts, almonds, pine nuts, and sesame seeds—all of which are requisites of the Mexican chef.

Nuts, of course, are available everywhere and will retain their fresh flavor for months if kept in tightly closed containers and stored in a cool, dry place. We, of course, use only the unsalted varieties.

ONIONS
We mention this universal vegetable not because it is unique to Mexican cuisine but only to point out that the yellow onion grown in this country is generally not as sharply flavored as the white onion produced in Mexico. In the recipes in this book, we have tried to compensate for this slight difference by using various other ingredients to enhance the onion.

OREGANO
Some call it wild marjoram. The Greeks named it "joy of the mountain." But by any name at all, this sweet herb of the mint family is delicious in any dish. Oregano is most commonly available in dried or ground form. If stored in a tightly closed container, it will keep indefinitely in a cool, dark place.

PAPRIKA
Spanish paprika is an often-used alternative to cayenne pepper, which, in turn, is an appropriate substitute for the pequín, a small, dried, very hot red pepper. For our purposes, commercially prepared paprika, which is generally of a milder order than its Spanish counterpart, will suffice.

PARSLEY
See Coriander.

PEPPERCORNS
Mexican cooks use only whole peppercorns both in cooking and to grind fresh at the table. Although black peppercorns are the most common, white, green, and the more exotic pink varieties can be used interchangeably, as desired.

RICE
Rice—that small white grain served in Mexico with as much frequency as the beloved beans—was a gift of the Spanish conquistadores. Today it is an integral part of Mexican cuisine. Rarely served plain, it is flavored with soup stocks, herbs, and spices, and is often cooked with vegetables, meat, fish, or poultry as well. Rice is almost as important to Mexican cooking as it is to Chinese. Stored in plastic containers or jars, it will keep indefinitely on the shelf.

RUM
Mexico makes its own rum (and vodka and gin as well), which is most popular in mixed drinks like the daiquiri and is also used more than occasionally in cooking.

SEVILLE ORANGES
Tart, and to some palates sour, the Seville orange is generally available in this country only in Spanish and Puerto Rican food stores. Thus, because

they are not easy to come by and are very expensive, throughout this book we have substituted a combination of our home-grown sweet oranges plus lemon or lime juice to approximate the taste of the Seville orange.

SHERRY (See Wine.)

Unknown in pre-Hispanic times, dry sherry and red and white wines now play a major role in the Mexican kitchen. They are often used in marinades to flavor or tenderize, as well as to impart a rich, heady flavor to foods as they cook. One important note: never use the cooking sherry or cooking wines you find on your supermarket shelves. They all contain salt. Instead, choose any inexpensive regular sherry or wine for your pantry. They will provide the flavor you need, without salt, and will keep indefinitely on the shelf.

TAMALES

Made from cornmeal, tamales date back to pre-Hispanic times. Their sticky surfaces are generally filled with a variety of chicken, meat, or sauce blends, then traditionally wrapped in corn husks or banana leaves and steamed. They are a staple in the Mexican diet; our recipe can be found on page 61.

TEQUILA

The best-known and most popular of those Mexican alcoholic beverages made from the century (or maguey) plant. Named for a major tequila-producing town in Jalisco, tequila is most commonly enjoyed straight with a lick of salt and a squeeze of lime between sips, or as the mixed favorite: the salt-rimmed margarita. However, for us, the charms of tequila will be reserved for the more exotic (and salt-free) tequila sunrise.

TOMATOES

For thousands of years, this luscious fruit, indigenous to Mexico, has been one of the four primary staples in Mexican cuisine (the others being beans, chiles, and corn). Not only are tomatoes an important ingredient in almost every dish, they are also the basis for many of the sauces, called *tingas*, so often and lavishly used. For cooking, Mexicans peel tomatoes by blanching them in boiling water, then submerging them in cold water. The skin practically cracks off with this method. However, to conserve time, in this book we irreverently use tomatoes skin and all. Although unorthodox, the results are equally delicious.

TORTILLAS

Except for the white-flour northern variety, these wafer-thin pancakes are most commonly corn-based and can be traced back to the Mayan and Aztec cultures. More than Mexico's staff of life, tortillas are also this country's most versatile food: they are alternately stuffed, baked, shredded, fried, rolled, crimped, served plain, filled, or piled with every imaginable food mixture and sauce. Until recently, tortillas were rhythmically slapped into shape by hand, following the ancient methods. Today homemade tortillas are prepared more quickly and easily with the help of a tortilla press (page 23). A recipe for this most basic of Mexican foods appears on page 48.

VANILLA
Mexico is famous for the rich aroma and flavor of this amber liquid, crushed and pressed from orchid pods in Papantla, and used primarily in baked goods. In fact, it was one of the delicacies Cortes's aides wrote home about, as it was then unknown outside the Americas. Today, bottled vanilla extract (though generally not the Mexican variety) is sold everywhere. Stored on a cool, dark shelf, it will keep its full-bodied flavor indefinitely.

VINEGAR
The red, white, and cider vinegars used throughout this book are widely available. You need only remember to be wary of herbed, spiced, or seasoned blends, which sometimes contain salt. Vinegar will keep indefinitely on the shelf.

WINE, RED or WHITE
See Sherry.

A Low-Sodium Pantry

BEETS, CANNED
Beets and, for that matter, a veritable cornucopia of other vegetables are widely available today canned in water for low-sodium consumption. You can find these items in the diet section of most supermarkets, as well as in health food stores. So popular have they become that, like their salty counterparts, they are usually available in two sizes (8 and 16 ounces), often produced by leading brand-name manufacturers. Because they are vacuum-packed, they have an indefinite shelf life. In addition, there is a bonus: because salt drains off the flavorful moisture of any food, the low-sodium products taste fresher and richer than the salty ones.

Note: Although frozen vegetables are also acceptable, they often have added salt, so before using them, read the labels carefully.

BOUILLON, BEEF and CHICKEN
Bouillon mixed with boiling water is a commonly used shortcut when a recipe calls for soup or stock. But there's a big difference between salted and unsalted bouillon. One teaspoon of salted beef or chicken bouillon contains 1,143 milligrams of sodium—more than some of us are allowed all day. Compare that to unsalted beef bouillon, which has only 10 milli-

grams of sodium per teaspoon, or unsalted chicken bouillon, which has only 5 milligrams of sodium per teaspoon—an amazingly healthy difference.

These low-sodium seasonings are widely available today in health food stores and supermarkets throughout the country. Some come in powdered form; others are granulated, packed in small jars. Low-sodium chicken bouillon is an instant "salty" pick-me-up for poultry, fish and shellfish, and vegetables. Low-sodium beef bouillon has the same effect on all meats. Low-sodium bouillon has the added benefits of being low in fat, carbohydrates, and calories, and high in potassium. It will keep indefinitely on the shelf.

CELERY SEED
These tiny brown seeds from the root of wild celery are similar in taste but actually no relation to the celery commonly found in supermarket produce sections. Celery seed is found on the spice racks of these same markets and will keep indefinitely on your shelf if stored in a tightly closed container in a cool, dry place. Since France is a primary source, celery seed was probably brought into Mexico during the brief reign of Maximilian and Carlota.

CHEESE (See also page 11.)
Low-sodium cheeses are so popular, you can find them in health food stores and supermarkets throughout the country. The variety is amazing and their flavor excellent. Although not as long-lasting as their salty cousins, low-sodium cheeses will stay fresh in your refrigerator up to one month. For nutritional content, consult the Tables of Nutritional Values (page 320).

CORN, CANNED
Corn, plain or creamed-style, is one of the many vegetables available canned for the low-sodium dieter. See Beets.

HOT CHERRY PEPPERS
Available in the pickle section of most supermarkets, low-sodium hot cherry peppers generally come in 16-ounce jars. Pickled in distilled vinegar, these spicy hot peppers contain only 7 milligrams of sodium per ounce compared to approximately 386.6 milligrams of sodium per ounce for their brine-packed counterparts. Once opened, low-sodium hot cherry peppers should be refrigerated and will keep indefinitely.

KETCHUP
Ketchup probably came to Mexico via Italy. This tomato-based condiment and its low-sodium counterpart are widely available in food stores throughout the country. One variation is low-sodium chili ketchup, which contains chopped onion and sometimes chopped pickle. Fortunately, low-sodium ketchup and chili ketchup have only 5 to 10 milligrams of sodium per tablespoon compared to 298 milligrams for the salted products. Once opened, these low-sodium items should be refrigerated where they will keep indefinitely.

LEMON PEEL POWDER
Ground from dried lemon peel, this spice concentrate adds zip to any dish. It is available in the spice sections of food stores throughout the country. If bottled or tightly sealed in a plastic bag and stored in a cool, dry place, it will keep its full, pungent flavor indefinitely.

MAYONNAISE
Available in a wide variety of sizes, low-sodium mayonnaise is marketed by several leading health manufacturers. Some brands are flavored with honey, others with egg yolks, and still others with lemon juice. All are delicious and, at only 4 milligrams sodium per tablespoon, a lot healthier than the salted commercial brands containing 85.5 milligrams sodium for the same tablespoon. Once opened, low-sodium mayonnaise should be refrigerated immediately and will keep indefinitely.

MUSTARD
Hot, mild, Dijon, deli, or salad style, low-sodium mustard can be found everywhere. Although it contains only 3 to 7 milligrams per ounce versus the 358 to 373 milligrams for the salty blends, low-sodium mustard has a pungent, zesty flavor that is every bit as tasty, if not tastier, than the salted varieties. Once opened, it should be refrigerated and will keep indefinitely.

ORANGE PEEL POWDER
Ground from dried orange peel. See Lemon Peel Powder.

SUGAR SUBSTITUTES
Natural sugar—whether raw or processed—is a simple carbohydrate. Diabetics, of course, should avoid it altogether, and too much of it is unhealthy for all of us. The sugar substitutes on the market come in packets containing one- or two-teaspoon equivalents, and are sold in boxes. They will keep indefinitely on the shelf. We recommend using only those made with calcium saccharine or aspartame (if it agrees with you) since these are low-sodium as well as sugar-free.

SWEET PEPPER HALVES
Available in the pickle section of most supermarkets, low-sodium sweet pepper halves generally come in 24-ounce jars. Made from sweet red peppers, these pickled delicacies, at only 7 milligrams of sodium per ounce, are the perfect salt-free alternative to pimientos, which are packed in salt, and contain approximately 203.4 milligrams of sodium per ounce. Once opened, low-sodium sweet pepper halves should be refrigerated and will keep indefinitely.

TOMATO PASTE
Low-sodium tomato paste, with only 3 milligrams of sodium per ounce, is widely available in supermarkets and health food stores across the country.

It is rich and better tasting than its salty counterpart, which contains 57 milligrams of sodium per ounce. Although tomato paste is sold in cans to preserve its freshness, once opened, it should be transferred to glass or plastic containers, leaving ½ inch of headspace; it can be stored up to two months in the refrigerator, or indefinitely in the freezer.

TOMATO PUREE
This thick, tomato-rich, subtly special blend is a great aid for perking up leftovers or freshening the flavor of a defrosted tomato-based dish. The low-sodium variety, containing only 3 milligrams sodium per ounce, is as readily available in supermarkets as the salty kind at 114 milligrams per ounce. Once opened, the puree should be stored in glass or plastic containers, leaving ½ inch of headspace. Refrigerated, it will keep up to 3 weeks; frozen, indefinitely.

TOMATO SAUCE
Although in Mexican cooking, tomato sauce is made from scratch with plump fresh tomatoes, low-sodium tomato sauce is a handy alternative to have in your pantry. Many major manufacturers produce this basic sauce in 8- and 16-ounce cans and distribute it in supermarkets throughout the country. With only 3 milligrams of sodium per ounce, compared to 86 for its salty counterpart, once opened, low-sodium tomato sauce should be stored in glass or plastic containers, leaving ½ inch of headspace. Refrigerated, it will keep up to 3 weeks; frozen, indefinitely.

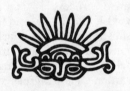

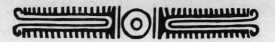

For Ease
of Preparation

Utensils

Although nothing is ever quite as good as the real thing, Mexican cooking equipment is not imperative to fine culinary results. In fact, in addition to a blender and heavy cast-iron skillets of varying sizes, your own kitchen is probably well-stocked for proper food preparation. However, because so many Mexican cooking utensils in practical use today date back to the Aztecs, we thought you would enjoy knowing a little about them.

Bean Masher. Made of wood, this utensil is much like a long-handled pestle. A metal potato masher is a reasonable and expedient substitute.

Comal. The traditional round cast-iron or earthenware griddle used for making tortillas. You may substitute any thick cast-iron skillet.

Flan Mold. The ingenious, all-in-one Mexican unit consisting of the mold, lid, and water bath pan. Any ovenproof custard cups placed in a tin baking dish will do as well.

Metate. A slab of volcanic rock set on three stubby legs, this is the traditional grinding stone for preparing corn, chiles, or any ingredient that must be pulverized to a fine powder. Mexicans call it an Aztec blender, and, in truth, a blender is the modern cook's time-saving substitute.

Metlalpil. The stone rolling pin used for grinding corn on the metate.

Molcajete and Tejolete. These are the Mexican mortar and pestle made of the black volcanic rock, basalt. Larger than a marble mortar, the molcajete is bowl-shaped and sits on three short legs. It is excellent both for preparing small amounts of spices and for blending sauces as well. What is more, once the sauce is made, the molcajete can be used as a serving dish. Of course, you may substitute any mortar and pestle or blender for grinding spices and pureeing sauces.

Tortilla Press. Available in varying sizes, the 6-inch press is standard and will eliminate the frustration of learning to pat tortillas into shape by hand. They are available in some gourmet shops, but you may have to do some searching.

Preparation and Assembly

There is no special magic, no specific requirements in Mexican cooking.

If you read my last book, *The Salt-Free Chinese Diet Cookbook,* you would know that the Chinese are exquisitely precise in their approach to food. They have numerous ways of slicing, cutting, and chopping ingredients, specific cooking times for each, and several cooking methods, some of which are distinct from one another only in degree.

In Mexico, cooking is a much more homely affair. That is not to say that the artistry is any less fine or the results any less heavenly. The Mexicans simply adhere to the axiom, "The whole is greater than the sum of its parts."

That is why, in Mexican cuisine, sauces play such an integral role and so many foods are simmered together. In both cases, a variety of textures and flavors combines to form totally new taste experiences.

The only real criterion for success is organization. A multitude of herbs, spices, and foods may be required for one simple dish. Some may be blended for sauces; others cooked separately and added later; and still others prepared to form the nucleus of a given recipe. Therefore, to avoid unnecessary confusion and frustration, you should first assemble all your ingredients, then read the directions to plan your time.

There is no need to worry, however. The recipes in this book have been developed to make them easy for you to follow and enjoy in minimum time. What is more, in Mexican cuisine, the wonderful blending of numerous tastes virtually guarantees success. So a little more of this, a little less of that, cooked a little too long or not quite long enough will not make one taste bit of difference.

The truth is that, in Mexican cooking, a glad heart produces joyous results.

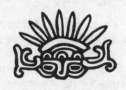

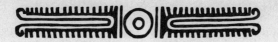

How to Adapt Your Favorite Mexican Recipes

When I first told friends I was writing a Mexican cookbook, they said, "Fabulous. Mexican food is so good, so spicy, so much fun." When I added that the book would be salt-free, they said, "Impossible."

When my friends said, "Impossible," they were jumping to two erroneous conclusions: first, that salt-free food is synonymous with bland; second, that Mexican food without salt is drained of its spicy bite. Neither is true.

For the last several years—since salt was publicly exposed as a potential health hazard—doctors, nutritionists, dieticians, this author, and others have offered countless suggested salt replacements both to add flavor and even to impart a "salty" taste. Allow me to enumerate them here:

- Any pungent or hot spice will give food a zesty flavor. These include: cayenne pepper, black pepper, hot pepper flakes, cumin, lemon peel powder, Chili Powder (page 210), garlic powder, paprika, and aniseed. You get the idea.
- Even sweet spices and herbs like basil, dill, cinnamon, cloves, nutmeg, and orange peel powder trick the mind and palate into thinking sweet rather than salty.
- Condiments that have an acid content really do give foods a salty flavor. Marinate or cook meat, fish, or poultry in vinegar, lemon juice, low-sodium ketchup, mustard, or wine, and you will be a believer.
- One final tip: Low-sodium bouillon, either beef- or chicken-flavored, will instantly give you the taste of salt. Just stir either the granulated or powdered form into any dish, and everyone will think you have added salt.

Coincidentally and happily, Mexican food preparation makes good use of all these salt alternatives. Indeed, many of the suggested salt options are generic to the cuisine.

So you see, my friends were wrong. Mexican food is not impossible to cook salt-free. Quite the contrary. Like every distinctive and highly seasoned cuisine, its generic herbs, spices, and condiments are so chock-full of flavor that salt is really unnecessary.

Once you try these tips you will discover that salt is not the only flavor enhancer. Nor is it the most interesting one. In adapting recipes, Mexican or otherwise, try to decide which flavors the salt is supposed to accent. Then use your cooking instincts, imagination, and palate to determine which salt replacement will work best.

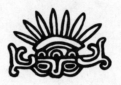

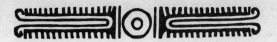

Other Diet Tips

Physical fitness is very much part of our lives today. Over the last ten years, all across the country, the number of people who work out, jog, and actively engage in sports has risen steadily, while the two biggest detriments to health—cigarette smoking and alcohol consumption—have declined.

Food Watching

No longer labeled craze, or trend, or fad, fitness and health have become an unself-conscious way of life for the majority. Diet, along with exercise, is, of course, key to the equation, with "caffeine-free," "sugar-free," and "salt-free" the buzz words of the Eighties.

Today, caffeine-free coffee, soft drinks, and even tea are abundantly displayed on every supermarket shelf throughout the country. Sugar-free products are equally accessible, but the controversy about sugar substitutes goes on.

In 1977, studies with laboratory rats indicated that saccharin—the best-known and most popular sugar replacement—was a carcinogen. When the FDA sought to ban it, however, public protest resulted in a congressional moratorium so that additional studies could be done. Over the years, consumer groups like the Community Nutrition Institute, a nonprofit organization dedicated to food safety and policy, have maintained that saccharin is a low-level carcinogen, not safe at any level. Nevertheless, the moratorium on saccharin has been extended continually because most research substantiates its safety.

Saccharin comes in two forms: sodium saccharin and calcium saccharin. The latter carries the label "sodium-free" and should be the choice of all salt-watchers.

Cyclamate, a sodium synthetic banned by the FDA in 1970, is under harsher attack than saccharin. Although each successive study weakens the link between cyclamate and cancer, several concerns remain. The April, 1985, issue of *Mademoiselle* cites John Schubert, Ph.D., chairman of the chemistry department at the University of Maryland-Baltimore County, whose work shows that, in the body, cyclamate changes to cyclohexylamine, which can cause male sterility. Other studies have shown that cyclamate can also cause the chromosome defect resulting in Down's Syndrome.

Because of its many potentially harmful effects, it is highly unlikely that cyclamate will be made available to consumers any time soon.

Although widely used in many products, especially candy, the artificial sweetener sorbital is clearly not acceptable to everyone. Up to 30 percent of whites and 52 percent of blacks with diabetes suffer severe reactions (including diarrhea) to this carbohydrate derivative. An article in the June, 1985, issue of *Glamour* states that, according to Dr. Naresh K. Jain, a gastroenterologist with Misericordia Hospital in New York, diabetics suffering from diarrhea cannot properly absorb their food, and therefore, could become hypoglycemic.

The newest sugar substitute is aspartame, commercially sold under the name NutraSweet. Aspartame is an amino acid compounds which produces the taste equivalent of sugar, without the bitter aftertaste of saccharin.

Only on the market since 1981, it is already creating a stir as reports surface of headaches, depression, and dizziness following its use. To date, studies at the Centers for Disease Control in Atlanta have been unable to corroborate any causal relationship between these disorders and aspartame. However, experts generally agree that some people exhibit a high sensitivity to the sweetener. In particular, those with the genetic disorder phenylketonuria could suffer mental retardation from aspartame because they must restrict their intake of one of its key components.

What all this means is that no artificial sweetener is 100 percent safe. Consult your doctor to determine which sugar substitutes you are allowed. Then read labels to be sure that the products flagged "dietetic" are truly all right for you.

Sugar substitutes aside, today many nutritionists believe that sugar itself, in very small doses, is not harmful to the diabetic. For that matter, its limited consumption will not obstruct the goals of the calorie conscious either. In the final analysis, the password for sugar and its many alternatives is "moderation," which we have scrupulously respected in this book.

Moderation is also critical where salt is concerned, but controlling intake requires more detective work than with sugar, primarily because salt can be present in foods in many disguises. The three-point guide detailed in *The Chinese Salt-Free Diet Cookbook* still applies and is given below:

- Avoid everything from saccharin to soda that contains salt or a sodium compound, such as sodium benzoate, disordium sulfate, sodium saccharin, brine, sodium bicarbonate (baking soda, baking powder), etc.
- Avoid products that still list "natural ingredients," which is often the deceptive label for, among other things, salt.
- Avoid all packaged goods and canned goods that are not labeled "low-sodium."

Do not be nervous. These rules are not as difficult as you think because today most manufacturers are complying with the federal government's request for full-disclosure ingredients listing. Equally important, in response to consumer demand, major marketers are producing and distributing every conceivable salt-free product, from pickles to nuts, to supermarkets everywhere.

Most of these salt-free products detail the sodium content as well as the fat, carbohydrates, and calories, either per serving or per 100 grams (equivalent to an approximate 3½ ounces). Others are not so specific, and their labeling needs some explaining, detailed below per government guidelines:

- *No salt added.* These products may have been processed with salt or sodium without extra salt added for flavor. No-salt-added products should be avoided by everyone on salt-free diets.
- *Low-sodium.* Containing at least 75 percent less salt than their salt counterparts, low-sodium products average 140 milligrams per serving. They are fine for those on moderately restricted diets, but should be avoided by those who must not exceed 1,000 milligrams sodium, or less, per day.
- *Very low-sodium.* At 35 milligrams sodium per serving, or less, these products are acceptable for those with even the most severe salt restrictions.
- *Sodium-free.* No one need worry about these products, which contain less than 5 milligrams of sodium per serving.

Salt restriction is necessary for some of us, healthy for all of us, and has some wonderful side benefits as well. We all know that salt retains water, so it only stands to reason that reducing salt consumption will help eliminate the unsightly and uncomfortable pounds of bloat and the pressure it puts on the vital organs. Salt also hampers the digestive process and has been linked to the formation of the dreaded fatty deposits we call cellulite.

Health and a little healthy vanity are two very good reasons for cutting back on salt. Thanks to consumer groups and public interest, living salt-free is easy today both for those who must and for those who want to subscribe to the safe and more than adequate range of 1,100 to 3,000 milligrams of sodium per day that the United States Department of Agriculture recommends.

Travel and Other Pleasures

In *The Chinese Salt-Free Diet Cookbook,* published in 1985, we enumerated several guides to help you maintain your salt-free diet outside the home. Readers have told us how helpful they are, how easy to remember and follow. So we think they bear repeating here.

The travel and hotel industries have always led the salt-free brigade. Indeed, these service businesses have consistently shown the greatest awareness of any special diet problems.

With 48 hours notice, any airline will provide one of a number of special diet meals, including low-calorie, vegetarian, seafood, kosher, diabetic, and low-sodium. These meals are special in more ways than one, for often they are much tastier than regulation airline fare.

Hotels will also try their best to accommodate your dietary needs. On request, they will install a refrigerator in your room (usually for a modest day rate) so you can have any special foods or medication at hand. What is more, if you explain your problem and requirements to room service, the restaurant maitre d', or the hotel manager, they will generally be understanding and helpful. But one word of caution: wherever you are and whatever the circumstances, if the food you get is not the food you ordered, send it back. Never, but never, settle for less than perfection when your health is at stake.

By the way, it is always a good idea to carry a few low-sodium snacks and canned goods when you travel, in case an emergency arises or boredom sets in. A small container of your favorite spices will also come in handy for perking up a meal "out."

Closer to home, you will have many more occasions to eat out. Today restaurants are much more sensitive to the special dieter than they were a decade ago. I used to carefully explain to the waiter or captain not only what I needed but why, trying to communicate how important my requests were. They would listen politely but with slightly bemused expressions, and would often reply, "Ah, yes, Madame is watching her figure." Funny to think about now, but maddening and often disastrous then. They did not take me seriously, and my food, when it arrived, was predictably unacceptable.

But times have changed. Today that same waiter in that same restaurant will nod with understanding as you describe your problem. He will also faithfully see that your order is prepared exactly as you like it.

Unfortunately, in Mexican restaurants, your needs cannot be so easily met. That is because the soups, sauces, dressings, and condiments, which play important roles in the cuisine, are prepared ahead of time and contain salt. In fact, these items should be avoided in any restaurant for the same reason.

The rule of thumb for dining out is simple: avoid all foods made in advance; stick to dishes broiled with nothing more than herbs and spices or a little wine; when in doubt, ask before you order or taste. You will be surprised how many dishes are available to you in Mexican restaurants or in any other.

As for visiting, do not be shy. Tell your friends the problem. Chances are they will want to prepare food you can enjoy. If that is not possible, brown-bag your own. It is as easy as that.

Always be aware, however, that even with the best intentions, people can make mistakes. Be glad they are receptive and want to be helpful, but, fortified with the tips outlined above, you should—and must—always be the questioner, the final judge of, and the last word on what is best for you.

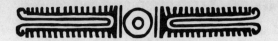

Recipes

The popular belief is that Mexican food is hot, spicy, and smothered in cheese or tomato sauce. While some dishes are, most are mild and delicately though distinctly flavored. Indeed, gourmets consider authentic Mexican cooking to be one of the three truly original cuisines of the world, displaying as much subtlety, variety, and complexity as its Chinese and French companions.

We believe the recipes in this book will demonstrate the truth of this accolade. You will sample succulent tropical fruits, contrasted with the snap of garlic, then cooked with meats or poultry, an example of the German influence on Mexican cooking. You will enjoy exotic dishes accented with one or more of the one hundred kinds of chiles for which Mexico is famous, ranging from the fiery to the lesser-known mild and sweet types.

Most of all, you will continually be delighted by the wide assortment of herbs, spices, and condiments that so beautifully enhance the food.

The warm, nutty flavor of cumin; the licorice refreshment of anise; the "salty" dash that comes from the acid in lemons, limes, wines, and vinegar; the sweet pungency of cinnamon and cloves; the aromatic nip of nutmeg; and, of course, the fiery blend of crushed chiles, paprika, and cumin, which we call chili powder. These and all the other seasonings generic to Mexican cuisine have such lively, rich, and highly individual flavors that they make salt not only unnecessary but totally extraneous.

In short, as we hope this book will prove, Mexican food can be adapted for the salt-free dieter without losing either the integrity of the style or the authenticity of the taste of the cuisine.

In addition to eliminating salt, we are also observing the spirit rather than the letter of the law in two other areas to promote better nutrition and health. First, we have reduced the amount of cooking fat (and, consequently, calories as well) by using very low heat for browning and frying. Second, to address the needs of the diabetic, we have tried to curtail the carbohydrate content of combination dishes, and have restricted the use of sugar (except in the Dessert section).

You may ask why we do not opt for salt and sugar substitutes. With regard to salt, the reasons are twofold. First, too much of anything is unhealthy, and indiscriminate use of salt substitutes (potassium chloride) can, over time, be just as harmful as overdosing on salt. Second, salt in any form masks the true flavor of food. Our purpose is to enhance it, which we can do most deliciously and easily with the extensive selection of Mexican seasonings so abundantly at our disposal.

We have avoided sugar substitutes for three reasons. First, as noted earlier in this book, some diabetics cannot tolerate sugar replacements. Second, sugar substitutes break down under the heat of cooking and produce a bitter, lingering aftertaste. Third, on a per-serving basis, the amount of sugar found in any of our recipes is fairly small and may be allowed even on the diabetic's diet.

"May be" is the key phrase and must be qualified, for whether your problem is sugar, salt, fat, or calories, you should never play guessing games with your health. Always check with your doctor before using this or any diet book.

Just two more reminders before you start your journey on one of the most historically diverse culinary paths in the food world:

1. The calorie, sodium, carbohydrate, and fat contents given for each recipe include all ingredients called for but do not include any of the suggested accompanying dishes.
2. For convenience, we have used dried rather than fresh herbs and spices in these recipes, unless otherwise noted. However, do use fresh whenever you can because nothing tastes quite as good. Just remember: because the flavor in dried, ground, or powdered herbs and spices is concentrated, you will need three times the amount if you use the fresh form.

There is nothing more to add, no more reason for delay. Just imagine caballeros serenading in the background, a soft, warm breeze caressing your cheek, the perfume of bougainvillea teasing your senses. And once you are in the mood, read on and begin to savor the artistry and virtuosity of Mexican cuisine.

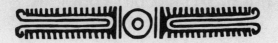

Appetizers
and Snacks

Perhaps because Mexicans love to nibble on food all day, perhaps because there are so many delectables to nibble on—whatever the reason, in Mexico there are almost as many names for appetizers as there are appetizers themselves. Call them *aperitivos, botanas, bocadillos, entremeses*, these tantalizing goodies to munch on and crunch on appear on the many push-carts and stands that pepper every town.

Tidbits of meat, fish, or poultry, marinated and deep-fried or sautéed, wait temptingly to be popped into your mouth, stuffed in a taco, or smothered in a succulent sauce. Enticing fresh-made dips beg to be scooped up with a crisp taco or a raw vegetable stick sprinkled with lime juice.

But you do not have to travel to Mexico to enjoy these finger foods. You can produce the heavenly smells and succulent tastes of Mexican appetizers in your own kitchen. See for yourself by sampling the delicious recipes in this chapter. And remember, small, bite-size pieces of meat, seafood, and poultry also make lovely snacks. One more thing: do not forget heaps of tacos and tostadas.

Imaginative and fanciful, Mexican snacks and appetizers are truly deserving of their most often-used name: *antojitos*, which means little whims.

Guacamole

MAKES 4 CUPS

Although we use this traditional international favorite primarily as a dip, technically Guacamole is a sauce. And it is equally delicious as a garnish for meat, fish, or poultry. Any way you try it, you will enjoy this zesty Mexican treat.

2 ripe avocados, peeled, pitted, and
  mashed
1 tomato, chopped
1 small onion, minced
¼ teaspoon garlic powder
½ green pepper, diced
2 green chiles, seeded and minced

2 tablespoons cider vinegar
½ teaspoon sugar
1 teaspoon low-sodium chicken
  bouillon
Black pepper to taste
¼ teaspoon Chili Powder (page 210)

1. In bowl, combine first 6 ingredients, blending thoroughly.
2. Stir in remaining ingredients. Cover and chill at least 2 hours to allow flavors to blend.

Per recipe: 1,293.4 calories; 83.0 mg. sodium; 82.0 gm. carbohydrates; 114.8 gm. fat.
Per cup: 323.4 calories; 20.8 mg. sodium; 20.5 gm. carbohydrates; 28.7 gm. fat.
Per tablespoon: 20.2 calories; 1.3 mg. sodium; 1.3 gm. carbohydrates; 1.8 gm. fat.

Avocado, Cucumber, and Beet Dip

MAKES 3 CUPS

A most refreshing and tangy dip that is simply wonderful with crudités, low-sodium crackers, potato chips, or crispy Tacos (page 50).

2 avocados, peeled, pitted, and
  mashed
1 cucumber, peeled and chopped
1 can (8 ounces) low-sodium beets,
  diced, including liquid
2 green chiles, seeded and chopped
1 onion, minced

1 tablespoon olive oil
2 tablespoons red wine vinegar
2 teaspoons lime juice
3 halves low-sodium sweet pepper
  slices, chopped
2 scallions, chopped, including
  greens

In bowl, combine all ingredients, blending thoroughly. Cover and chill at least 2 hours to allow flavors to blend.

Per recipe: 1,590.8 calories; 233.6 mg. sodium; 110.6 gm. carbohydrates; 128.9 gm. fat.
Per cup: 530.3 calories; 77.9 mg. sodium; 36.9 gm. carbohydrates; 43.0 gm. fat.
Per tablespoon: 33.1 calories; 4.9 mg. sodium; 2.3 gm. carbohydrates; 14.3 gm. fat.

Chile-Cheddar Dip

MAKES 4 CUPS

A fabulous and unusual dip for shrimp or any leftover cooked meats and wonderful with crudités. You will love this versatile taste-pleaser.

2 cups Basic Salsa (page 210)
3 serrano chiles, seeded and minced
  (or ¼ teaspoon hot pepper flakes)
1 onion, chopped
1 green pepper, diced

6 ounces low-sodium Cheddar
  cheese, shredded
1 cup low-sodium cottage cheese
1 teaspoon dried oregano
2 teaspoons paprika

1. In saucepan, combine first 5 ingredients. Turn heat to low. Cover and cook ½ hour, stirring occasionally.
2. Add remaining ingredients. Cook 20 minutes more, stirring often.

Per recipe: 1,124.0 calories; 162.8 mg. sodium; 83.8 gm. carbohydrates; 60.0 gm. fat.
Per cup: 281.0 calories; 40.7 mg. sodium; 21.0 gm. carbohydrates; 15.0 gm. fat.
Per tablespoon: 17.6 calories; 2.5 mg. sodium; 1.3 gm. carbohydrates; 0.9 gm. fat.

Salmon and Caper Dip

MAKES 2¾ CUPS

Bursting with Mexican spices, this zesty, refreshing dip is just as good made with sardines (two 3¾-ounce cans). Serve with low-sodium crackers.

1 teaspoon olive oil
1 onion, minced
2 cloves garlic, minced
3 carrots, steamed* and diced
4 green chiles, seeded and minced
1 can (7¾ ounces) low-sodium salmon, including liquid
2 tablespoons dry white wine
¼ teaspoon ground cumin
⅟₁₆ teaspoon ground nutmeg
½ teaspoon dried dill
1½ tablespoons dried parsley
2 teaspoons capers† (or 1 tablespoon white vinegar)
6 scallions, chopped, including greens
½ cup sour cream

1. In skillet, heat oil over low heat. Add onion and garlic and cook 5 minutes, or until onion is golden.
2. Stir in carrots, chiles, and salmon, including liquid. Cook 10 minutes more, stirring often.
3. Stir in remaining ingredients, except sour cream, blending thoroughly. Cook 5 minutes more.
4. Transfer salmon mixture to blender. Add sour cream. Blend 30 seconds. Cover and chill at least 1 hour to allow flavors to blend.

With salmon. Per recipe: 1,047.2 calories; 350.0 mg. sodium; 72.3 gm. carbohydrates; 63.1 gm. fat.
Per cup: 380.8 calories; 127.3 mg. sodium; 26.3 gm. carbohydrates; 22.9 gm. fat.
Per tablespoon: 23.8 calories; 8.0 mg. sodium; 1.6 gm. carbohydrates; 1.4 gm. fat.
With sardines. Per recipe: 1,206.1 calories; 425.0 mg. sodium; 74.3 gm. carbohydrates; 86.0 gm. fat.
Per cup: 438.2 calories; 154.5 mg. sodium; 27.0 gm. carbohydrates; 31.2 gm. fat.
Per tablespoon: 27.4 calories; 9.7 mg. sodium; 1.6 gm. carbohydrates; 1.9 gm. fat.

* Do not add salt to water.
† Preserved in vinegar only.

Sour Cream Dip

Sour cream is found in many Mexican dishes. Here it is the base for a tangy dip for tacos, potato chips, or crudités. This spicy blend is also a wonderful topping for fish, meat, and potatoes.

½ cup boiling water
2½ teaspoons low-sodium beef
  bouillon
2 onions, minced
2 cups sour cream
½ teaspoon low-sodium Dijon
  mustard

2 tomatoes, chopped
2 hot cherry peppers, seeded and
  minced
3 scallions, chopped, including
  greens
1 tablespoon dried parsley

1. Preheat oven to 350°.
2. In bowl, combine first 2 ingredients, stirring to dissolve bouillon. Set aside.
3. On baking sheet, place onions. Bake 10 minutes, or until onions are toasted. Transfer to bowl.
4. Stir in remaining ingredients, including bouillon mixture, blending thoroughly. Cover and chill at least 2 hours to allow flavors to blend.

Per recipe: 1,836.5 calories; 210.5 mg. sodium; 79.9 gm. carbohydrates; 175.0 gm. fat.
Per cup: 612.1 calories; 70.2 mg. sodium; 26.2 gm. carbohydrates; 58.3 gm. fat.
Per tablespoon: 38.3 calories; 4.4 mg. sodium; 1.7 gm. carbohydrates; 3.6 gm. fat.

Eggplant and Apple Dip
MAKES 7 CUPS

Mexican in spirit if not in fact. Once you taste this delicious blend, both sweet and mildly piquant, you will be glad to have so much on hand. This dip is great with everything. It is also a lovely and unusual condiment with any main dish.

1 tablespoon vegetable (or peanut) oil
2 onions, minced
4 cloves garlic, minced
½ teaspoon aniseed
1 eggplant (about 1½ pounds), peeled and diced
4 tomatoes, chopped
1 teaspoon Chili Powder (page 210)
¼ teaspoon orange peel powder
1 green pepper, chopped

4 apples, peeled, cored, and diced
½ cup low-sodium tomato juice
1 teaspoon dried basil
1 tablespoon dried parsley
1 tablespoon dry sherry
Black pepper to taste
1 cucumber, peeled and diced
3 scallions, chopped, including greens

1. In skillet, heat oil over low heat. Add onions, garlic, and aniseed. Cook 10 minutes, or until onion is golden, stirring often.
2. Add eggplant, tomatoes, chili powder, and orange peel powder. Cover and cook ½ hour, or until eggplant is soft, stirring often.
3. Add green pepper, apples, tomato juice, basil, parsley, sherry, and black pepper. Cover and simmer ½ hour more.
4. Transfer eggplant mixture to blender. Grind briefly to blend all ingredients. (Mixture will be slightly lumpy.) Transfer to bowl.
5. Stir in cucumber and scallions. Cover and chill at least 1 hour to allow flavors to blend.

Per recipe: 1,242.8 calories; 177.1 mg. sodium; 261.2 gm. carbohydrates; 24.1 gm. fat.
Per cup: 177.5 calories; 25.3 mg. sodium; 37.3 gm. carbohydrates; 3.4 gm. fat.
Per tablespoon: 11.1 calories; 1.6 mg. sodium; 2.3 gm. carbohydrates; 0.2 gm. fat.

Tuna-Stuffed Mushrooms   MAKES 24 CANAPES

These mouth-watering canapés will have your guests asking for more. Equally scrumptious with 1 cup of cooked and minced chicken substituted for the tuna.

1 teaspoon olive oil
1 onion, minced
2 cloves garlic, minced
1/16 teaspoon cayenne pepper
1 can (6½ ounces) low-sodium tuna, including liquid
2 tablespoons lemon juice
1 teaspoon low-sodium chicken bouillon

¾ teaspoon dried oregano
1/16 teaspoon clove powder
1/16 teaspoon ground cumin
4 tablespoons sour cream
24 medium-size mushrooms, stems reserved for future use
2 tablespoons unsalted margarine

1. In skillet, heat oil over low heat. Add onion and garlic. Cook 10 minutes, or until onion is lightly browned, stirring often.
2. Stir in cayenne pepper, tuna, including liquid, lemon juice, bouillon, oregano, clove powder, and cumin. Cook 5 minutes more, stirring often.
3. Transfer tuna mixture to blender. Add sour cream. Blend for 30 seconds.
4. Preheat oven to 350°.
5. Dot bottoms of mushrooms with margarine. Place on baking sheet.
6. Stuff mushrooms with tuna mixture. Bake 15 minutes.

Per canapé with tuna: 43.1 calories; 8.6 mg. sodium; 2.0 gm. carbohydrates; 3.1 gm. fat.
Per canapé with chicken: 43.9 calories; 8.8 mg. sodium; 2.0 gm. carbohydrates; 3.1 gm. fat.

Chile-Chicken Canapés MAKES 48 CANAPES

So easy and so sure to please. Experiment by substituting any shellfish for the chicken. Just remember, shellfish get tough and lose their flavor when cooked too long, so if they are your choice, add them to the sauce during the last 5 minutes of cooking.

2 cups Chile-Tomato Sauce (page 213)   **3 cups cooked chicken, cut in 1½-inch chunks**

1. In saucepan, combine both ingredients. Turn heat to medium-low. Cover and cook ½ hour, stirring occasionally. Transfer mixture to platter.
2. Skewer chicken chunks with toothpicks.

Per canapé: 14.5 calories; 4.5 mg. sodium; 1.1 gm. carbohydrates; 0.4 gm. fat.

Avocado and Caper Canapés MAKES 16 CANAPES

Yogurt and avocados mellow the bite of the cherry peppers in this tangy dish. The capers add an elegant touch. You may replace the green pepper with any crunchy vegetables for a different taste experience.

2 avocados, halved, pitted, and peeled
½ cup plain yogurt
2 tablespoons lime juice
3 low-sodium hot cherry peppers, seeded and minced

4 scallions, chopped, including greens
1 tablespoon capers* (or 1 tablespoon white vinegar)
4 green peppers, seeded and quartered

1. In bowl, mash together avocados, yogurt, and lime juice.
2. Stir in hot cherry peppers, scallions, and capers, blending thoroughly. Cover and chill at least 2 hours to allow flavors to blend.
3. Spoon avocado mixture onto green pepper quarters.

Per canapé: 101.9 calories; 21.1 mg. sodium; 8.6 gm. carbohydrates; 7.6 gm. fat.

* Preserved in vinegar only.

Cucumber and Chorizo Canapés

MAKES 24 CANAPES

Cool, crispy cucumber is the perfect complement for spicy chorizo, but feel free to substitute whatever fresh vegetable strikes your fancy. Three zucchini cut in 1½-inch rounds and 3 red peppers cut in sixths are two options.

¾ pound Chorizo (page 158)
3 scallions, chopped, including
** greens**
¹⁄₁₆ teaspoon ground cinnamon
1 teaspoon paprika

2 carrots, steamed* and chopped
3 cucumbers, peeled and cut in
** ½-inch rounds**

1. In skillet, over medium-low heat, fry chorizo until browned all over.
2. In blender, combine chorizo, scallions, cinnamon, paprika, and carrots. Grind briefly.
3. Top cucumber rounds with chorizo mixture.

Per canapé with cucumber: 60.4 calories; 22.1 mg. sodium; 3.3 gm. carbohydrates;
    2.2 gm. fat.
Per canapé with zucchini: 51.0 calories; 16.4 mg. sodium; 3.2 gm. carbohydrates;
    2.2 gm. fat.
Per canapé with red pepper: 54.5 calories; 22.4 mg. sodium; 4.1 gm. carbohydrates;
    2.3 gm. fat.

* Do not add salt to water.

Sweet Pepper and Mackerel Canapés
MAKES 24 CANAPES

Any fish can replace the mackerel in this uniquely elegant dish.

1 can (3¾ ounces) low-sodium
  mackerel in tomato sauce
1 teaspoon paprika
1 small onion, minced
½ teaspoon dried oregano
1 package (8 ounces) low-sodium
  cream cheese

6 slices low-sodium bread, crusts
  trimmed, bread toasted
6 halves low-sodium sweet peppers,
  quartered

1. In bowl, combine first 4 ingredients, thoroughly mashing the fish.
2. Blend in cream cheese. Cover and chill at least ½ hour to allow flavors to blend.
3. Quarter each slice of bread by cutting it on both diagonals.
4. Spread each bread quarter with fish mixture. Top with a piece of sweet pepper.

Per canapé: 75.3 calories; 15.3 mg. sodium; 6.3 gm. carbohydrates; 4.6 gm. fat.

Minced Veal Canapés
MAKES 40 CANAPES

This is not a typically Mexican approach to veal for two reasons. First, veal is not widely available in Mexico, and second, ground meat of any kind is almost always formed into balls and poached to absorb the flavor of the sauce. Nonetheless, we think you will very much enjoy the Mexican style of the recipe which follows. So much so, in fact, that we urge you to try it with beef as well as with veal.

1 tablespoon unsalted margarine
1 pound ground veal
1 onion, minced
2 cloves garlic, minced
1 teaspoon low-sodium chicken
  bouillon

Black pepper to taste
1 tablespoon dried parsley
2 tomatoes, chopped
2 tablespoons dry sherry
⅓ cup heavy cream
40 low-sodium wheat crackers

1. In skillet, heat margarine over medium-low heat. Add veal, onion, and garlic. Cook until veal is browned all over, stirring often.

2. Stir in bouillon, pepper, parsley, and tomatoes. Cook 2 minutes more, stirring often. Transfer mixture to blender. Blend 1 minute, or until mixture is smooth but not mushy.
3. Stir in sherry and cream. Cover and chill ½ hour to allow flavors to blend.
4. Top crackers with veal mixture.

Per canapé with veal: 46.3 calories; 12.4 mg. sodium; 2.0 gm. carbohydrates; 3.3 gm. fat.
Per canapé with beef: 51.6 calories; 7.4 mg. sodium; 2.0 gm. carbohydrates; 3.6 gm. fat.

Pickled Ceviche
SERVES 8

One of the most famous Latin American dishes, ceviche actually originated in the Orient. It is a dish of succulent delicacy, perfect as an appetizer. We have strayed somewhat from more orthodox versions, primarily by choosing not to use a more fatty fish like mackerel, which the Mexicans prefer, and substituting a sweeter white fish instead. In addition, we have added pickling spice for a slightly piquant flavor. No matter, for any way at all, fish "cooked" in lime juice is habit-forming.

2 pounds haddock, flounder, or sole
    fillets
1¼ cups lime juice
1 onion, minced
1 tablespoon pickling spice
½ teaspoon dried oregano

2 teaspoons dried parsley
2 teaspoons low-sodium chicken
    bouillon
⅓ cup boiling water
Black pepper to taste

1. In bowl, combine first 6 ingredients. Cover and refrigerate ½ hour.
2. While fish is marinating, in small bowl, combine remaining ingredients, stirring to dissolve bouillon. Let stand 20 minutes to cool.
3. Add bouillon mixture to fish mixture. Cover and refrigerate at least 4 hours to allow flavors to blend.

Per serving with haddock: 109.5 calories; 72.8 mg. sodium; 6.2 gm. carbohydrates;
    0.4 gm. fat.
Per serving with flounder: 109.5 calories; 92.2 mg. sodium; 6.2 gm. carbohydrates;
    1.2 gm. fat.
Per serving with sole: 109.5 calories; 92.2 mg. sodium; 6.2 gm. carbohydrates;
    1.2 gm. fat.

Marinated Beef

MAKES 24 CANAPES

In this Mexican version of steak tartare, the ground beef is "cooked" in lime juice. It is absolutely marvelous.

½ pound ground London broil
⅛ teaspoon ground cumin
1/16 teaspoon cayenne pepper
1/16 teaspoon ground cinnamon
2 green chiles, seeded and minced
1 tablespoon dried parsley

1 onion, minced
1 tomato, chopped
½ cup lime juice
1 tablespoon cider vinegar
24 low-sodium crackers

1. In bowl, combine first 6 ingredients, blending thoroughly.
2. Stir in onion and tomato, blending thoroughly.
3. Stir in lime juice and vinegar, blending thoroughly. Cover and refrigerate at least 8 hours to allow meat to "cook" and flavors to blend.
4. Serve with low-sodium crackers.

Per canapé: 57.9 calories; 9.0 mg. sodium; 5.0 gm. carbohydrates; 3.3 gm. fat.

Fruit Juice Chicken Wings

MAKES 48 CANAPES

Chicken wings have never tasted so good. The blend of citrus, cayenne pepper, cumin, and chili ketchup gives the fruit juice its uniquely Mexican tang and makes the chicken wings deliciously unforgettable.

48 chicken wings
1 recipe Fruit Juice Dressing
   (page 226), oil deleted, divided

1. Preheat broiler.
2. On baking sheet, place chicken wings. Pour half the dressing over all. Broil 4 inches from heat 5 minutes.
3. Turn wings. Pour on remaining dressing. Broil 5 minutes more, or until wings start to brown.

Per canapé: 75.5 calories; 21.8 mg. sodium; 0.4 gm. carbohydrates; 4.3 gm. fat.

Sweet Hot Apple Relish　　MAKES 14 CUPS

The chiles give a Mexican flavor to this south-of-the-border version of chutney. The relish, with its intermingling hot and sweet and spicy and pungent flavors, is tantalizingly delicious whether served as a dip or a side-dish condiment.

10 Granny Smith apples, cored and
　chopped
2 lemons, seeded and chopped
3 onions, minced
4 green chiles, seeded and minced
2 cups light brown sugar
1¼ cups cider vinegar

¾ cup apple juice
1½ cups water
2 teaspoons mustard powder
1¼ cups dark raisins*
¼ teaspoon cayenne pepper
½ teaspoon ginger powder

1. In Dutch oven, combine first 7 ingredients. Simmer over low heat ½ hour.
2. While apple mixture is cooking, in small bowl, combine water and mustard powder, blending thoroughly. Stir into apple mixture.
3. Add remaining ingredients. Cover and simmer 2 hours more. Remove from heat. Let cool ½ hour.
4. Pour mixture into jars, leaving 1-inch headspace. Cover tightly and refrigerate or freeze. Will keep up to 3 months in refrigerator and indefinitely in freezer.

Per recipe: 4,024.5 calories; 286.1 mg. sodium; 1,071.3 gm. carbohydrates; 14.0 gm. fat.
Per cup: 287.5 calories; 20.4 mg. sodium; 76.5 gm. carbohydrates; 1.0 gm. fat.
Per tablespoon: 18.0 calories; 1.3 mg. sodium; 4.8 gm. carbohydrates; 0.1 gm. fat.

* Preserved in non-sodium ingredient.

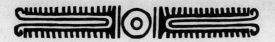

Tortillas, Tacos, and the Like

Slap, pat, slap, pat. In towns and villages throughout Mexico, you can still hear the rhythm of hands stamping out tortillas while the comal heating nearby stands ready to receive them. Although this ancient technique, which can be traced back to Mexico's earliest civilizations, is fast giving way to the modern technology of mass production, the foundation—corn—will forever be solid and sure. For if tortillas are the bread which nourishes Mexico, corn is its very soul.

To the Mayans, corn was the life force from which man sprang; to the Aztecs, corn was a god. While it is no longer an object of worship, today corn is still the single most important ingredient in Mexican cuisine.

Wheat was unknown in Mesoamerica until the Spanish Conquest. It flourished in the flatlands of northern Mexico to such an extent that white flour tortillas are now as much a part of Mexican cuisine as the corn variety.

Whether it's white or yellow, you are sure to become a devotee of the versatile tortilla and its offspring.

Tortillas

Corn Tortillas
MAKES 20

Corn, ground and pulverized, is the basis for the flat bread known as the tortilla, which has been the national bread of Mexico for centuries, dating back to the Mayans and the Aztecs. Although the ingredients are few, and the directions simple, tortillas take practice, so do not be discouraged if your first batch is not perfect. The next one will be, and then you will agree that homemade tortillas are well worth the effort.

2 cups masa harina
1 tablespoon low-sodium chicken
  bouillon

1⅓ cups warm water

1. In bowl, combine first 2 ingredients, blending thoroughly.
2. Add water gradually, working with fingers to make a soft, but not sticky, dough. Cover and let stand ½ hour.
3. Form dough into 20 balls. Place each ball between 2 sheets of waxed paper and flatten to discs about 4 inches in diameter.
4. Remove top sheet of waxed paper. If dough sticks, work in a little more masa harina, 1 teaspoon at a time.
5. Heat cast-iron skillet (or comal*) over medium heat. Cook tortillas, one at a time, 2 to 3 minutes, or until edges curl slightly and tops are spotted brown.
6. Turn and cook 2 minutes more.
7. Stack tortillas between paper towels. Wrap in damp cloth. Then wrap in aluminum foil.
   Note: If they are to be served within 2 hours, keep warm in oven or dry place until ready to use. Otherwise, store in refrigerator up to 2 days, or in freezer up to 1 month, and reheat by warming about 20 minutes in oven at 200°.

Per tortilla: 86.1 calories; 1.2 mg. sodium; 17.3 gm. carbohydrates; 0.2 gm. fat.

* Tortilla press.

White Flour Tortillas

MAKES 20

The Spanish conquerors brought white flour to Mexico, and the white flour tortilla was born. Today it is the foundation for many Mexican favorites, including the burritos found later in this chapter.

2 cups all-purpose flour
1½ tablespoons low-sodium chicken bouillon
1½ teaspoons low-sodium baking powder

2 tablespoons shortening
⅞ cup slightly warm water

1. In bowl, combine first 3 ingredients, blending thoroughly.
2. Cut in shortening and water to form a stiff dough.
3. Form dough into 20 balls. Turn onto lightly floured board and roll to ⅛-inch thickness.
4. Heat cast-iron skillet over medium heat. Cook tortillas, one at a time, 2 to 3 minutes, or until edges curl slightly and tops are spotted brown.
5. Turn and cook 2 minutes more.
6. Stack tortillas between paper towels. Wrap in damp cloth. Then wrap in aluminum foil.

Note: If they are to be served within 2 hours, keep warm in oven or dry place until ready to use. Otherwise, store in refrigerator up to 2 days, or in freezer up to 1 month and reheat by warming in oven at 200°.

Per tortilla: 98.1 calories; 3.8 mg. sodium; 17.6 gm. carbohydrates; 1.4 gm. fat.

Tacos and Tostadas

Tacos are miniature tortillas, stuffed with the same fillings and skewered with toothpicks to make the finger foods so popular at cocktail parties. Tacos may also be fried—plain or filled—in hot oil or vegetable shortening.

Tostadas are tortillas that have been fried in hot oil or vegetable shortening and then smothered in the combination of your choice.

Any of the tortilla recipes in this book can magically become a taco or tostada at the snap of your fingers.

Burritos

Burritos I   MAKES 20

Burritos are white flour tortillas, filled and rolled with beans, chicken, or meat mixtures. Deep-fried, they are called chimichangas. Two versions follow:

1 recipe White Flour Tortillas
  (page 49)
1 double recipe Shredded Pork
  (page 163)

2 cups iceberg lettuce, shredded
2 cups Basil-Tomato Sauce (page 212)

1. On center of each tortilla, place 3 tablespoons pork, some shredded lettuce, and 1½ tablespoons tomato sauce.
2. Fold two sides of tortilla toward center. Then fold over both open ends.
3. Repeat until all ingredients are gone.

Per burrito: 311.8 calories; 65.3 mg. sodium; 26.5 gm. carbohydrates; 11.8 gm. fat.

Burritos II

MAKES 20

1 tablespoon unsalted margarine
6 half chicken breasts, poached,
   flesh shredded
2 leeks, minced, including greens
1 cup Almond Sauce (page 218)

1 recipe White Flour Tortillas
   (page 49)
¾ cup vegetable oil

1. In skillet, heat margarine over medium-low heat. Add chicken and leeks. Fry 2 minutes, stirring often.
2. Add sauce and cook 5 minutes more, stirring often.
3. On center of each tortilla, place 2 tablespoons chicken mixture.
4. Fold two sides of tortilla toward center. Then fold over both open ends.
5. In skillet, heat oil over medium heat. When crackling hot, add tortillas, 5 at a time, seam side down, and fry until golden brown. Drain on paper towels.
6. Repeat Step 5 with remaining tortillas.

Per burrito: 171.2 calories; 21.3 mg. sodium; 20.7 gm. carbohydrates; 5.2 gm. fat.

Chicken Chilaquiles
in Chile-Tomato Sauce

SERVES 4

Chilaquiles offer the cleverest, most delicious way of freshening up stale tortillas. Derived from the Mexican expression meaning broken old sombrero, chilaquiles consist of tortilla pieces prepared in cheese sauce, with vegetables, poultry, or meats. The recipe below is only one possibility. For variety, substitute ⅓ pound cooked and shredded pork for the chicken. Or make up your own recipe. You cannot miss. Chilaquiles are sure to be a favorite in your home.

½ cup vegetable oil
4 stale Corn Tortillas (page 48), cut
  into pieces
2 cups Chile-Tomato Sauce (page 213)

2 chicken breasts, poached, flesh
  shredded
2 ounces low-sodium mozzarella
  cheese, shredded

1. Preheat oven to 375°.
2. In skillet, heat oil over medium heat. Add tortillas and fry 2 minutes. Drain on paper towels. Transfer to 5 x 9-inch baking pan.
3. Pour tomato sauce over tortillas. Add chicken. Then top with cheese and bake 15 minutes.

Per serving with chicken: 350.0 calories; 66.5 mg. sodium; 31.3 gm. carbohydrates;
    13.3 gm. fat.
Per serving with pork: 336.7 calories; 43.2 mg. sodium; 31.3 gm. carbohydrates;
    16.3 gm. fat.

Empanadas

Empanada Dough   MAKES 24

Mexico owes thanks to their Spanish conquerors for these tender, flaky, versatile turnovers made with white flour. Stuff them with chicken or meat or vegetables, and you will have an elegant meal. Fill them with fruit or jam, and you will never enjoy a sweeter dessert. The basic dough recipe appears below, followed by several favorite variations.

2 cups all-purpose flour
1½ teaspoons low-sodium baking
   powder
1 teaspoon sugar
1 tablespoon low-sodium chicken
   bouillon

⅟₁₆ teaspoon cayenne pepper
6 tablespoons shortening
¼ cup ice water

1. In bowl, combine first 5 ingredients, blending thoroughly.
2. Cut in shortening and add water to form a stiff dough.
3. Turn dough onto lightly floured board and roll to ⅛-inch thickness.
4. With cookie cutter, cut dough into 24 2-inch circles.
5. Stuff with your favorite filling. Then bake or fry.

Per empanada: 98.5 calories; 1.7 mg. sodium; 14.7 gm. carbohydrates; 3.0 gm. fat.

Chicken and Shrimp Empanadas MAKES 24

For a slightly different taste, substitute 3 ounces of low-sodium minced Cheddar cheese for the chili ketchup.

1 tablespoon unsalted margarine
2 half chicken breasts, skinned, boned, and diced
¼ teaspoon dried thyme
1 leek, chopped, including greens
¼ pound fresh shrimp, shelled, deveined, and minced

1 tablespoon dry sherry
3 tablespoons low-sodium chili ketchup
1 recipe Empanada Dough (page 53)
1 egg, lightly beaten
2 tablespoons low-fat milk

1. In skillet, heat margarine over low heat. Add chicken and sauté 2 minutes.
2. Stir in thyme and leek. Sauté 2 minutes more.
3. Add shrimp, sherry, and chili ketchup. Cook 5 minutes, or until shrimp are pink all over, stirring often. Set aside.
4. Preheat oven to 375°.
5. Prepare dough by following Steps 1 through 4 of the basic recipe.
6. On center of each circle of dough, place 1 teaspoon chicken and shrimp mixture.
7. Fold circles in half and crimp edges together. Place on greased and floured baking sheet.
8. In bowl, beat together egg and milk. Brush mixture over empanadas and bake 15 minutes, or until empanadas are lightly browned.

Per empanada with chili ketchup: 124.6 calories; 16.4 mg. sodium; 15.6 gm. carbohydrates; 4.0 gm. fat.
Per empanada with cheese: 137.8 calories; 16.4 mg. sodium; 15.6 gm. carbohydrates; 5.1 gm. fat.

Meat and Cheese Empanadas   MAKES 24

Fabulous accompanied by Guacamole (page 34).

1 recipe Empanada Dough (page 53)
1 cup Picadillo with Vegetables
  (page 169)
4 ounces low-sodium Muenster
  cheese, diced

1 egg, lightly beaten
2 tablespoons low-fat milk

1. Preheat oven to 375°.
2. Prepare dough by following Steps 1 through 4 of the basic recipe.
3. On center of each circle of dough, place 2 teaspoons of picadillo. Then sprinkle on cheese.
4. Fold circles in half and crimp edges together. Place on greased and floured baking sheet.
5. In bowl, beat together egg and milk. Brush mixture over empanadas and bake 15 minutes, or until empanadas are lightly browned.

Per empanada: 134.5 calories; 8.8 mg. sodium; 16.6 gm. carbohydrates; 5.2 gm. fat.

Vegetable Empanadas   MAKES 24

A vegetarian's delight.

2 carrots, steamed* and diced
3 halves low-sodium sweet pepper
  slices, minced
1 tablespoon unsalted margarine
1 zucchini, peeled and diced
1 teaspoon low-sodium beef bouillon
1 onion, minced
2 cloves garlic, minced
1 teaspoon paprika

1 green pepper, diced
1 cup Tomato Sauce with Cayenne
  (page 212)
1 recipe Empanada Dough (page 53)
1 egg
¼ cup low-fat milk
1 pint sour cream

1. In blender, combine first 2 ingredients. Grind for 30 seconds. Set aside.
2. In skillet, heat margarine over low heat. Add zucchini, bouillon, onion, and garlic. Stir to blend. Cover and cook 20 minutes, stirring occasionally. Stir in paprika and green pepper.
3. Add carrot mixture and tomato sauce. Stir to blend.
4. Raise heat to medium and cook 10 minutes, stirring often.
5. Preheat oven to 375°.
6. Prepare dough by following Steps 1 through 4 of the basic recipe.
7. On center of each circle of dough, place 2 teaspoons of vegetable mixture.
8. Fold circles in half and crimp edges together. Place on greased and floured baking sheet.
9. In bowl, beat together egg and milk. Brush mixture over empanadas and bake 15 minutes, or until empanadas are lightly browned.
10. Serve 1 tablespoon of sour cream with each empanada.

Per empanada: 187.4 calories; 17.3 mg. sodium; 19.6 gm. carbohydrates; 10.9 gm. fat.

* Do not add salt to water.

Dessert Empanadas I

MAKES 24

Totally addictive, and low-calorie, too.

1 recipe Empanada Dough (page 53)
2 cups Sweet Hot Apple Relish
  (page 45)

1 egg, lightly beaten
2 tablespoons low-fat milk

1. Preheat oven to 375°.
2. Prepare dough by following Steps 1 through 4 of the basic recipe.
3. On center on each circle of dough, place 1 rounded tablespoon of relish.
4. Fold circles in half and crimp edges together. Place on greased and floured baking sheet.
5. In bowl, beat together egg and milk. Brush mixture over empanadas and bake 15 minutes, or until empanadas are lightly browned.

Per empanada: 126.2 calories; 6.3 mg. sodium; 21.2 gm. carbohydrates; 3.3 gm. fat.

Dessert Empanadas II

MAKES 24

When you taste these flaky morsels, you will swear "nirvana" is a Spanish word.

½ cup golden raisins*
¼ cup unsalted walnuts, minced
4 tablespoons shredded coconut
½ cup peach (or strawberry)
  preserves†

1 recipe Empanada Dough (page 53)
1 egg, lightly beaten
2 tablespoons low-fat milk

1. In blender, combine first 2 ingredients. Grind. Transfer to bowl.
2. Stir in coconut and preserves, blending thoroughly.
3. Preheat oven to 375°.
4. Prepare dough by following Steps 1 through 4 of the basic recipe.
5. On center of each circle of dough, place 1 scant tablespoon of raisin mixture.
6. Fold circles in half and crimp edges together. Place on greased and floured baking sheet.
7. In bowl, beat together egg and milk. Brush mixture over empanadas and bake 15 minutes, or until empanadas are lightly browned.

Per empanada: 151.3 calories; 6.5 mg. sodium; 22.8 gm. carbohydrates; 4.7 gm. fat.

* Preserved in non-sodium ingredient.
† Preserved without pectin or sodium.

Enchiladas

Meat Enchiladas in Pungent Chile Sauce SERVES 24

Enchiladas are corn tortillas rolled around any desired filling—usually chicken- or meat-based—and baked in a sauce, then garnished with chopped and shredded vegetables and cheese. They are, quite simply, marvelous and make delightful, finger-licking hors d'oeuvres or light meals. The tortillas are fried briefly so they will be soft enough to roll without crumbling, but there is very little oil residue in the final dish.

What follows are three examples of this wonderful Mexican classic.

¼ cup vegetable oil
24 Corn Tortillas (page 48)
2 cups Sweet-and-Hot Chile Sauce (page 215)
3 cups Picadillo with Vegetables (page 169)

1 cup shredded low-sodium Muenster cheese
1 head iceberg lettuce, shredded

1. Preheat oven to 350°.
2. In skillet, heat oil over medium heat. With tongs, add tortillas, one at a time, and fry very briefly. Drain on paper towels.
3. Dip tortillas in chile sauce.
4. On center of tortillas, spoon 2 tablespoons of picadillo.
5. Fold 2 sides of tortillas toward center and place, seam side down, in 9-inch-square ovenproof casserole.
6. Repeat Step 5 until enchiladas are layered in the casserole.
7. Pour remaining chile sauce over all. Cover and bake 15 minutes.
8. Cut enchiladas in half. Garnish with cheese and lettuce and serve.

Per serving: 206.9 calories; 22.4 mg. sodium; 27.3 gm. carbohydrates; 7.9 gm. fat.

Avocado and Cheese Enchiladas   SERVES 16

Creamy and crunchy and mouth-wateringly good.

¼ cup vegetable oil
16 Corn Tortillas (page 48)
2 cups Chile-Vegetable Sauce
   (page 214)
1½ cups Chile-Avocado Sauce
   (page 214)

6 ounces low-sodium Cheddar cheese,
   minced
2 onions, minced

1. Preheat oven to 350°.
2. In skillet, heat oil over medium heat. With tongs, add tortillas, one at a time, and fry very briefly. Drain on paper towels.
3. Dip tortillas in vegetable sauce.
4. On center of tortillas, spoon 1½ tablespoons of avocado sauce. Then sprinkle with cheese and onions.
5. Fold 2 sides of tortillas toward center, and place, seam side down, in 9-inch-square ovenproof casserole.
6. Repeat Step 5 until enchiladas are layered in the casserole.
7. Pour remaining vegetable sauce over all and bake 15 minutes.

Per serving: 150.7 calories; 13.4 mg. sodium; 25.7 gm. carbohydrates; 10.1 gm. fat.

Sour Cream-Chicken Enchiladas SERVES 8

Four ounces of leftover flounder is a terrific substitute for the chicken.

1 tablespoon olive oil
8 scallions, chopped, including
  greens
8 mushrooms, chopped
2 cups cooked chicken, shredded
Black pepper to taste
1 teaspoon paprika
1 teaspoon low-sodium chicken
  bouillon

½ teaspoon dried oregano
⅛ teaspoon celery seed*
¼ cup vegetable oil
16 Corn Tortillas (page 48)
2 cups Chile-Cheddar Dip (page 35)
8 tablespoons sour cream

1. In skillet, heat olive oil over low heat. Add scallions, mushrooms, and chicken. Sauté 3 minutes, stirring often.
2. Stir in pepper, paprika, bouillon, oregano, and celery seed, blending thoroughly. Set aside.
3. Preheat oven to 350°.
4. In skillet, heat vegetable oil over medium heat. With tongs, add tortillas, one at a time, and fry very briefly. Drain on paper towels.
5. On center of tortillas, spoon 2 tablespoons of chicken mixture.
6. Fold 2 sides of tortillas toward center and place, seam side down, in 9-inch-square ovenproof casserole.
7. Repeat Step 6 until enchiladas are layered in the casserole.
8. Pour dip over all and bake 15 minutes.
9. Divide enchiladas among 8 plates. Garnish with sour cream.

Per serving with chicken: 377.3 calories; 35.8 mg. sodium; 43.0 gm. carbohydrates; 16.2 gm. fat.
Per serving with flounder: 367.0 calories; 37.0 mg. sodium; 43.0 gm. carbohydrates; 15.5 gm. fat.

* Do not use celery flakes, which contain salt.

Tamales

Tamale Dough

Like tortillas, plain tamales are often substitutes for bread at the Mexican table. And like tortillas, tamales can be stuffed with any filling imaginable. In every other way, however, tamales are unique unto themselves.

First, tamale dough, although more complex, is easier to prepare than its tortilla counterpart. Second, tamales are always steamed, usually in corn husks, although we will rely on the more readily available aluminum foil. Third, for centuries, tamales have been holiday food—eaten at ceremonies and on special occasions.

The basic dough recipe below is followed by two filling options.

2 cups masa harina
5 teaspoons low-sodium chicken bouillon, divided
Black pepper to taste
3½ teaspoons low-sodium baking powder
1¼ cups warm water
⅓ cup vegetable shortening

1. In bowl, combine masa harina, 1 teaspoon bouillon, pepper, and baking powder, blending thoroughly.
2. In second bowl, combine remaining bouillon and water stirring to dissolve bouillon.
3. To masa harina mixture, add bouillon mixture gradually, working with fingers to make a soft dough.
4. Beat in shortening, a little at a time, until dough is spongy.
5. Divide dough into 16 parts.
6. In center of 8 x 10-inch piece of aluminum foil, place 1 part tamale dough. Spread slightly.
7. Fold foil in half and crimp edges together to seal in dough.
8. Repeat Steps 6 and 7 until all tamales are prepared.
9. Over Dutch oven, place rack. Add water, up to 2 inches from top of pot. Turn heat to high and bring to a boil.
10. Place tamales, crimped side down, on rack. Cover and steam 1 hour, or until dough pulls away from foil without sticking.

Per tamale: 145.1 calories; 3.3 mg. sodium; 22.2 gm. carbohydrates; 4.2 gm. fat.

Chicken and Cheese Tamales

MAKES 16

These tamales are equally delicious if you substitute ½ pound of ground beef or pork or veal for the chicken.

1 tablespoon unsalted margarine
1 onion, minced
2 cloves garlic, minced
2 green chiles, seeded and minced
½ pound ground chicken
⅛ teaspoon ground cumin
2 tablespoons golden raisins*

1 teaspoon low-sodium beef bouillon
3 ounces low-sodium Swiss cheese, minced
1 teaspoon dried basil
1 recipe Tamale Dough (page 61)

1. In skillet, heat margarine over low heat. Add onion, garlic, and chiles and cook 5 minutes, or until onion is golden, stirring often.
2. Add chicken and cumin, stirring to blend. Raise heat to medium and cook 10 minutes, or until chicken loses all pink color, stirring constantly.
3. Stir in raisins, bouillon, cheese, and basil, blending thoroughly. Cook 3 minutes more, stirring occasionally. Set aside.
4. Prepare dough by following Steps 1 through 4 of the basic recipe.
5. In center of 8 x 10-inch piece of aluminum foil, place 1 tablespoon dough. Spread with fingers.
6. On top of dough, place 1 tablespoon of chicken mixture.
7. Top with a second tablespoon of dough.
8. Fold foil in half and crimp edges together to seal in tamale.
9. Repeat Steps 5 through 8 until all tamales are prepared.
10. Over Dutch oven, place rack. Add water, up to 2 inches from top of pot. Turn heat to high and bring to a boil.
11. Place tamales, seam side down, on rack. Cover and steam 1 hour, or until dough pulls away from foil without sticking.

Per tamale with chicken: 193.0 calories; 11.0 mg. sodium; 25.4 gm. carbohydrates; 7.0 gm. fat.
Per tamale with beef: 223.1 calories; 12.7 mg. sodium; 25.4 gm. carbohydrates; 9.4 gm. fat.
Per tamale with pork: 218.5 calories; 16.0 mg. sodium; 25.4 gm. carbohydrates; 8.5 gm. fat.
Per tamale with veal: 216.5 calories; 18.9 mg. sodium; 25.4 gm. carbohydrates; 9.1 gm. fat.

* Preserved in non-sodium ingredient.

Seafood Tamales

MAKES 16

A fabulous rival to the American shrimp roll.

1 tablespoon olive oil
½ pound red snapper fillets, chopped
4 scallions, chopped, including
　greens
¼ pound fresh shrimp, shelled,
　deveined, and minced
¼ teaspoon Chili Powder (page 210)

1 teaspoon low-sodium chicken
　bouillon
¹⁄₁₆ teaspoon clove powder
1 tablespoon dried parsley
1 recipe Tamale Dough (page 61)

1. In skillet, heat oil over low heat. Add snapper and scallions. Cover and cook 10 minutes, stirring occasionally.
2. Stir in shrimp, chili powder, bouillon, clove powder, and parsley. Cover and cook 10 minutes more, or until shrimp are pink, stirring occasionally. Set aside.
3. Prepare dough by following Steps 1 through 4 of the basic recipe.
4. In center of 8 x 10-inch piece of aluminum foil, place 1 tablespoon of dough. Spread with fingers.
5. On top of dough, place 1 tablespoon of seafood mixture.
6. Top with a second tablespoon of dough.
7. Fold foil in half and crimp edges together to seal in tamale.
8. Repeat Steps 4 through 7 until all tamales are prepared.
9. Over Dutch oven, place rack. Add water, up to 2 inches from top of pot. Turn heat to high and bring to a boil.
10. Place tamales, crimped side down, on rack. Cover and steam 1 hour, or until dough pulls away from foil without sticking.

Per tamale: 175.9 calories; 24.1 mg. sodium; 22.8 gm. carbohydrates; 5.4 gm. fat.

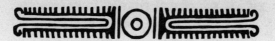

Breads

Although tortillas are the bread most identified with Mexico, they are by no means your only choice. The influence of French and German baking traditions, introduced by way of Spain, combine with the spices and herbs indigenous to Mexico to produce a selection of rolls and breads which rivals the finest from Europe. One taste of Orange-Banana Wheat Rolls (page 69), Glazed Crescent Rolls (page 71), Comb Bread (page 67), or Mexican Sweet Bread (page 68) will convince you more satisfactorily than words. So preheat your oven and let the sweet aroma of Mexican breads seduce your senses.

Bread of the Dead   SERVES 36

Bread of the Dead is really a cake, traditionally served on All Soul's Day as a respectful remembrance of those loved ones who have died. But this special cake marks an occasion of joy rather than sorrow. Families troop, in resplendent colors, to visit and tend graves, after which they picnic and make macabre fun of the inevitable future. Candy skulls are popular, and cheers greet those who parade in skeleton costumes. For, in actuality, this ceremonial day is a tribute to life and to the endurance of the human spirit.

1 package active dry yeast
½ cup warm water
3¾ cups all-purpose flour
⅓ cup sugar
¼ pound unsalted margarine, melted

4 eggs, lightly beaten
1½ teaspoons orange peel powder
½ teaspoon aniseed, ground
¼ cup low-fat milk

1. In bowl, combine first 2 ingredients. Set aside.
2. In second bowl, combine flour and sugar, blending thoroughly.
3. Cream in margarine.
4. Beat in yeast mixture plus remaining ingredients, except milk.
5. Turn dough onto lightly floured board and knead until dough is spongy and elastic.
6. Turn dough into greased bowl. Cover and let stand in warm, dry place until doubled in bulk.
7. Turn dough onto lightly floured board. Knead 5 minutes.
8. Divide dough in half and shape into 2 loaves. Take 1 fistful of dough from each loaf. Set aside. Cover loaves and both small dough pieces and let stand in warm place until doubled in bulk.
9. Preheat oven to 350°.
10. Turn small dough pieces onto floured board. Roll to ½-inch thickness.
11. Cut 2 strips from each small dough piece and lay them, crisscrossed, on top of loaves to symbolize cross bones.
12. Shape each remaining small dough piece into a ball. Place atop crisscrosses in center of large loaves to symbolize tears.
13. Place loaves on lightly floured baking sheet. Brush loaves with milk and bake ½ hour, or until loaves are lightly browned.
14. Loaves should be refrigerated to prevent spoilage.

Per serving: 125.0 calories; 8.0 mg. sodium; 19.3 gm. carbohydrates; 3.1 gm. fat.

Comb Bread

SERVES 36

The Mexican name for this simple bread is peineta, which means a special, fancy comb.

1 package active dry yeast
⅓ cup warm water
¼ cup low-fat milk
½ cup cold water
4 tablespoons shortening
4 cups all-purpose flour, divided

3 tablespoons sugar
¼ teaspoon vanilla extract
½ teaspoon lemon peel powder
1 egg

1. In bowl, combine first 2 ingredients. Set aside.
2. In saucepan, combine milk and cold water. Turn heat to medium and cook 5 minutes.
3. Stir in shortening. Transfer mixture to second bowl. Let stand 20 minutes.
4. Beat in 2 cups flour, sugar, vanilla, and lemon peel powder.
5. Beat in yeast mixture and egg.
6. Beat in remaining flour.
7. Turn dough onto lightly floured board and knead until dough is spongy and elastic.
8. Turn dough into greased bowl. Cover and let stand in warm, dry place until doubled in bulk.
9. Turn dough onto lightly floured board. Knead 5 minutes.
10. Divide dough into 3 parts.
11. Roll each part into an 8-inch circle. With scissors, make 1-inch cuts, 1 inch apart, around the circumference of each dough part.
12. Place loaves on greased and floured baking sheets. Cover and let stand in warm place until doubled in bulk.
13. Preheat oven to 350°.
14. Bake 20 minutes, or until loaves are lightly browned on top.

Per serving: 110.5 calories; 3.2 mg. sodium; 19.9 gm. carbohydrates; 1.4 gm. fat.

Mexican Sweet Bread

SERVES 32

This delightful bread is tasty in any language. Use it for sandwiches, and you may never eat plain white bread again.

1 package active dry yeast
¼ cup warm water
½ cup low-fat milk
½ cup plus 1 tablespoon cold water, divided
4 tablespoons unsalted margarine

⅓ cup sugar
1 teaspoon almond extract
4 cups all-purpose flour, divided
2 eggs, separated
½ teaspoon lemon peel powder

1. In bowl, combine first 2 ingredients. Set aside.
2. In saucepan, combine milk and ½ cup cold water. Turn heat to medium-low and cook 5 minutes, or until mixture bubbles around the edges.
3. Stir in margarine, sugar, and almond extract. Transfer mixture to second bowl.
4. Beat 2 cups flour into milk mixture.
5. Beat in yeast mixture.
6. Beat in remaining flour.
7. Beat in both egg yolks, 1 egg white, and lemon peel powder.
8. Turn dough onto lightly floured board and knead until dough is spongy and elastic.
9. Turn dough into greased bowl. Cover and let stand in warm, dry place until doubled in bulk.
10. Turn dough onto lightly floured board. Knead 5 minutes.
11. Divide dough in half.
12. Roll each half into a 6-inch circle. Place on greased and floured baking sheets. Cover and let stand in warm place until doubled in bulk.
13. Preheat oven to 350°.
14. In third bowl, combine remaining tablespoon of cold water and remaining egg white. Brush mixture on top of loaves.
15. Pierce loaves with fork and bake 20 minutes, or until loaves are lightly browned on top.

Per serving: 133.1 calories; 6.3 mg. sodium; 24.0 gm. carbohydrates; 1.8 gm. fat.

Orange-Banana Wheat Rolls MAKES 24 ROLLS

On a cold day, these scrumptious delicacies will warm you. On a hot day, they will refresh you. At any time, they are a delight. For an elegant light lunch, serve with Squid Salad with Peppers (page 106).

1 package active dry yeast	**2 cups all-purpose flour**
½ cup warm water	**2 eggs, lightly beaten**
¼ cup low-fat milk	**1 ripe banana, mashed**
½ cup orange juice	**1 tablespoon brandy**
¼ cup sugar	**¼ cup crushed, unsalted almonds**
½ teaspoon vanilla extract	
2 cups whole wheat flour	

1. In bowl, combine first 2 ingredients. Set aside.
2. In saucepan, combine milk, orange juice, sugar, and vanilla. Turn heat to medium and cook until mixture just starts to boil. Remove from heat.
3. In second bowl, combine wheat and all-purpose flours.
4. Beat in milk mixture. Then beat in eggs.
5. Beat in yeast mixture and remaining ingredients, blending thoroughly to form a stiff dough.
6. Turn dough onto lightly floured board. Knead until dough is spongy and elastic.
7. Place dough in greased bowl. Cover and let stand in warm, dry place until doubled in bulk.
8. Punch down dough. Turn onto lightly floured board and knead again.
9. Preheat oven to 350°.
10. Divide dough into 24 pieces. Shape dough pieces into balls and place on greased and floured baking sheet. Cover and let stand in warm, dry place until doubled in bulk.
11. Bake 20 minutes, or until rolls are lightly browned.

Per roll: 171.3 calories; 6.9 mg. sodium; 32.4 gm. carbohydrates; 1.2 gm. fat.

Crescent Rolls

MAKES 36 ROLLS

A heartier version of French croissants and just as tasty.

1 package active dry yeast
½ cup warm water
1 cup low-fat milk, divided
4 tablespoons unsalted margarine, melted

4½ cups all-purpose flour
¼ cup sugar
1½ teaspoons lemon peel powder
2 eggs

1. In bowl, combine first 2 ingredients. Set aside.
2. In saucepan, heat ½ cup milk over medium heat. Stir in margarine. Transfer mixture to second bowl.
3. Beat in flour, yeast mixture, sugar, lemon peel powder, and eggs.
4. Turn dough onto lightly floured board and knead until dough is spongy and elastic.
5. Turn dough into greased bowl. Cover and let stand in warm, dry place until doubled in bulk.
6. Turn dough onto lightly floured board. Knead 5 minutes.
7. Divide dough in 3 parts.
8. Roll each part into a 9-inch circle. Quarter each circle. Then divide each quarter into 3 triangles.
9. With fingers, mold each triangle into a crescent shape.
10. On greased and floured baking sheet, place crescents. Cover and let stand in warm place until doubled in bulk.
11. Preheat oven to 350°.
12. Brush crescents with remaining milk and bake 15 minutes, or until rolls are golden brown on top.

Per roll: 126.9 calories; 7.3 mg. sodium; 22.8 gm. carbohydrates; 1.6 gm. fat.

Sugar-Glazed Crescent Rolls MAKES 36 ROLLS

The perfect breakfast sweet roll.

1 recipe Crescent Rolls (page 70)
¼ cup dark brown sugar
2 tablespoons unsalted margarine

2½ teaspoons lemon peel powder
¼ cup water

1. Prepare rolls by following Steps 1 through 10 of the basic recipe.
2. While rolls are rising for the second time, in saucepan, combine remaining ingredients. Turn heat to medium and bring to a slow boil, stirring often.
3. Preheat oven to 350°.
4. Brush each roll with sugar mixture and bake 15 minutes, or until rolls are golden brown.

Per roll: 138.6 calories; 7.9 mg. sodium; 24.3 gm. carbohydrates; 2.2 gm. fat.

Fruit Logs

MAKES 24 ROLLS

Any preserve or jam gives these treats the sweet surprise that makes them extra-special.

1 package active dry yeast
¼ cup warm water
¾ cup boiling water
1 tea bag
2 tablespoons molasses
¼ cup brown sugar
2 tablespoons shortening

1½ cups whole wheat flour
1 teaspoon orange peel powder
1 egg
3 cups all-purpose flour
⅓ cup orange marmalade*
⅓ cup dried apricots, diced

1. In bowl, combine first 2 ingredients. Set aside.
2. In second bowl, combine water and tea bag. Let stand 20 minutes. Discard tea bag.
3. In third bowl, combine molasses, sugar, and shortening. Pour tea over all. Stir until sugar is dissolved. Set aside.
4. Beat wheat flour, orange peel powder, and egg into tea mixture.
5. Beat in yeast mixture.
6. Beat in flour.
7. Turn dough onto lightly floured board and knead until dough is spongy and elastic.
8. Place dough in greased bowl. Cover and let stand in warm place until doubled in bulk.
9. Turn dough onto lightly floured board and knead briefly.
10. Divide dough into 4 equal parts.
11. Roll each part to ⅛-inch-thick rectangle.
12. Spoon marmalade off-center down the length of each roll. Then sprinkle apricots on top of marmalade.
13. Starting from the marmalade side, roll up dough and place logs on a greased and floured baking sheet. Cover and let stand in warm place until doubled in bulk.
14. Preheat oven to 350°.
15. Bake logs 20 minutes, or until lightly browned on top.
16. Let cool 20 minutes. Then divide logs into 6 equal pieces

Per roll: 195.1 calories; 3.9 mg. sodium; 37.0 gm. carbohydrates; 1.2 gm. fat.

* Preserved without pectin or sodium.

Golden Cinnamon Rolls

MAKES 24 ROLLS

These sweet rolls are equally wonderful for breakfast or for a dinner dessert when spread with honey or jam.

1 package active dry yeast
½ cup warm water
4 tablespoons unsalted margarine, melted, divided
¾ cup low-fat milk, divided

3½ cups all-purpose flour
1 tablespoon ground cinnamon
½ cup dark raisins*
1/16 teaspoon ground nutmeg
2 eggs, lightly beaten

1. In bowl, combine first 2 ingredients. Set aside.
2. In saucepan, combine 2 tablespoons margarine and ½ cup milk. Turn heat to medium and cook until mixture just starts to boil. Remove from heat. Let stand 20 minutes.
3. In second bowl, combine flour and cinnamon, blending thoroughly.
4. Beat in milk mixture.
5. Stir in raisins and nutmeg. Then beat in yeast mixture and eggs, blending to form a stiff dough.
6. Turn dough onto lightly floured board. Knead until dough is spongy and elastic.
7. Place dough in greased bowl. Cover and let stand in warm, dry place until doubled in bulk.
8. Punch down dough. Turn onto lightly floured board and knead again.
9. Preheat oven to 350°.
10. Divide dough into 24 pieces. Shape dough pieces into ovals and place on greased and floured baking sheet.
11. In third bowl, combine remaining margarine and milk. Brush mixture over rolls and bake 20 minutes, or until rolls are golden brown.

Per roll: 162.5 calories; 10.8 mg. sodium; 29.1 gm. carbohydrates; 2.4 gm. fat.

* Preserved in non-sodium ingredient.

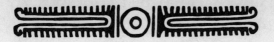

Soups

The scintillating flavors and colors of Mexican cuisine are brought to zesty fruition in the Mexican stock pot, for soups are the heart and soul of this country's diet.

No meal would be complete without soup, and the stock pot simmers and bubbles all day long, its contents changing in texture and flavor as different bits of food are added at the whim of the cook.

Thus, it should come as no surprise that many Mexican soups are meals in themselves, bursting with an extravagant array of the vegetables this country produces so prodigiously. Some offer a combination of Mexico's excellent fresh seafood and others contain succulent pieces of poultry or meat.

But whatever the final delicacy, all Mexican soups start with a good basic stock, made with the freshest ingredients. So important is this vital element that the first lesson in every Mexican cookbook is devoted to the proper preparation of stock. The results, as you will taste for yourself, make the effort very worthwhile.

This love of soups did not originate in Mesoamerica. Indeed, all available documents indicate that the Mayans and Aztecs were indifferent to the temptations of the stock pot. Rather, it was the Spanish who introduced the flavorful goodness of soups to the Mexican culinary repertoire.

No matter how they got there, we are all fortunate that soups are now an integral part of the cuisine. Refreshing on the one hand, like the delicious Fruit Soup (page 80) or heartwarming and invigorating on the other, like Lamb, Tomato, and Bean Soup (page 91), Mexican soups merit a rousing *Olé*.

Chicken Stock

SERVES 16
MAKES 12 CUPS

There is no cuisine that does not have its own definitive recipe for chicken soup. Mexico is no exception, but here an entire stewing fowl is used: head, neck, feet, and all. Although ours is not that all-inclusive, what follows is a true adaptation of the rich, delicious stock which is used so often in Mexican cooking. You will want to keep a freezer supply on hand.

4 quarts water
1 3-pound chicken
Giblets
1 onion, sliced
2 cloves garlic
10 black peppercorns
½ teaspoon celery seed*

1 carrot
4 tablespoons low-sodium chicken
   bouillon
4 sprigs parsley (or 2 tablespoons
   dried parsley)
1 leek, chopped, including greens

1. In Dutch oven, combine first 8 ingredients. Turn heat to medium and cook ½ hour, or until mixture bubbles around the edges.
2. Stir in bouillon. Reduce heat to low and cook ½ hour more. Remove from heat and let stand 20 minutes.
3. Transfer chicken to warm platter. Slice meat and refrigerate for future use.
4. Skim fat off stock. Return stock to medium heat. Stir in remaining ingredients and cook 20 minutes more, stirring occasionally.
5. Strain if you desire a clear consommé or wish to use the stock in other recipes.
6. May be refrigerated in tightly closed jars up to 1 week, or frozen in plastic containers indefinitely.

Per serving: 44.4 calories; 22.5 mg. sodium; 4.9 gm. carbohydrates; 1.3 gm. fat.
Per cup: 59.2 calories; 30.1 mg. sodium; 6.5 gm. carbohydrates; 1.7 gm. fat.

* Do not use celery flakes, which contain salt.

Fish Stock

SERVES 12
MAKES 8 CUPS

A lovely stock which clearly and tastily acknowledges its French origins.

2 quarts water
1 pound fish heads and tails
1 onion, chopped
2 cloves
1 teaspoon celery seed*
Black pepper to taste
1 bay leaf

¼ cup dry vermouth
1 tablespoon white vinegar
1 tablespoon lime juice
6 tablespoons low-sodium chicken
   bouillon

1. In Dutch oven, combine all ingredients. Turn heat to medium and cook ½ hour, or until mixture bubbles around the edges.
2. Reduce heat to low. Cover and cook 45 minutes more, stirring occasionally. Strain.
3. May be refrigerated in tightly closed jars up to 1 week, or frozen in plastic containers up to 1 month.

Per serving: 41.1 calories; 14.7 mg. sodium; 5.0 gm. carbohydrates; 1.6 gm. fat.
Per cup: 61.7 calories; 22.0 mg. sodium; 7.5 gm. carbohydrates; 2.4 gm. fat.

* Do not use celery flakes, which contain salt.

Meat Stock

SERVES 16
MAKES 12 CUPS

Although most often used strained as a stock base for other recipes, unstrained Mexican Meat Stock is hardy fare. Add your favorite soup greens, beans, peas, or squash to the recipe below for a warming main dish. To complete your meal, serve with Baked Rice with Chicken and Chorizo (page 185).

2 pounds short ribs
2 pounds marrow bones
5 quarts water
2 onions, minced
2 bay leaves
3 carrots, cut in ½-inch rounds
1 tablespoon dried parsley

10 black peppercorns
1 teaspoon paprika
1 teaspoon celery seed*
⅛ teaspoon garlic powder
5 tablespoons low-sodium beef
  bouillon

1. In skillet, over high heat, sear short ribs. Transfer to Dutch oven.
2. Add marrow bones and water. Turn heat to high and bring to a boil. Continue boiling 5 minutes.
3. Add all remaining ingredients, except bouillon. Reduce heat to medium-low and cook 1 hour, stirring occasionally.
4. Stir in bouillon and cook 15 minutes more, stirring often.
5. Strain if you desire a clear consommé or wish to use the stock in other recipes.
6. May be refrigerated in tightly closed jars up to 1 week, or frozen in plastic containers indefinitely.

Per serving: 74.7 calories; 34.1 mg. sodium; 6.3 gm. carbohydrates; 5.9 gm. fat.
Per cup: 99.6 calories; 45.5 mg. sodium; 8.3 gm. carbohydrates; 7.8 gm. fat.

* Do not use celery flakes, which contain salt.

Black Bean Soup

SERVES 8

This traditional soup is an absolutely fabulous first course for a meal featuring Snapper Yucatan (page 121). Mixed Salad San Miguel (page 101) is the perfect companion.

1 cup black beans
3 quarts water
1 tablespoon olive oil
2 onions, minced
2 cloves garlic, minced
2 green chiles, seeded and minced
2 tablespoons paprika
¼ cup dry vermouth

1 tablespoon dried oregano
4 tablespoons low-sodium beef
  bouillon
1 teaspoon orange peel powder
½ cup grated low-sodium Gouda
  cheese

1. In Dutch oven, combine first 2 ingredients. Turn heat to high and bring to a boil. Reduce heat to low. Cover and simmer 2 hours, or until beans are soft.
2. While beans are cooking, in skillet, heat oil over low heat. Add onions, garlic, and chiles and cook 10 minutes, or until onions are golden, stirring occasionally. Add to Dutch oven.
3. Stir in paprika and vermouth. Then stir in all remaining ingredients, except cheese. Raise heat to medium and cook 10 minutes, or until mixture starts to bubble around the edges.
4. Stir in cheese and cook 5 minutes more, or until cheese starts to melt.

Per serving: 145.6 calories; 22.9 mg. sodium; 22.6 gm. carbohydrates; 8.3 gm. fat.

Fruit Soup

SERVES 4

Tasty and unique; this soup is zesty served hot, delightful when chilled.

1 teaspoon unsalted margarine
1 leek, chopped, including greens
Black pepper to taste
1 apple, peeled, cored, and cubed
3 cups Chicken Stock (page 76)

1 stick cinnamon
1 pear, cored and cubed
8 dried apricots, diced
¼ cup dry red wine

1. In skillet, heat margarine over low heat. Add leek, pepper, and apple. Cook 5 minutes, stirring occasionally.
2. Add remaining ingredients, except wine. Cover and cook ½ hour, stirring occasionally.
3. Add wine, cook, uncovered, 20 minutes more. Discard cinnamon.

Per serving: 173.5 calories; 30.8 mg. sodium; 32.0 gm. carbohydrates; 2.9 gm. fat.

Melon Soup

SERVES 4

An unexpected but exquisite way to serve the juicy, sweet fruit of the cantaloupe. This soup will lend elegance to your table and is a wonderful opener for a menu that includes Chicken and Chorizo (page 134) and Bean-Stuffed Chiles (page 192).

¼ cup dry sherry
½ cantaloupe, flesh chopped
1 cup boiling water
1 tablespoon low-sodium chicken bouillon

Black pepper to taste
1 cup low-fat milk
Dash of clove powder
1 tablespoon unsalted margarine

1. In blender, combine all ingredients, except margarine. Puree.
2. In saucepan, melt margarine over low heat. Add puree and cook 10 minutes, stirring occasionally.

Per serving: 93.4 calories; 43.3 mg. sodium; 10.4 gm. carbohydrates; 3.8 gm. fat.

Gazpacho

SERVES 8

This classic, spicy but refreshing soup is such a universal favorite it is often found on the menus of the most elegant continental restaurants. It makes a lovely light lunch and is especially appealing in spring and summer. Garnish with chopped onion, green pepper, cucumber, toasted low-sodium bread cubes, and almonds.

½ cup water, divided
1 onion, chopped
½ green pepper, chopped
1 green chile, seeded and minced
1 cucumber, peeled, seeded, and chopped
1 clove garlic, chopped
4 slices low-sodium wheat (or white) bread, crusts trimmed

¼ cup red wine vinegar
¼ cup vegetable oil
5 tomatoes, chopped
2 teaspoons low-sodium chicken bouillon
1½ teaspoons Chili Powder (page 210)
8 cups low-sodium tomato juice

1. In blender, combine ¼ cup water with onion, green pepper, chile, cucumber, and garlic. Grind to a paste. Transfer mixture to bowl.
2. Stir in bread, vinegar, and oil, blending thoroughly.
3. Stir in tomatoes and bouillon.
4. Stir in remaining water and chili powder, blending thoroughly.
5. Stir in tomato juice. Chill at least 2 hours before serving to allow flavors to blend.

Per serving: 202.7 calories; 30.2 mg. sodium; 27.2 gm. carbohydrates; 8.7 gm. fat.

Garlic Soup

SERVES 8

The Spanish influence is temptingly offered in this soup, which has a delicate, nutty flavor—not "garlicky" at all. It is also a perfect soup for dunking tasty slices of Mexican Sweet Bread (page 68).

1 tablespoon olive oil
1 large onion, minced
10 cloves garlic, minced
6 cups Chicken Stock (page 76)
¼ cup dry red wine

2 teaspoons low-sodium beef
   bouillon
2 tablespoons dried parsley
Black pepper to taste
⅟₁₆ teaspoon ground nutmeg

1. In saucepan, heat oil over medium-low heat. Add onion and garlic and cook 10 minutes, or until garlic is lightly browned, stirring often.
2. Stir in remaining ingredients. Raise heat to medium and bring to a slow boil. Continue boiling 5 minutes.
3. Reduce heat to medium-low and cook 20 minutes more, stirring occasionally.

Per serving: 95.4 calories; 31.6 mg. sodium; 13.7 gm. carbohydrates; 3.5 gm. fat.

Corn Soup

SERVES 8

Every Mexican region and town has its own special version of this soup, featuring that most precious ingredient—corn. The combination of pureed corn and cream in the recipe below provides an especially rich consistency and flavor. Serve as a prelude to any fish or poultry dish such as Flounder in Green Garlic Sauce (page 110) or Almond-Sherry Chicken (page 132).

1 tablespoon unsalted margarine
1 large onion, minced
Black pepper to taste
5 cups Chicken Stock (page 76)
1 leek, chopped, including greens
3 cans (24 ounces) low-sodium corn
   niblets, drained, divided, liquid
   reserved

⅟₁₆ teaspoon ground cinnamon
1 tablespoon dry sherry
4 tablespoons heavy cream

1. In skillet, heat margarine over low heat. Add onion. Season with pepper and cook 10 minutes, or until onion is lightly browned, stirring often.

2. While onion is cooking, in Dutch oven, over medium heat, bring stock to a slow boil.
3. Reduce heat to medium-low. Add onion, leek, half the corn, cinnamon, and sherry. Cook 10 minutes, stirring occasionally.
4. While soup is cooking, in blender, combine remaining corn and reserved liquid. Puree. Transfer to Dutch oven.
5. Stir in cream and cook 10 minutes more.

Per serving: 145.6 calories; 26.9 mg. sodium; 23.0 gm. carbohydrates; 5.8 gm. fat.

Creamy Carrot Soup SERVES 4

The sweet leek and hot tang of cayenne pepper make this carrot soup memorable indeed.

1 teaspoon unsalted margarine
1 leek, chopped, including greens
8 mushrooms, chopped
4 cups Chicken Stock (page 76)
1/16 teaspoon cayenne pepper
1 teaspoon paprika

1 tablespoon dry sherry
4 carrots, steamed* and mashed
1/2 cup low-fat milk
2 tablespoons heavy cream
1/16 teaspoon ground nutmeg

1. In skillet, heat margarine over low heat. Add leek and mushrooms and cook 5 minutes, stirring often. Transfer to saucepan.
2. Add stock, pepper, and paprika. Cook over medium-low heat 15 minutes, or until mixture bubbles around the edges.
3. Add sherry, carrots, and milk, stirring to blend. Cook 15 minutes more.
4. Stir in cream. Cook 2 minutes more.
5. Stir in nutmeg.

Per serving: 174.9 calories; 96.7 mg. sodium; 23.3 gm. carbohydrates; 5.8 gm. fat.

* Do not add salt to water.

Broccoli and Corn Soup
SERVES 8

As flavorful as it is colorful, this soup is a beautiful predecessor for a fish dish like Baked Salmon in Mustard Sauce (page 116) or a poultry specialty like Chicken and Spiced Fruit (page 135). Either main choice results in a delightful meal.

1½ tablespoons unsalted margarine, divided
1 onion, minced
4 stalks broccoli, chopped, divided
5 cups Chicken Stock (page 76)

1 teaspoon Chili Powder (page 210)
2 cans (16 ounces) low-sodium corn niblets, including liquid
¹⁄₁₆ teaspoon ground nutmeg
1 teaspoon dry sherry

1. In skillet, heat ½ tablespoon margarine over low heat. Add onion and cook 5 minutes, or until onion is golden, stirring often.
2. Add remaining margarine and half the broccoli. Cook 2 minutes more, stirring occasionally. Transfer mixture to blender. Puree.
3. Transfer mixture to saucepan. Add stock, chili powder, corn including liquid, and nutmeg. Turn heat to medium and cook 15 minutes, or until mixture bubbles around the edges, stirring occasionally.
4. Stir in sherry. Reduce heat to medium-low and cook 5 minutes more.
5. Add remaining broccoli. Cover and cook 5 minutes more.

Per serving: 101.9 calories; 26.9 mg. sodium; 15.7 gm. carbohydrates; 3.7 gm. fat.

Cabbage Soup Veracruz
SERVES 4

A hearty soup which becomes a warming lunch on a chilly day.

¼ pound pork, diced
1 teaspoon olive oil
1 leek, chopped, including greens
1 clove garlic, minced
Black pepper to taste
2 cups Meat Stock (page 78)

1 can (8 ounces) low-sodium tomato sauce
1 teaspoon sugar
1 teaspoon red wine vinegar
1 cup cabbage, shredded

1. In saucepan, cook pork in own fat over medium heat 3 minutes, stirring often.

2. Add oil, leek, and garlic. Reduce heat to low and cook 2 minutes more, stirring often.
3. Add all remaining ingredients, except cabbage, stirring to blend. Cover and cook 10 minutes.
4. Uncover. Raise heat to medium-low. Add cabbage and cook 15 minutes more.

Per serving: 171.5 calories; 55.6 mg. sodium; 16.5 gm. carbohydrates; 7.9 gm. fat.

Cheddar Cheese Soup   SERVES 8

A wonderful way to enjoy the combination of tomatoes and cheese found so often in Mexican cuisine. Shrimp Salad Mazatlan (page 106) is a very tasty follow-up.

6 cups Chicken Stock (page 76)
1 leek, chopped, including greens
2 tomatoes, chopped
¼ cup dry sherry
¼ cup grated low-sodium Cheddar
  cheese

Black pepper to taste
2 tablespoons dried parsley
¼ cup heavy cream

1. In Dutch oven, combine first 4 ingredients. Turn heat to medium and bring to a slow boil. Reduce heat to medium-low and continue cooking 10 minutes, stirring occasionally.
2. Add cheese, pepper, and parsley. Reduce heat to low. Cover and cook 15 minutes more, stirring occasionally.
3. Stir in cream. Cook, uncovered, 5 minutes more.

Per serving: 122.8 calories; 29.7 mg. sodium; 9.5 gm. carbohydrates; 6.4 gm. fat.

Three-Color Festival Soup

SERVES 8

This soup sparkles with the cornucopia of flavors its name implies. One bowl will have you shouting *"Viva México."*

2 tablespoons olive oil
2 potatoes, peeled and diced
2 onions, minced
2 cloves garlic, minced
2 green chiles, seeded and minced
1 leek, chopped, including greens
1 teaspoon paprika

5 cups boiling water
⅓ cup dry red wine
2 tomatoes, chopped
1/16 teaspoon clove powder
3 tablespoons low-sodium chicken bouillon

1. In Dutch oven, heat oil over medium-low heat. Add potatoes, onions, garlic, and chiles. Cook 5 minutes, or until potatoes are lightly browned, stirring occasionally.
2. Add leek and cook 3 minutes more, stirring often.
3. Stir in paprika. Then add water and wine. Cook 10 minutes, stirring often.
4. Stir in remaining ingredients. Cook 15 minutes more, stirring occasionally.

Per serving: 118.8 calories; 12.3 mg. sodium; 18.3 gm. carbohydrates; 5.1 gm. fat.

Cucumber Soup

SERVES 8

This refreshing soup is delicious hot or cold.

½ tablespoon unsalted margarine
1 onion, minced
1 clove garlic, minced
Black pepper to taste
4 cucumbers, peeled and cubed
1 tablespoon all-purpose flour
5 cups boiling water

1 teaspoon celery seed*
2 potatoes, parboiled,† peeled and mashed
3 tablespoons low-sodium chicken bouillon
1 tablespoon lemon (or lime) juice
4 tablespoons sour cream

1. In skillet, heat margarine over low heat. Add onion and garlic and cook 5 minutes, stirring often.

2. Add pepper and cucumbers. Cook 5 minutes more, stirring often.
3. Stir in flour, blending thoroughly. Add water gradually. Then stir in celery seed and potatoes. Cover and simmer 20 minutes, stirring occasionally.
4. Stir in bouillon. Cover and simmer 10 minutes more.
5. Stir in lemon juice. Then stir in sour cream. Cook, uncovered, 10 minutes more, stirring occasionally.

Per serving: 147.4 calories; 34.3 mg. sodium; 16.7 gm. carbohydrates; 4.8 gm. fat.

* Do not use celery flakes, which contain salt.
† Do not add salt to water.

Mexican Vegetable Soup
SERVES 8

Vegetable soup in any cuisine is generally an ingenious and flavorful way to serve the odds and ends in the vegetable bin. For example, in this recipe you might replace the carrots with butternut squash; some broccoli, cauliflower, or green beans for the green peppers; and a cucumber for the zucchini. In other words, there are no rules for vegetable soup, so make your own. But before you do, try the tasty one below along with Flounder with Walnut-Orange Sauce (page 111).

6 cups Chicken Stock (page 76)
1 large onion, chopped
⅛ teaspoon garlic powder
3 carrots, cut in ¼-inch rounds
1/16 teaspoon clove powder
1 tablespoon dried oregano
1/16 teaspoon celery seed*

2 green chiles, seeded and chopped
2 tomatoes, chopped
1 can (8 ounces) low-sodium tomato sauce
1 green pepper, chopped
2 zucchini, chopped
1 tablespoon dry sherry

1. In Dutch oven, combine first 4 ingredients. Turn heat to high and bring to a boil. Reduce heat to medium and cook 10 minutes, stirring occasionally.
2. Add clove powder, oregano, celery seed, and chiles. Reduce heat to medium-low and cook 10 minutes more.
3. Add remaining ingredients, stirring to blend. Cook ½ hour more, stirring occasionally.

Per serving: 106.9 calories; 49.2 mg. sodium; 21.1 gm. carbohydrates; 1.7 gm. fat.

* Do not use celery flakes, which contain salt.

Puree of Avocado Soup SERVES 8

Garnished with lemon or lime slices, this soup is a subtly elegant dish that will lend sophistication to any meal. Serve with Tortillas (pages 48, 49).

4 cups Chicken Stock (page 76)
1 ripe avocado, peeled, pitted, and
  mashed
¼ cup dry sherry
Black pepper to taste

½ cup low-fat milk
2 teaspoons lime juice
½ tablespoon low-sodium chicken
  bouillon
2 tablespoons heavy cream

1. In saucepan, combine stock and avocado. Turn heat to medium-low and cook 15 minutes, stirring occasionally.
2. Stir in sherry, pepper, and milk. Reduce heat to low. Cover and simmer 20 minutes, stirring occasionally.
3. Stir in lime juice and bouillon. Simmer, uncovered, 10 minutes more.
4. Stir in cream. Cook 5 minutes more, stirring occasionally.

Per serving: 128.7 calories; 26.7 mg. sodium; 76.0 gm. carbohydrates; 9.4 gm. fat.

Puree of Spinach Soup SERVES 4

For a lovely change of pace, serve this soup instead of salad. You might follow it with a meal consisting of Pork Stew (page 161).

1 teaspoon unsalted margarine
1 leek, chopped, including greens
1 clove garlic, minced
½ pound spinach
1 cup boiling water
4 cups cold water
Black pepper to taste

3 tablespoons low-sodium chicken
  bouillon
1⁄16 teaspoon ground nutmeg
1⁄16 teaspoon clove powder
4 tablespoons sour cream
¼ cup dry sherry

1. In skillet, heat margarine over low heat. Add leek and garlic and cook 5 minutes, stirring occasionally.
2. While leek and garlic are cooking, in saucepan, blanch spinach in boiling water. Drain. Transfer spinach to blender.
3. To blender, add leek and garlic mixture. Puree. Transfer mixture to saucepan.

4. Add cold water. Turn heat to medium and cook 5 minutes, stirring occasionally.
5. Stir in remaining ingredients. Cook 15 minutes more, stirring occasionally.

Per serving: 147.5 calories; 59.4 mg. sodium; 12.5 gm. carbohydrates; 8.9 gm. fat.

Puree of Squash Soup   SERVES 8

Squash—any kind of squash—is exceedingly popular in Mexico. The soup below is just one reason why. Serve with Mexican Pot Roast (page 153) or Shrimp with Peppers and Peanuts (page 127) and boiled white rice to complete your meal.

½ tablespoon unsalted margarine
3 pearl onions, halved
1 clove garlic, minced
2 yellow squash, cubed
1/16 teaspoon ground nutmeg
4 cups boiling water

6 tablespoons low-sodium chicken bouillon
Black pepper to taste
¼ cup dry sherry
¼ cup heavy cream

1. In skillet, heat margarine over low heat. Add onions, garlic, and squash. Cover and simmer 10 minutes, stirring occasionally. Transfer mixture to blender. Puree. Transfer mixture to Dutch oven.
2. Add water, bouillon, pepper, and sherry, stirring to blend. Turn heat to low and simmer ½ hour, stirring occasionally.
3. Stir in cream and simmer 15 minutes more.

Per serving: 97.6 calories; 16.9 mg. sodium; 11.2 gm. carbohydrates; 5.8 gm. fat.

Lentil with Okra Soup

SERVES 8

A full-bodied, heartwarming soup which beautifully blends the Aztec and Spanish influences.

1½ quarts water
1 cup dried lentils
10 black peppercorns
1 tablespoon unsalted margarine
1 onion, chopped
¼ pound okra, chopped
¼ cup dry red wine

1 tablespoon dried basil
1/16 teaspoon cayenne pepper
6 cups Meat Stock (page 78)
2 carrots, diced
½ teaspoon ground cumin

1. In Dutch oven, combine first 3 ingredients. Turn heat to low. Cover and simmer 1 hour, or until lentils are soft.
2. While lentils are cooking, in skillet, heat margarine over low heat. Add onion and okra and cook 5 minutes, stirring occasionally.
3. Stir in wine, basil, and cayenne. Stir to blend. Transfer mixture to Dutch oven.
4. Add remaining ingredients. Cover and simmer ½ hour more, stirring occasionally.

Per serving: 187.6 calories; 53.8 mg. sodium; 25.4 gm. carbohydrates; 7.6 gm. fat.

Lamb, Tomato, and Bean Soup   SERVES 8

A perfect example of a Mexican stock pot, with this dish you can add or substitute any herbs or vegetables you choose and always have a delectable soup. Perfect with Cucumber Salad La Jolla (page 100).

1 cup white beans
1 pound lamb shoulder, cubed
2 onions, minced
4 cloves garlic, minced
Black pepper to taste
4 cups Meat Stock (page 78)
1 can (14 ounces) low-sodium
    tomatoes, chopped, including juice
¼ teaspoon orange peel powder

¼ teaspoon ground cinnamon
⅟₁₆ teaspoon clove powder
1½ teaspoons ground cumin
2 zucchinis, cubed
¼ cup dry red wine
2 tablespoons dry sherry
1½ teaspoons dried basil
2 tablespoons dried parsley

1. In Dutch oven, combine beans with enough water to cover. Let stand overnight. Drain. Add fresh water to cover. Turn heat to low. Cover and simmer 2 hours, or until beans are fork tender, adding water if necessary to prevent sticking.
2. While beans are cooking, in skillet, combine lamb, onions, and garlic. Turn heat to medium and brown lamb on all sides, stirring often.
3. Add lamb mixture to cooked beans along with pepper, stock, tomatoes, orange peel powder, cinnamon, clove powder, and cumin. Stir to blend. Cover and simmer 1½ hours, or until lamb is fork tender, stirring occasionally.
4. Add remaining ingredients. Cover and simmer 15 minutes more.

Per serving: 314.5 calories; 78.7 mg. sodium; 32.6 gm. carbohydrates; 10.9 gm. fat.

Shrimp Soup

SERVES 8

Shrimp (*camarones* in Mexico) are plump, sweet, and tender sea morsels so delicious they are habit-forming. In this recipe, their subtle yet distinct flavor punctuates the succulent blend of the other ingredients to produce a truly superb dish. A simple salad and boiled white rice are the only accompaniments you need.

1 teaspoon vegetable oil
1 onion, minced
¼ cup unsalted almonds, crushed
4 tomatoes, chopped
¼ cup cold water
1 teaspoon mustard powder
5 cups boiling water
1 bay leaf
1 tablespoon cider vinegar
¹⁄₁₆ teaspoon allspice

1 clove
4 black peppercorns
2 teaspoons dried oregano
1 pound fresh shrimp, shelled,
  deveined, and chopped
2 tablespoons low-sodium chicken
  bouillon
3 tablespoons sour cream

1. In skillet, heat oil over low heat. Add onion and almonds and cook 5 minutes, or until onion is golden, stirring occasionally.
2. Add tomatoes and cook 5 minutes more, stirring occasionally.
3. While tomatoes are cooking, in bowl, combine cold water and mustard powder. Stir into tomato mixture, blending thoroughly. Transfer mixture to saucepan.
4. Add boiling water, bay leaf, vinegar, allspice, clove, peppercorns, and oregano. Cook ½ hour.
5. Reduce heat to low. Add shrimp and bouillon and cook 10 minutes, stirring occasionally.
6. Stir in sour cream. Raise heat to medium and cook 5 minutes more, stirring often.

Per serving: 133.0 calories; 93.0 mg. sodium; 9.4 gm. carbohydrates; 5.8 gm. fat.

Fish Soup

SERVES 8

A hearty, wonderfully tasty dish—a meal in itself. If you want to vary the flavor, substitute ¼ pound shrimp, shelled, deveined, and chopped, for the snapper. Just one thing: add the shrimp during the last 5 minutes of cooking. Serve with Green Bean and Sweet Pepper Salad (page 100).

1 tablespoon olive oil
1 onion, chopped
3 cloves garlic, minced
1 tablespoon all-purpose flour
3 tomatoes, chopped
7 cups Fish Stock (page 77)
1 tablespoon dried oregano
2 tablespoons low-sodium chicken
  bouillon

Dash of ground nutmeg
1 tablespoon dry sherry
½ pound halibut fillets, cut in 1-inch
  chunks
½ pound red snapper fillets, cut in
  1-inch chunks
Parsley for garnish

1. In skillet, heat oil over low heat. Add onion and garlic and cook 10 minutes, or until onion is lightly browned, stirring often.
2. Stir in flour, blending thoroughly.
3. Add tomatoes and cook 2 minutes more. Transfer mixture to Dutch oven.
4. Add stock. Turn heat to medium and cook 10 minutes, or until mixture bubbles around the edges.
5. Stir in oregano, bouillon, nutmeg, and sherry. Cook 15 minutes more, stirring occasionally.
6. Reduce heat to medium-low. Add fish. Cover and cook 15 minutes more, or until fish flakes easily.
7. Garnish with parsley.

Per serving with snapper: 167.3 calories; 61.3 mg. sodium; 15.3 gm. carbohydrates;
  5.5 gm. fat.
Per serving with shrimp: 153.7 calories; 62.2 mg. sodium; 15.5 gm. carbohydrates;
  5.4 gm. fat.

Chicken-Walnut Soup

SERVES 8

German-inspired, this dish will lend an elegant flavor to any meal. One suggestion is Salad of Colors (page 102) and Meat-Stuffed Chiles (page 194).

½ tablespoon unsalted margarine	⅓ cup unsalted crushed walnuts
1 onion, minced	1 stick cinnamon
1 tablespoon paprika	2 tablespoons sour cream
6 cups Chicken Stock (page 76)	1 tablespoon dry red wine

1. In Dutch oven, heat margarine over low heat. Add onion and cook 5 minutes, or until onion is golden, stirring occasionally.
2. Stir in paprika.
3. Add stock, walnuts, and cinnamon. Turn heat to medium and bring to a slow boil. Continue boiling 10 minutes.
4. Stir in sour cream and wine. Reduce heat to low and cook 15 minutes more. Discard cinnamon.

Per serving: 130.2 calories; 25.7 mg. sodium; 9.0 gm. carbohydrates; 9.0 gm. fat.

Peppercorn Chicken Soup

SERVES 4

Cinnamon is the special flavor that gives this soup its irresistible appeal. For a truly sumptuous meal, follow with a main course of Chile Rice with Shrimp and Cheese (page 184) or Mexican Lasagna (page 183).

1 teaspoon olive oil	1 teaspoon dried sage
1 onion, minced	1 stick cinnamon
2 cloves garlic, minced	3 tablespoons low-sodium chicken bouillon
5 cups water	
1 half chicken breast, shredded	1 teaspoon cider vinegar
2 bay leaves	4 black peppercorns, ground

1. In skillet, heat oil over low heat. Add onion and garlic and cook 10 minutes, or until onion is lightly browned, stirring often.
2. Transfer to saucepan. Add water, chicken, bay leaves, sage, and cinna-

mon. Turn heat to high and bring to a boil. Reduce heat to medium-low and cook 20 minutes, stirring occasionally.
3. Add remaining ingredients, stirring to blend. Cook 20 minutes more, stirring occasionally. Discard cinnamon.

Per serving: 94.5 calories; 27.4 mg. sodium; 10.7 gm. carbohydrates; 4.1 gm. fat.

Pork and Avocado Soup   SERVES 4

An unusual but flavorful combination of ingredients, this soup makes a wonderful meal when followed by Shrimp Salad Mazatlan (page 106).

4 cups Meat Stock (page 78)   ¹⁄₁₆ teaspoon ground mace
1 potato, peeled and diced   1 avocado, peeled, pitted, and cut
¼ pound pork, cut into thin strips   into thin slices
1 red chile, halved and seeded

1. In Dutch oven, combine first 2 ingredients. Turn heat to medium-low and cook 15 minutes, stirring occasionally.
2. While soup is cooking, in skillet, over medium heat, cook pork in its own juices 3 minutes, stirring often.
3. Add pork to soup, along with chile and mace. Cook 15 minutes more, stirring occasionally.
4. Pour soup into bowls. Garnish with avocado slices.

Per serving: 164.3 calories; 36.2 mg. sodium; 10.2 gm. carbohydrates; 12.2 gm. fat.

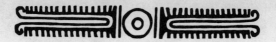

Salads

If you walked through a Mexican market, your eyes would be dazzled by the kaleidoscope of richly colored, oversize vegetables that crowd every stall. Your mouth would start to water as visions of crisp, crunchy, cool salads teased your mind. But fresh, raw vegetable medleys, served as separate courses, are not the rule in Mexico.

Of course, there are beautiful exceptions like Christmas Eve Salad (page 103)—a delicious, festive concoction of beets, lettuce, fruit, and nuts—served as part of the midnight feast following Christmas Eve mass. In general, however, the Mexican *ensalada* is descriptive of the vegetables which are part of virtually every dish, whether strewn decoratively on top or used as the sauce.

Think of the tortillas and tacos bursting with ribbons of shredded lettuce and plump, succulent nuggets of tomato. Whether it is Spiced Chicken and Vegetable Stew (page 148), smothered in a delectable garden mélange, or Cinnamon-Chile Pork Chops (page 159), lovingly bathed in a rich tomato sauce, to Mexicans, the vegetables in these dishes are salads all.

Nevertheless, there are countless ways to add a Mexican flair to the raw combinations we Americans so enjoy. This chapter provides what, we hope you will agree, are some delicious examples.

Avocado, Tomato, and Cheese Salad

SERVES 8

An unusual and delightful coming-together of two of the most popular vegetables in Mexico. A lovely start to any meal.

½ cup Lemon Dressing (page 226)
1 head romaine lettuce, shredded
2 scallions, chopped, including greens
1 avocado, peeled, pitted, and sliced

2 tomatoes, sliced
2 ounces low-sodium Cheddar
   cheese, sliced very thin

1. In bowl, combine first 2 ingredients. Toss to blend.
2. Garnish with scallions, avocado, tomatoes, and cheese.

Per serving: 159.8 calories; 13.1 mg. sodium; 8.3 gm. carbohydrates; 13.4 gm. fat.

Bean Salad

SERVES 8

Beans are a favorite in Mexico, the more the better. So feel free to use whichever kind you prefer in this wonderfully flavorful salad. We promise you that after trying it you will want to have beans a lot more often. A nice companion would be Shrimp in Creamy Wine Sauce (page 126) or Parsley Chicken (page 144).

2 cups cooked kidney beans*
2 cups cooked pink beans*
2 tablespoons cider vinegar
1 onion, minced
20 slices low-sodium butter pickles,
   chopped
1 red pepper, diced
¼ cup cold water
1 teaspoon mustard powder
¼ cup heavy cream

¼ cup red wine vinegar
¼ cup dry sherry
¼ teaspoon Chili Powder (page 210)
¼ teaspoon orange peel powder
1 head Boston lettuce, chopped
1 head iceberg lettuce, shredded
4 ounces low-sodium Cheddar
   cheese, chopped
4 scallions, chopped, including greens

1. In bowl, combine first 6 ingredients. Toss to blend. Cover and chill at least ½ hour.
2. In second bowl, combine water and mustard powder, blending thoroughly.

3. Add cream, vinegar, sherry, chili powder, and orange peel powder blending thoroughly.
4. In third bowl, combine all lettuce, cheese, and scallions. Toss to blend. Divide among 8 plates.
5. Combine bean mixture with mustard mixture. Spoon over lettuce mixture.

Per serving: 237.1 calories; 34.4 mg. sodium; 26.4 gm. carbohydrates; 11.0 gm. fat.

* Do not add salt to water.

Cauliflower Salad   SERVES 8

A mouth-watering combination of mellow avocado, tangy Swiss cheese, and distinctly nutty-flavored cauliflower. Especially good with Steak with Chile Strips (page 156).

1 ripe avocado, peeled, pitted, and
  mashed
¼ teaspoon garlic powder
¼ teaspoon onion powder
⅛ teaspoon ground nutmeg
1 ounce low-sodium Swiss cheese,
  grated

1 cup boiling water
1 tablespoon low-sodium chicken
  bouillon
Cayenne pepper to taste
4 cups cauliflowerettes, steamed*
2 heads Boston lettuce

1. In bowl, combine first 4 ingredients, blending thoroughly.
2. Stir in cheese. Cover and chill at least 1 hour to allow flavors to blend.
3. In second bowl, combine water, bouillon, and cayenne pepper, stirring to dissolve bouillon. Let cool.
4. In blender, combine avocado mixture and ½ cup bouillon mixture. Puree. Transfer to bowl. Stir in remaining bouillon mixture.
5. Add cauliflower. Toss to blend.
6. Divide lettuce among 8 plates. Top with cauliflower mixture.

Per serving: 137.8 calories; 26.9 mg. sodium; 12.5 gm. carbohydrates; 9.0 gm. fat.

* Do not add salt to water.

Cucumber Salad La Jolla SERVES 8

One of the most refreshing salads it will ever be your pleasure to savor. Wonderful with fish.

3 cucumbers, peeled and chopped
⅛ teaspoon garlic powder
1 teaspoon paprika
⅛ teaspoon ground cinnamon
½ green pepper, chopped
1 teaspoon dried parsley

½ teaspoon dried oregano
5 tablespoons red wine vinegar
½ teaspoon sugar
3 tablespoons low-sodium
   mayonnaise
2 tomatoes, chopped

1. In bowl, combine first 7 ingredients. Toss to blend.
2. In second bowl, combine vinegar, sugar, and mayonnaise. stirring to blend thoroughly. Pour over cucumber mixture. Toss to blend.
3. Garnish with chopped tomatoes.

Per serving: 98.3 calories; 22.6 mg. sodium; 6.0 gm. carbohydrates; 4.3 gm. fat.

Green Bean and Sweet Pepper Salad SERVES 8

Nutmeg is the unexpected and pleasing note in this elegantly simple dish. The cumin and cayenne pepper make it sparkle with Mexican flair. Perfect with Veal Loaf (page 167), or any other main dish for that matter.

1 pound green beans, steamed*
1 onion, minced
2 halves low-sodium sweet peppers, chopped
⅓ cup Oil and Vinegar Dressing (page 227)

1/16 teaspoon ground nutmeg
1/16 teaspoon ground cumin
Cayenne pepper to taste

In bowl, combine all ingredients. Toss to blend. Cover and chill at least 2 hours to allow flavors to blend.

Per serving: 75.5 calories; 12.7 mg. sodium; 8.8 gm. carbohydrates; 4.6 gm. fat.

* Do not add salt to water.

Mixed Salad San Miguel

SERVES 4

Hot-and-Sweet Dressing is the key to this imaginative and very Mexican answer to our own tossed salad. Feel free to use any selection of vegetables you prefer. Needless to say, this salad is great with any meal.

1 head romaine lettuce, chopped	3 radishes, sliced
2 tomatoes, chopped	2 scallions, chopped, including greens
1 cup fresh peas,* steamed†	½ cup Hot-and-Sweet Dressing
4 mushrooms, sliced	(page 228)
2 carrots, cut in ½-inch rounds and steamed†	

1. In bowl, combine all but last ingredient. Toss to blend.
2. Pour dressing over all. Toss to blend.

Per serving: 157.8 calories; 44.8 mg. sodium; 19.4 gm. carbohydrates; 8.6 gm. fat.

* Do not use frozen, which contain salt. If fresh are not available, substitute 1 can (8 ounces) low-sodium peas.
† Do not add salt to water.

Salad of Colors   SERVES 8

The tangy combination of oranges, onion, and beets is found in many cuisines: German and French to name only two. This Mexican variation is sure to tantalize. Chicken Ancho (page 133) is a lovely follow-up.

2 oranges, peeled and sectioned
1 small onion, sliced in rings
1 can (8 ounces) low-sodium beets, including juice
2 carrots, julienned
⅛ cup olive oil
⅓ cup boiling water
1 teaspoon low-sodium beef bouillon

1 teaspoon low-sodium Dijon mustard
¼ cup cider vinegar
½ teaspoon sugar
1 head iceberg lettuce, shredded
1 avocado, peeled, pitted, and sliced
2 tomatoes, sliced
2 limes, cut in wedges

1. In bowl, combine first 4 ingredients. Toss to blend. Cover and chill at least 2 hours to allow flavors to blend.
2. In second bowl, combine oil, water, bouillon, and mustard, blending thoroughly.
3. Stir in vinegar and sugar. Let stand 1 hour.
4. Divide lettuce among 8 plates. Top with orange and onion mixture. Garnish with avocado and tomato slices and lime wedges.
5. Serve oil and vinegar mixture on the side.

Per serving: 186.0 calories; 38.2 mg. sodium; 23.3 gm. carbohydrates; 11.4 gm. fat.

Fruit Salad Picante   SERVES 8

Long before health foods were the rage, Mexicans were enjoying delectable salads such as this one.

2 oranges, peeled and sectioned
1 grapefruit, peeled, sectioned, and chopped
2 pears, cored and sliced
2 apples, cored and sliced
2 bananas, peeled and sliced

¼ cup dark raisins*
¾ cup Honey-Lime Dressing (page 229) or Sweet Dressing (page 230)
1 head iceberg lettuce, shredded

1. In bowl, combine first 6 ingredients. Toss to blend.

2. Add dressing and toss to blend.
3. Divide lettuce among 8 plates. Top with fruit mixture.

Per serving with Honey-Lime Dressing: 198.0 calories; 12.8 mg. sodium; 45.8 gm. carbohydrates; 2.8 gm. fat.
Per serving with Sweet Dressing: 216.8 calories; 15.5 mg. sodium; 43.0 gm. carbohydrates; 5.9 gm. fat.

* Preserved in non-sodium ingredient.

Christmas Eve Salad   SERVES 8

One look at this spectacular salad will tell you it is very special indeed. It
fairly sparkles with color and gaiety. Indeed, it is generally reserved, as
its name suggests, for the midnight supper following mass on Christmas
Eve. But there is no reason for you not to enjoy this joyous dish whenever
you want to add a festive touch to your meal.

1 can (8 ounces) low-sodium beets,
   drained, liquid reserved
2 oranges, peeled, sectioned, and
   chopped
2 green apples, peeled, cored, and
   chopped
2 scallions, minced, including greens

1 head iceberg lettuce, shredded
1 can (8 ounces) pineapple chunks,
   liquid reserved
2 bananas, peeled and sliced
¼ cup chopped unsalted walnuts
1¼ cups Sweet Dressing (page 230)

1. In bowl, combine first 4 ingredients. Toss to blend. Cover and chill at
   least 1 hour to allow flavors to blend.
2. In second bowl, combine lettuce, pineapple, bananas, and walnuts. Toss
   to blend.
3. In third bowl, combine dressing, reserved beet liquid, and reserved
   pineapple liquid. Stir to blend thoroughly.
4. Stir beet mixture into lettuce mixture. Divide among 8 plates.
5. Serve dressing mixture on the side.

Per serving: 233.8 calories; 28.1 mg. sodium; 33.2 gm. carbohydrates; 11.6 gm. fat.

Chicken Salad Cozumel

SERVES 4

Once you sample this dish, "ordinary" chicken salad will lose its appeal.

2 half chicken breasts, poached* and
  cubed
1 apple, peeled, cored, and diced
¼ cup unsalted peanuts, crushed
2 scallions, chopped, including greens

½ cup Sweet Dressing (page 230)
1 tablespoon dry sherry
½ teaspoon dried tarragon
1 head romaine lettuce, chopped
2 limes, cut in wedges

1. In bowl, combine all but last 2 ingredients. Cover and chill at least 1 hour to allow flavors to blend.
2. Divide lettuce among 4 plates. Top with chicken mixture.
3. Garnish with lime wedges.

Per serving: 253.3 calories; 45.8 mg. sodium; 22.5 gm. carbohydrates; 12.7 gm. fat.

* Do not add salt to water.

Stuffed Avocado Salad

SERVES 4

Any cooked meat or fish will be just as delicious in this marvelous and very Mexican dish. Terrific for lunch or dinner.

2 avocados, halved and pitted
1 cup cooked chicken, cubed
¼ cup unsalted cashews, chopped
1 apple, peeled, cored, and diced

8 dried apricots, diced
⅓ cup Fruit Juice Dressing (page 226)
  or Honey-Lime Dressing (page 229)

1. Scoop out avocado pulp, leaving ½ inch all around. Transfer pulp to bowl. Chop.
2. Add remaining ingredients, except avocado halves. Toss to blend thoroughly.
3. Stuff avocado halves with chicken mixture. Cover and chill at least 1 hour to allow flavors to blend.

Per serving with Fruit Juice Dressing: 426.6 calories; 26.0 mg. sodium; 28.3 gm. carbohydrates; 35.1 gm. fat.
Per serving with Honey-Lime Dressing: 440.5 calories; 25.9 mg. sodium; 28.3 gm. carbohydrates; 34.8 gm. fat.

Jicama and Chorizo Salad   SERVES 8

The crunchy sweetness of jicama is an exotic treat set off to advantage in this lovely dish. But you should also enjoy jicama the way the Mexicans do: accented with nothing more than lime juice and a dash of Chili Powder (page 210).

1 head iceberg lettuce, shredded
1 head romaine lettuce, chopped
2 scallions, chopped, including greens
2 cups peeled, thinly sliced jicama
2 ounces low-sodium Swiss cheese, minced
12 cherry tomatoes, halved

1 cucumber, peeled and diced
1 teaspoon olive oil
4 ounces Chorizo (page 158)
2 red peppers, halved
½ cup Oil and Vinegar Dressing (page 227)

1. Preheat oven to broil.
2. In bowl, combine first 7 ingredients. Toss to blend. Set aside.
3. In skillet, heat oil over low heat. Add chorizo and cook 10 minutes, or until browned all over, stirring often.
4. While chorizo is cooking, on baking sheet, place peppers cut side down. Broil 6 inches from heat 5 minutes, or until pepper skins are browned. Transfer to platter. Chop.
5. To lettuce mixture, add chorizo and peppers. Toss to blend.
6. Pour dressing over all. Toss to blend.

Per serving: 192.1 calories; 55.6 mg. sodium; 21.9 gm. carbohydrates; 7.7 gm. fat.

Shrimp Salad Mazatlan

SERVES 4

This truly delicate meal is as wonderful to see as it is to eat, a marvelous assault on the senses: pungent and creamy white yogurt, spicy green chile, sweet, moist orange, and delectable bites of shrimp. Serve with Rice with Tomatoes (page 188).

1 pint plain yogurt
½ teaspoon dried basil
1 green chile, seeded and minced
3 tablespoons lime juice
1 cucumber, peeled and diced
1 orange, peeled and sectioned

½ pound fresh shrimp, shelled,
   deveined, steamed,* and chopped
16 leaves of romaine lettuce
2 hard-cooked eggs, halved
   lengthwise

1. In bowl, combine first 4 ingredients, stirring to blend thoroughly.
2. Stir in cucumber and orange. Cover and chill at least 1 hour to allow flavors to blend.
3. Stir in shrimp.
4. Divide lettuce among 4 plates. Top with shrimp mixture.
5. Garnish with eggs.

Per serving: 220.5 calories; 126.5 mg. sodium; 16.5 gm. carbohydrates; 6.7 gm. fat.

* Do not add salt to water.

Squid Salad with Peppers

SERVES 4

Squid is not the first thing that comes to mind when talking about seafood, but once you try this dish, you are bound to think of it more often.

1 cup Lemon Dressing (page 226)
1 green chile, seeded and minced
1 onion, sliced
½ pound cleaned squid, chopped
1 tablespoon dried parsley

1 teaspoon paprika
¼ teaspoon dried thyme
1 large green pepper, sliced
1 large red pepper, sliced
1 head Boston lettuce, chopped

1. In bowl, combine first 4 ingredients. Toss to blend.
2. Stir in parsley, paprika, and thyme. Stir to blend thoroughly. Cover and chill at least 1 hour to allow flavors to blend.

3. In second bowl, combine green and red peppers and lettuce. Toss to blend.
4. Divide lettuce mixture among 4 plates. Top with squid mixture.

Per serving: 286.4 calories; 66.8 mg. sodium; 26.1 gm. carbohydrates; 16.5 gm. fat.

Chili-Tuna Salad   SERVES 4

The distinctly sweet taste of tuna makes it especially suitable for mixing and mingling with other flavors. This salad is a notable example.

1 can (6½ ounces) low-sodium tuna
3 low-sodium hot cherry peppers, seeded and minced
½ teaspoon celery seed*
1 teaspoon dried oregano
1 cucumber, peeled, seeded, and chopped
⅓ cup low-sodium chili ketchup
½ teaspoon Chili Powder (page 210)

¼ teaspoon ground cumin
2 teaspoons lime juice
¼ cup orange juice
2 tablespoons low-sodium mayonnaise
1 head iceberg lettuce, shredded
Parsley sprigs for garnish

1. In bowl, break tuna into flakes. Add hot cherry peppers, celery seed, oregano, and cucumber. Toss to blend. Cover and chill at least ½ hour to allow flavors to blend.
2. In second bowl, combine chili ketchup, chili powder, cumin, and lime juice, blending thoroughly.
3. In third bowl, combine orange juice and mayonnaise, blending thoroughly.
4. Stir mayonnaise mixture into chili ketchup mixture, blending thoroughly. Cover and chill at least ½ hour to allow flavors to blend.
5. In fourth bowl, combine lettuce and tuna mixture. Toss to blend.
6. Add ketchup-mayonnaise mixture. Toss to blend.
7. Garnish with parsley.

Per serving: 183.2 calories; 61.8 mg. sodium; 11.5 gm. carbohydrates; 6.5 gm. fat.

* Do not use celery flakes, which contain salt.

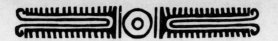

Fish and Shellfish

Hundreds of inland rivers and lakes, thousands of miles of seemingly endless coastline which winds and stretches down one side of Mexico and up the other—all teem with a staggeringly abundant variety of fish and shellfish.

Thus, wherever you go in Mexico, fish is a specialty of the house: shrimp in Mazatlan, snapper in Veracruz, fish on a stick and the internationally popular ceviche on every pushcart, and oysters, sea bass, flounder, and tuna in every port of call.

In Mexico, fish is generally poached in a fish or chicken stock, often flavored with wine and herbs. Sauces are important, too, and be they pungent or mild, Mexican sauces never obscure but, rather, raise the delicate perfection of the seafood to sublime gastronomic heights. What is more, because there is so little distance between coasts, fresh fish from the Caribbean, Pacific, and Gulf coasts can be quickly transported and enjoyed in the interior.

As you may have guessed, Mexico is famous for its seafood. Guaymas, Mazatlan, Puerto Vallarta, Acapulco, Veracruz, and Matamoros all contribute to this reputation. And now you are the happy recipient of this expertise.

As you savor such succulent delights as Oysters in Sherry-Tomato Sauce (page 129) and Salmon with Vegetables Veracruz (page 117), close your eyes. You can almost believe you are enjoying your meal as the sun sprinkles gold over the gently lapping surf which yielded its bounty for your pleasure.

Flounder in Chile-Corn Sauce SERVES 4

A marvelous multi-taste experience. Complement this dish with Melon Soup (page 80) and Mixed Salad San Miguel (page 101).

1 pound flounder fillets
¼ cup cider vinegar
½ cup orange juice
1 stick cinnamon
¹⁄₁₆ teaspoon cayenne pepper
1 teaspoon olive oil
1 onion, minced
2 green chiles, seeded and minced

2 cloves garlic, minced
1 can (8 ounces) low-sodium corn
 niblets, including liquid
½ teaspoon dried oregano
1 teaspoon dried parsley
2 teaspoons low-sodium chicken
 bouillon
2 tablespoons heavy cream

1. In bowl, combine first 5 ingredients. Cover and chill at least 4 hours, turning fish occasionally.
2. Preheat oven to 325°.
3. In skillet, heat oil over low heat. Add onion, chiles, and garlic. Sauté 5 minutes, or until onion is golden, stirring often.
4. Add onion mixture and all remaining ingredients, except cream, to fish mixture. Cover and bake 20 minutes.
5. Stir in cream. Bake, uncovered, 10 minutes more, or until fish flakes easily. Discard cinnamon.

Per serving: 202.2 calories; 101.3 mg. sodium; 29.4 gm. carbohydrates; 5.9 gm. fat.

Flounder in Green Garlic Sauce SERVES 4

Do not be put off by the garlic. Fried in olive oil, it takes on a sweet and nutty flavor. Once you try this dish, you will appreciate this humble bulb. Cheesy Hot Noodles (page 182) and Broiled Tomatoes with Avocado (page 200) round out the menu nicely.

1 pound flounder fillets
¼ cup lime juice
2 tablespoons dry white wine
2 tablespoons olive oil, divided

6 cloves garlic, chopped
2 green chiles, seeded and minced
2 tablespoons dried parsley

1. In bowl, combine first 3 ingredients. Let stand 20 minutes.
2. While fish is marinating, in skillet, heat 2 teaspoons oil over low heat.

Add garlic and simmer 10 minutes. Transfer garlic to small bowl and mash. Set aside.

3. To skillet, add chiles and simmer 5 minutes, stirring often. Add to garlic.
4. In skillet, heat remaining oil over low heat.
5. Drain fish, reserving marinade. Add fish to skillet. Sauté 5 minutes.
6. While fish is cooking, in blender, combine garlic, chiles, reserved marinade, and parsley. Puree.
7. Turn fish and sauté 3 minutes. Add parsley mixture and cook 5 minutes more.

Per serving: 183.6 calories; 95.0 mg. sodium; 6.1 gm. carbohydrates; 8.4 gm. fat.

Flounder with Walnut-Orange Sauce

SERVES 8

French and German influences work their magic in this wonderful dish. Lovely with Peas and Almonds (page 206) and boiled noodles or white rice.

2 pounds flounder fillets
1/8 teaspoon cayenne pepper
2 tablespoons lemon juice
3/4 cup orange juice
1 small orange, sliced in 1/4-inch rounds
1/4 cup dry sherry
1 teaspoon unsalted margarine
1 onion, minced

1 clove garlic, minced
1/4 cup crushed unsalted walnuts
2 teaspoons cider vinegar
8 fresh mushrooms, sliced
1 teaspoon dried basil
1 teaspoon paprika
2 ounces low-sodium Swiss cheese, sliced thin

1. In 9 x 13-inch ovenproof casserole, combine first 6 ingredients. Cover and refrigerate 1 hour.
2. Preheat oven to 350°.
3. While flounder is marinating, in skillet, heat margarine over low heat. Add onion and garlic and cook 10 minutes, or until onion is lightly browned.
4. Add walnuts and cook 1 minute more.
5. Stir in vinegar, blending thoroughly.
6. Spoon onion mixture around fish. Add mushrooms, basil, and paprika. Bake 20 minutes.
7. Remove fish from oven. Top with cheese.
8. Turn on broiler. Broil fish 4 inches from heat 2 minutes, or until cheese melts.

Per serving: 182.8 calories; 95.3 mg. sodium; 9.1 gm. carbohydrates; 6.2 gm. fat.

Haddock in Walnut Sauce

SERVES 8

A traditional Mexican combination of ingredients with delicious results. Serve with your favorite rice recipe.

1 cup water
½ cup dry white wine
2 onions, chopped
2 carrots, cut in 1-inch rounds
1 clove garlic, minced
6 black peppercorns, ground

⅟₁₆ teaspoon clove powder
3 tomatoes, chopped
2 tablespoons dried parsley
2 pounds haddock steak
½ cup unsalted walnuts

1. In skillet, combine first 7 ingredients. Turn heat to medium and bring to a slow boil. Reduce heat. Cover and simmer 20 minutes.
2. Add remaining ingredients. Cover and simmer 20 minutes more, or until fish flakes easily. Transfer fish to warm platter.
3. In blender, puree cooking sauce a little at a time.
4. Return sauce to skillet. Raise heat to medium-low. Cook 10 minutes, or until sauce bubbles around the edges.
5. Pour sauce over fish.

Per serving: 194.5 calories; 87.7 mg. sodium; 12.4 gm. carbohydrates; 5.9 gm. fat.

Tomato Fried Haddock

SERVES 8

Absolutely scrumptious with Green Beans, Mushrooms, and Sweet Peppers (page 203) served alongside.

½ cup all-purpose flour
2 teaspoons dried basil
2 tablespoons low-sodium chicken
    bouillon
¼ teaspoon cayenne pepper
2 eggs, lightly beaten

⅓ cup water
½ cup salad oil
2 pounds haddock fillets
2 cups Sweet Tomato Sauce
    (page 211)
1 teaspoon paprika

1. In small bowl, combine first 4 ingredients. Set aside.
2. In second bowl, beat together eggs and water. Set aside.

3. In skillet, heat oil over medium heat until it starts to crackle.
4. Dip fish, first in flour mixture, then in egg mixture.
5. Lower fish into skillet. Reduce heat to medium-low and fry 5 minutes, or until bottom is golden brown.
6. Turn fish and fry 5 minutes more, or until second side is golden brown. Remove fish and drain on paper towels.
7. Drain off any oil remaining in skillet. Then add tomato sauce and paprika, stirring to blend. Cook 10 minutes, stirring occasionally.
8. Return fish to skillet. Raise heat to medium and cook until sauce bubbles around the edges.

Per serving: 225.5 calories; 90.6 mg. sodium; 17.1 gm. carbohydrates; 5.8 gm. fat.

Honey Fish SERVES 4

Rice with Tomatoes (page 188) and Baked Squash with Raisins (page 197) do this succulent dish proud.

1 pound flounder, red snapper, or
  salmon fillets
¾ cup cold water
¼ cup dry sherry
⅛ teaspoon aniseed
½ teaspoon lemon peel powder
1 tablespoon low-sodium beef
  bouillon

3 tablespoons red wine vinegar
⅛ teaspoon ground cumin
2 teaspoons mustard powder
⅓ cup boiling water
2 tablespoons honey

1. Place fish in 9 x 13-inch ovenproof casserole. Add cold water, sherry, aniseed, lemon peel powder, and bouillon. Cover and refrigerate ½ hour.
2. Add vinegar, cumin, and mustard powder. Let stand 20 minutes.
3. While fish is marinating, in bowl, combine last 2 ingredients. Let stand 20 minutes.
4. Preheat oven to 325°.
5. Pour honey mixture over fish. Cover and bake 20 minutes, or until fish flakes easily.

Per serving with flounder: 139.2 calories; 98.5 mg. sodium; 8.6 gm. carbohydrates; 1.7 gm. fat.
Per serving with red snapper: 155.2 calories; 85.9 mg. sodium; 8.6 gm. carbohydrates; 2.4 gm. fat.
Per serving with salmon: 296.9 calories; 82.5 mg. sodium; 8.6 gm. carbohydrates; 16.1 gm. fat.

Fish-Stuffed Eggplant　　　　SERVES 8

A tossed salad and Simple Beans (page 174) turn this humble dish into a memorable meal.

2 1-pound eggplants	1 teaspoon brandy
1 teaspoon peanut (or vegetable) oil	1 teaspoon lemon juice
1 onion, chopped	1 tablespoon heavy cream
1 clove garlic, minced	1 ounce low-sodium Swiss cheese,
2 tomatoes, chopped	shredded
2 teaspoons dried parsley	2 ounces low-sodium Cheddar
1 teaspoon Chili Powder (page 210)	cheese, sliced thin
1 pound scrod or halibut fillets, cut in	
1-inch chunks	

1. Preheat oven to broil.
2. Place eggplants on aluminum foil 4 inches from heat. Broil, turning often, until skins start to blacken. Remove to warm platter.
3. Split eggplants in half. Scoop out pulp, leaving ½ inch around the edges. Mash pulp and set aside. Set eggplant shells aside.
4. In skillet, heat oil over low heat. Add onion and garlic. Cook until onion is golden, stirring occasionally.
5. Add tomatoes, parsley, and chili powder. Stir to blend. Push onion mixture to sides of skillet.
6. Add fish and cook 5 minutes, stirring occasionally.
7. Stir in brandy, lemon juice, cream, and mashed eggplant pulp. Cook 2 minutes more.
8. Stir in Swiss cheese, blending thoroughly.
9. Spoon fish mixture into eggplant shells. Top with Cheddar cheese.
10. Place shells on cookie sheet. Reduce oven to 325° and bake stuffed eggplants 25 minutes, or until cheese melts and starts to brown on top.
11. Cut each shell in half.

Per serving with scrod: 145.9 calories; 50.3 mg. sodium; 11.7 gm. carbohydrates; 5.2 gm. fat.
Per serving with halibut: 158.5 calories; 41.2 mg. sodium; 11.7 gm. carbohydrates; 5.7 gm. fat.

Scrod and Potatoes in Spicy Cheese Sauce

SERVES 8

Both Spanish and German influences can be noted here, and the resulting combination tantalizes the tongue. A mixed green salad is all you need to complete this meal.

¼ cup all-purpose flour
Black pepper to taste
2 teaspoons low-sodium beef
  bouillon
1 tablespoon dried parsley
2 pounds scrod fillets
4 tablespoons olive oil, divided
6 pasilla chiles (or 6 dried chiles)
1 onion, chopped
2 cloves garlic, chopped
1 green pepper, chopped
¼ teaspoon dried marjoram
¼ teaspoon dried thyme
½ teaspoon dried oregano

⅛ teaspoon ground cinnamon
1⁄16 teaspoon clove powder
⅛ teaspoon ground cumin
2 tablespoons cider vinegar
1 teaspoon sugar
2 tomatoes, chopped
3 potatoes, parboiled,* peeled, and
  sliced
¼ cup dry white wine
2 tablespoons low-sodium
  mayonnaise
2 ounces low-sodium Cheddar
  cheese, grated

1. In bowl, combine first 4 ingredients, blending thoroughly.
2. Add fish and dust both sides with flour mixture.
3. In skillet, heat 2 tablespoons oil over medium-low heat. Add fish and sauté 5 minutes, or until bottom is golden brown.
4. Turn fish. Add remaining oil and sauté 5 minutes more, or until second side is golden brown. Transfer to warm platter.
5. While fish is cooking, in blender, combine chiles, onion, garlic, pepper, marjoram, thyme, oregano, cinnamon, clove powder, cumin, vinegar, sugar, and tomatoes. Puree.
6. Transfer puree to skillet and sauté in oil residue 3 minutes, stirring often.
7. Add potatoes, wine, and mayonnaise. Top with fish, then with cheese. Reduce heat to low. Cover and cook 20 minutes more, or until fish flakes easily.

Per serving with pasilla chiles: 311.7 calories; 93.5 mg. sodium; 23.3 gm. carbohydrates; 13.4 gm. fat.
Per serving with dried chiles: 330.7 calories; 120.2 mg. sodium; 26.6 gm. carbohydrates; 14.0 gm. fat.

* Do not add salt to water.

Baked Salmon in Mustard Sauce

SERVES 4

Mexican cuisine is the product of many European cooking traditions, blended to produce exquisite results. The recipe below is one example, the mustard signaling the Germanic influence. Serve it with Yellow Rice (page 190) and Asparagus in Crumb Sauce (page 196) for a truly superior meal.

1 teaspoon unsalted margarine
1 leek, chopped, including greens
1 clove garlic, minced
2 teaspoons all-purpose flour
2 cups Fish Stock (page 77)
¼ teaspoon dried thyme

2 tablespoons low-sodium Dijon
 mustard
1 pound salmon fillets
¼ cup heavy cream
2 teaspoons dried parsley

1. Preheat oven to 325°.
2. In saucepan, heat margarine over low heat. Add leek and garlic and sauté 2 minutes, or until leek is wilted, stirring often.
3. Stir in flour and blend thoroughly.
4. Add stock, thyme, and mustard. Raise heat to medium and cook 5 minutes, or until mixture bubbles around the edges.
5. While sauce is cooking, place salmon in 9-inch-square ovenproof casserole.
6. Pour sauce over salmon and bake 10 minutes.
7. Add cream and parsley. Cover and bake 10 minutes more, or until fish flakes easily.

Per serving: 365.6 calories; 91.0 mg. sodium; 10.4 gm. carbohydrates; 22.8 gm. fat.

Salmon with Vegetables Veracruz SERVES 4

Veracruz is noted for its fine seafood, and no better example exists than the dish below. It is lavishly replete with good tastes and needs only boiled white rice for accompaniment.

1 teaspoon olive oil
1 onion, minced
2 cloves garlic, minced
1 leek, chopped, including greens
1 pound salmon fillets
½ cup dry sherry
1 tablespoon tequila
½ teaspoon dried basil
1 teaspoon dried parsley
Black pepper to taste

½ teaspoon aniseed
¼ cup boiling water
1 teaspoon low-sodium chicken
  bouillon
2 halves low-sodium sweet peppers,
  sliced
2 carrots, steamed* and sliced
2 tomatoes, chopped

1. In skillet, heat oil over low heat. Add onion and garlic and cook 5 minutes, or until onion turns golden, stirring often.
2. Add leek and cook 2 minutes more. Transfer to 9 x 13-inch ovenproof casserole.
3. Add salmon, sherry, tequila, basil, parsley, black pepper, and aniseed. Let stand 5 minutes.
4. While salmon is marinating, in bowl, combine water and bouillon, stirring until bouillon is dissolved.
5. Pour bouillon mixture over salmon. Cover and chill 1 hour to allow flavors to blend, turning salmon once.
6. Preheat oven to 350°.
7. To casserole, add remaining ingredients. Cover and bake 25 minutes, or until fish flakes easily.

Per serving: 383.4 calories; 117.8 mg. sodium; 23.6 gm. carbohydrates; 17.4 gm. fat.

* Do not add salt to water.

Scrod in Pecan Sauce SERVES 4

The Kahlua makes this dish especially noteworthy. Creamed Chile Corn (page 204) is one delicious dish you might consider as an accompaniment.

2 cups Fish Stock (page 77)
2 leeks, chopped, including greens
2 teaspoons paprika
1 teaspoon low-sodium beef bouillon

1 tablespoon dried parsley
1 pound scrod fillets
¼ cup unsalted chopped pecans
1 teaspoon Kahlua

1. In skillet, combine first 5 ingredients. Turn heat to medium and bring to a slow boil.
2. Reduce heat to low. Add scrod and pecans. Cover and cook 20 minutes, or until fish flakes easily. Transfer fish to warm platter.
3. In blender, puree sauce a little at a time.
4. Return sauce to skillet. Stir in Kahlua. Raise heat to medium-low and cook until sauce bubbles around the edges.
5. Pour sauce over fish.

Per serving: 221.9 calories; 96.5 mg. sodium; 13.1 gm. carbohydrates; 8.1 gm. fat.

Sea Bass in Red Wine Sauce SERVES 8

This savory meal is just as tasty cold. Spicy Potato Casserole (page 180) and Cucumber Salad La Jolla (page 100) nicely balance the menu.

½ cup all-purpose flour
⅛ teaspoon ground nutmeg
2½ teaspoons low-sodium beef bouillon
⅛ teaspoon cayenne pepper
1 tablespoon dried parsley
1 3-pound sea bass, cleaned and gutted, head and tail intact

3 tablespoons unsalted margarine, divided
2 onions, minced
1 orange, chopped, including rind
1 cup water
¼ cup low-sodium chili ketchup
½ cup dry red wine

1. In bowl, combine first 5 ingredients, blending thoroughly.
2. Add sea bass and coat on both sides. Remove and set aside.

3. In skillet, heat half the margarine over medium-low heat. Add sea bass and sauté 10 minutes, or until fish is golden brown.
4. Turn fish. Add remaining margarine and onions. Sauté 10 minutes more.
5. Add remaining ingredients. Stir to blend. Reduce heat to low. Cover and simmer ½ hour, or until fish flakes easily.

Per serving: 216.2 calories; 69.2 mg. sodium; 20.1 gm. carbohydrates; 6.0 gm. fat.

Sea Bass and Tomatoes
SERVES 8

A sumptuous and elegant meal, beautifully enhanced with Sweet Rice with Green Beans (page 189).

4 tablespoons olive oil, divided
4 cloves garlic, minced
2 pounds sea bass fillets
2 onions, minced
⅛ teaspoon ground cumin
2 green chile peppers, seeded and
  minced
½ cup dry white wine
2 teaspoons low-sodium chicken
  bouillon

Black pepper to taste
½ teaspoon dried oregano
¼ teaspoon dried thyme
1 teaspoon paprika
3 tomatoes, chopped
8 mushrooms, chopped
½ teaspoon sugar

1. In skillet, heat 1 tablespoon oil over low heat. Add garlic and sauté 5 minutes, or until garlic is lightly browned, stirring often.
2. Add 2 tablespoons oil. Then add fish and onions. Raise heat to medium-low and sauté 3 minutes, stirring onions occasionally.
3. Turn fish. Add remaining oil and cook 3 minutes more.
4. Season fish with cumin. Add remaining ingredients. Reduce heat to low. Cover and simmer 15 minutes, or until fish flakes easily.

Per serving: 220.0 calories; 88.1 mg. sodium; 10.9 gm. carbohydrates; 10.3 gm. fat.

Snapper with
Prunes and Avocado

SERVES 8

The sweetness of prunes, the subtle nuttiness of avocado and the succulent delicacy of snapper combine to make this dish a gastronomic delight. Mexican White Rice (page 186) is the only side dish you will need.

10 prunes, pitted and chopped
1 lemon, chopped, including rind
2 cups water
2 tablespoons dried parsley
2 teaspoons dried oregano
1 tablespoon low-sodium beef
  bouillon
1 tablespoon dry sherry

1 avocado, peeled, pitted, and
  mashed
1½ pounds red snapper fillets
2 tablespoons heavy cream
⅛ teaspoon ground cumin
1 teaspoon paprika

1. Preheat oven to 350°.
2. In saucepan, combine first 5 ingredients. Turn heat to medium and bring to a slow boil, stirring occasionally.
3. Reduce heat to low. Stir in bouillon and sherry and cook 5 minutes more, stirring occasionally.
4. Add avocado and cook 10 minutes more, stirring frequently.
5. While sauce is cooking, place fish in 9-inch-square ovenproof casserole.
6. Pour sauce over fish. Cover and bake 10 minutes.
7. While fish is baking, in small bowl, combine cream, cumin, and paprika, stirring to blend thoroughly.
8. Pour cream sauce over fish. Bake, uncovered, 5 minutes more, or until fish flakes easily.

Per serving: 206.7 calories; 67.4 mg. sodium; 12.9 gm. carbohydrates; 9.6 gm. fat.

Snapper Yucatan

SERVES 8

The spicy tingle so popular in Yucatan is wonderfully evident in this dish. Serve with a mixed green salad vinaigrette and a baked potato.

½ cup lemon juice
2 tablespoons red wine vinegar
1 apple, cored and sliced
1 orange, sliced, including rind
4 halves low-sodium sweet peppers, sliced
1 onion, sliced
½ teaspoon Chili Powder (page 210)
½ cup boiling water

⅟₁₆ teaspoon hot pepper flakes
2 teaspoons low-sodium chicken bouillon
½ teaspoon aniseed
2 tablespoons olive oil
2 pounds red snapper fillets
1 tablespoon dried parsley
1 teaspoon dried basil

1. In 9 x 13-inch ovenproof casserole, combine all but last 3 ingredients, stirring to blend thoroughly.
2. Add fish. Cover and refrigerate at least 6 hours, turning fish occasionally, to allow flavors to blend.
3. Preheat oven to 325°.
4. Bake fish 15 minutes.
5. Add parsley and basil. Cover and bake 15 minutes more, or until fish flakes easily.

Per serving: 198.4 calories; 94.4 mg. sodium; 14.8 gm. carbohydrates; 5.4 gm. fat.

Swordfish and Capers
SERVES 8

This stylish meal tastefully exhibits its Veracruz inspiration. Christmas Eve Salad (page 103) and Potatoes with Chiles (page 180) are worthy companions.

1½ pounds swordfish steaks
1 cup dry red wine
2 tablespoons low-sodium beef bouillon
1 bay leaf
1½ teaspoons lemon peel powder
1 teaspoon olive oil

2 cloves garlic, minced
4 scallions, chopped, including greens
2 tablespoons capers* (or 2 tablespoons white vinegar)
4 tomatoes, chopped

1. In 9-inch-square ovenproof casserole, combine first 5 ingredients. Cover and refrigerate 1 hour, turning fish occasionally.
2. While fish is marinating, in small skillet, heat oil over low heat. Add garlic and cook 5 minutes, stirring often.
3. Preheat oven to broil.
4. Add scallions and cook 2 minutes more, stirring often.
5. Add capers and tomatoes and cook 1 minute more, stirring constantly.
6. Spoon tomato mixture around swordfish and broil 6 inches from heat 5 minutes.
7. Turn fish and broil 5 minutes more.

Per serving: 171.7 calories; 11.8 mg. sodium; 7.4 gm. carbohydrates; 5.3 gm. fat.

* Preserved in vinegar only.

Swordfish with Grapefruit   SERVES 8

In this exotic offering, the acid in the grapefruit starts the "cooking" process, and the end result is unforgettably delicious. Goes well with everything.

1 cup boiling water
2 teaspoons low-sodium beef
   bouillon
½ teaspoon paprika
1 teaspoon low-sodium Dijon
   mustard
2 pounds swordfish steaks

1 grapefruit, peeled and sectioned
1 leek, chopped, including greens
8 mushrooms, sliced
1 cup Sweet-and-Hot Chile Sauce
   (page 215)
2 limes, cut in wedges

1. In bowl, combine first 4 ingredients, stirring to blend thoroughly. Let stand ½ hour.
2. Preheat oven to broil.
3. In 9 x 13-inch ovenproof casserole, place fish. Surround with grapefruit, leek, and mushrooms. Pour mustard mixture over all.
4. Broil 6 inches from heat 5 minutes.
5. Turn fish and broil 5 minutes more.
6. Pour on chile sauce. Broil 5 minutes more, or until fish flakes easily.
7. Garnish with lime wedges.

Per serving: 203.0 calories; 13.3 mg. sodium; 14.8 gm. carbohydrates; 6.3 gm. fat.

Tuna and Apricots

SERVES 4

Once again, the traditions of French and German cookery combine to produce a Mexican recipe so fabulous that any accompaniment will taste like the perfect choice.

2 teaspoons olive oil
1 pound tuna steaks
1 clove garlic, minced
2 leeks, chopped, including greens
¼ cup dry white wine
Black pepper to taste
1 cup hot water
1 tablespoon low-sodium chicken
  bouillon

10 dried apricots, chopped
¹⁄₁₆ teaspoon ground nutmeg
1 tablespoon dried parsley
2 tablespoons low-sodium cream
  cheese

1. In skillet, heat oil over medium heat. Add fish and garlic and cook 3 minutes.
2. Turn fish and cook 3 minutes more.
3. Add leeks and cook 2 minutes more.
4. Add all remaining ingredients, except cream cheese. Reduce heat to low. Cover and simmer 15 minutes.
5. Add cream cheese. Cover and simmer 10 minutes more, or until fish flakes easily.

Per serving: 317.5 calories; 57.5 mg. sodium; 22.0 gm. carbohydrates; 10.9 gm. fat.

Tuna Casserole SERVES 8

Tuna casserole, Mexican style, is a one-dish meal everyone will love. It is an easy and excellent party pleaser, great with Beans with Cheese (page 175).

1 tablespoon olive oil
2 onions, minced
2 cloves garlic, minced
2 potatoes, boiled,* peeled, and
   sliced
Black pepper to taste
¼ teaspoon ground cumin
2 cans (13 ounces) low-sodium tuna
2 green chiles, seeded and minced
½ teaspoon celery seed†
1 tablespoon cider vinegar
1 tablespoon dry sherry

2 tablespoons raisins‡
1 teaspoon dried oregano
2 potatoes, boiled,* peeled, and
   mashed
1½ teaspoons low-sodium mustard
1 teaspoon dried parsley
1½ teaspoons low-sodium chicken
   bouillon
2 ounces low-sodium Cheddar
   cheese, sliced thin
2 teaspoons paprika

1. In skillet, heat oil over low heat. Add onions and garlic and cook 5 minutes, stirring occasionally.
2. Push onions and garlic to sides of skillet. To well created in center, add potatoes. Add pepper and cumin. Cook 5 minutes, or until potatoes are lightly browned on bottom.
3. Turn potatoes and cook 5 minutes more, or until lightly browned on bottom.
4. Transfer onions, garlic, and potatoes to 9-inch-square ovenproof casserole.
5. Preheat oven to 350°.
6. In bowl, combine tuna, chiles, celery seed, vinegar, sherry, raisins, and oregano, blending thoroughly. Spoon over onion and potato mixture.
7. In second bowl combine mashed potatoes, mustard, parsley, and bouillon, blending thoroughly. Spoon on top of tuna mixture.
8. Top mashed potatoes with cheese. Sprinkle with paprika. Bake ½ hour, or until top is crusty and browned.

Per serving: 185.8 calories; 34.8 mg. sodium; 22.3 gm. carbohydrates; 5.2 gm. fat.

* Do not add salt to water.
† Do not use celery flakes, which contain salt.
‡ Preserved in non-sodium ingredient.

Shrimp in Creamy Wine Sauce   SERVES 8

Serve Puree of Avocado Soup (page 88) and the rice of your choice with this special dish for a memorable meal.

1 tablespoon unsalted margarine
1 green pepper, chopped
1½ pounds fresh shrimp, shelled, deveined, and halved diagonally
1¾ cups Creamy Wine Sauce (page 221)

1 teaspoon dried parsley
½ teaspoon paprika
2 lemons, cut in wedges

1. In skillet, heat margarine over medium heat. Add pepper and shrimp and sauté 2 minutes, or until shrimp are pink all over, stirring constantly.
2. Stir in wine sauce, parsley, and paprika. Cook 5 minutes more, or until sauce bubbles around the edges.
3. Garnish with lemon wedges.

Per serving: 220.9 calories; 134.6 mg. sodium; 6.7 gm. carbohydrates; 14.0 gm. fat.

Shrimp in Spice Sauce   SERVES 4

Spicy and definitely addictive. For contrast, try this with Refried Beans (page 177) or Salad of Colors (page 102).

¾ pound fresh shrimp
3 cups water
1 onion
3 cloves
1 bay leaf
½ teaspoon garlic powder
4 tablespoons lemon juice

2 cups Chile-Vegetable Sauce (page 214)
2 tablespoons low-sodium ketchup
1 cucumber, peeled and diced
1 tablespoon dried parsley

1. In saucepan, combine first 7 ingredients. Turn heat to medium and bring to a slow boil. Continue boiling 3 minutes. Strain, reserving half the liquid. Let shrimp stand 5 minutes.
2. Shell, devein, and halve shrimp diagonally.
3. In bowl, combine reserved shrimp liquid and shrimp. Cover and refrigerate at least 1 hour to allow flavors to blend.

4. While shrimp is marinating, in second bowl, combine remaining ingredients.
5. Strain shrimp again. Then stir shrimp into vegetable sauce.

Per serving: 176.8 calories; 154.3 mg. sodium; 20.5 gm. carbohydrates; 0.6 gm. fat.

Shrimp with
Peppers and Peanuts

SERVES 4

Two products Mexico can claim as her own—peppers and peanuts—achieve culinary distinction in this lovely dish. Serve with steamed broccoli and boiled potatoes.

1 teaspoon olive oil
1 onion, minced
2 green chiles, seeded and minced
1 clove garlic, minced
¼ cup unsalted peanuts, crushed
¾ cup boiling water
1 teaspoon low-sodium chicken
   bouillon
½ teaspoon paprika
1 tablespoon dry red wine

½ can (3 ounces) low-sodium tomato
   paste
¹⁄₁₆ teaspoon cayenne pepper
1 green pepper, chopped
2 halves low-sodium sweet peppers,
   sliced
¾ pound fresh shrimp, shelled and
   deveined

1. In skillet, heat oil over low heat. Add onion, chiles, garlic, and peanuts. Cook 10 minutes, or until onion is lightly browned, stirring often.
2. While onion mixture is cooking, in bowl, combine water, bouillon, paprika, wine, tomato paste, and cayenne pepper, blending thoroughly. Stir into onion mixture.
3. Stir in green pepper and sweet peppers. Cover and simmer 10 minutes, stirring occasionally.
4. Add shrimp. Raise heat to medium-low. Cook, uncovered, 10 minutes more, or until shrimp turn pink all over.

Per serving: 230.0 calories; 55.6 mg. sodium; 18.9 gm. carbohydrates; 9.5 gm. fat.

Mixed Seafood in Lime Sauce   SERVES 8

A sophisticated version of ceviche that is mouth-wateringly delicious.

¾ cup Lime Sauce (page 217)
½ pound fresh shrimp, shelled,
    deveined, and halved diagonally
½ pound squid, cut in 1-inch chunks
1 pint shucked oysters, liquid reserved
1 tablespoon unsalted margarine

2 leeks, chopped, including greens
1 zucchini, chopped
3 tomatoes, chopped
2 teaspoons dry sherry

1. In bowl, combine first 4 ingredients, stirring to blend. Cover and refrigerate at least 4 hours to allow flavors to blend.
2. In skillet, heat margarine over low heat. Add seafood mixture, leeks, zucchini, tomatoes, and sherry. Cover and simmer 10 minutes.
3. Stir in reserved oyster liquid. Raise heat to medium and cook, uncovered, 2 minutes more.

Per serving: 183.8 calories; 131.0 mg. sodium; 22.7 gm. carbohydrates; 4.4 gm. fat.

Oysters in
Mayonnaise-Wine Sauce   SERVES 4

Perfectly elegant for lunch or dinner. Avocado, Tomato, and Cheese Salad (page 98) is a lovely accompaniment.

1 cup water
2 teaspoons low-sodium chicken
    bouillon
1 teaspoon lime juice
1 pint shucked oysters, liquid reserved
1 teaspoon unsalted margarine
1 onion, minced
Black pepper to taste

2 tablespoons dry white wine
2 teaspoons dried parsley
½ teaspoon dried thyme
½ teaspoon dried oregano
Cayenne pepper to taste
2 tablespoons low-sodium
    mayonnaise

1. In saucepan, combine first 3 ingredients. Turn heat to medium-low and cook until mixture bubbles around the edges, stirring often.
2. Add oysters and cook 1 minute. With slotted spoon transfer oysters to warm platter. Set aside.

3. To saucepan, add reserved oyster liquid, stirring to blend. Set aside.
4. In second saucepan, heat margarine over low heat. Add onion and cook 5 minutes, or until onion turns golden, stirring often.
5. Add remaining ingredients, except oyster liquid mixture and oysters. Cook 5 minutes, stirring until mayonnaise is thoroughly blended.
6. Stir in oyster liquid mixture. Raise heat to medium and cook 5 minutes more, or until sauce bubbles around the edges.
7. Add oysters and cook 2 minutes more.

Per serving: 142.5 calories; 71.5 mg. sodium; 9.5 gm. carbohydrates; 8.6 gm. fat.

Oysters in Sherry-Tomato Sauce   SERVES 4

After sampling this dish you will know why oysters are considered a delicacy by so many. This dish may be accented with Rice with Mushrooms and Cheese (page 188).

1 teaspoon olive oil
1 leek, minced, including greens
2 cloves garlic, minced
1/16 teaspoon ground cumin
2 tomatoes, chopped
1 teaspoon dried oregano
Black pepper to taste

1 cup Chicken Stock (page 76)
1/4 cup dry sherry
1 bay leaf
1 pint shucked oysters, including
   liquid

1. In saucepan, heat oil over low heat. Add leek and garlic and sauté 3 minutes, stirring often.
2. Stir in cumin, tomatoes, oregano, and pepper. Cook 2 minutes more, stirring often.
3. Add stock, sherry, and bay leaf. Raise heat to high and bring to a boil. Reduce heat to medium-low and cook 20 minutes, stirring occasionally.
4. Add oysters, including liquid, and cook 2 minutes more.

Per serving: 133.3 calories; 75.5 mg. sodium; 13.6 gm. carbohydrates; 3.5 gm. fat.

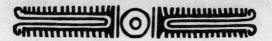

Poultry

Wild turkeys and domestic hens are indigenous to Mexico, so the number of poultry dishes in every Mexican home is infinite. Most recipes make delicious use of one or another of the chile sauces, passed on from generation to generation since the days of the Aztecs and changed ever so slightly to maximize the European seasonings and foods introduced to Mexico during and after the Spanish Conquest.

Italy, France, Germany, and, of course, Spain have all added gastronomic excitement to Mexico's prodigious poultry repertoire. Some delicious examples of their influence include Festival Chicken in Wine (page 142), Chicken and Spiced Fruit (page 135), and Poached Chicken in Chile Cream Sauce (page 144), which you will find in this chapter.

Almond-Sherry Chicken   SERVES 4

The Spanish influence is put on tasty display in this elegant dish. Guaranteed to please, Almond-Sherry Chicken is a perfect party dish.

1 tablespoon olive oil
2 onions, chopped
6 cloves garlic, minced
¼ cup unsalted slivered almonds
8 mushrooms, chopped
1 teaspoon all-purpose flour
2 cups Chicken Stock (page 76)
1 bay leaf

1 can (6 ounces) low-sodium tomato paste
4 half chicken breasts
⅛ teaspoon cayenne pepper
½ teaspoon orange peel powder
⅓ cup dry sherry
2 tablespoons dried parsley
½ teaspoon dried thyme

1. In Dutch oven, heat oil over low heat. Add onions, garlic, and almonds. Cover and cook 10 minutes, or until onions are lightly browned, stirring occasionally.
2. Add mushrooms and cook 2 minutes more, stirring constantly.
3. Stir in flour, blending well.
4. Stir in stock. Then add bay leaf, tomato paste, chicken, cayenne pepper, and orange peel powder. Raise heat to medium and bring to a slow boil. Continue boiling 5 minutes.
5. Add remaining ingredients. Reduce heat to low. Cover and cook 40 minutes, stirring occasionally.
6. Discard bay leaf.

Per serving: 331.7 calories; 85.9 mg. sodium; 29.9 gm. carbohydrates; 12.2 gm. fat.

Cheese-Stuffed Chicken   SERVES 4

Outrageously delicious.

½ cup low-sodium ricotta cheese
1 teaspoon dried basil
1 teaspoon Chili Powder (page 210)
1 green pepper, chopped
4 chicken cutlets
½ teaspoon garlic powder

Black pepper to taste
1 can (29 ounces) low-sodium tomato puree
¼ cup dry white wine
1 tablespoon paprika

1. Preheat oven to 325°.
2. In bowl, combine first 4 ingredients, blending thoroughly.

3. On cutting board, pound cutlets with knife handle to tenderize. Pierce one side with fork. Season with garlic powder and pepper.
4. Spoon equal amounts of cheese mixture on pierced side of cutlets. Roll up cutlets and skewer with toothpicks.
5. Place cutlets, skewered side down, in 9-inch-square ovenproof casserole.
6. Pour tomato puree and white wine over all. Sprinkle paprika over all.
7. Cover and bake 25 minutes. Uncover and bake 15 minutes more.

Per serving: 269.1 calories; 78.1 mg. sodium; 22.5 gm. carbohydrates; 7.1 gm. fat.

Chicken Ancho   SERVES 4

This dish uses the typically Mexican paste of ground chiles, but the savory flavor is anything but typical. Sweet Rice with Green Beans (page 189) and Cucumber Salad La Jolla (page 100) are two of the many possible accompaniments.

4 half chicken breasts	¼ teaspoon ground cinnamon
2 onions, minced	¼ cup dry sherry
2 cloves garlic, minced	1 tablespoon low-sodium chicken
Black pepper to taste	bouillon
6 ancho chiles (or 3 tablespoons	
sweet paprika)	
2 cups Chicken Stock (page 76)	
divided	

1. In large skillet, place chicken skin side down. Add onions and garlic. Season with black pepper. Turn heat to low and cook 15 minutes.
2. Raise heat to medium-low and cook 15 minutes more.
3. Turn chicken and cook 15 minutes more.
4. While chicken is cooking, in blender, combine chiles and ½ cup stock. Puree. Transfer to skillet.
5. Add remaining stock, cinnamon, and sherry. Reduce heat to low. Cover and simmer 15 minutes.
6. Stir in bouillon. Cover and simmer 15 minutes more.

Per serving: 199.9 calories; 75.9 mg. sodium; 18.4 gm. carbohydrates; 4.2 gm. fat.

Chicken and Bananas

SERVES 4

Only a Mexican chef would think to combine chicken with bananas. How lucky for us that he did. Some plain boiled white rice is all you need to complete this wonderful meal.

4 half chicken breasts	1 teaspoon dried oregano
½ cup lime juice	1⁄16 teaspoon ground nutmeg
¼ cup dry red wine	½ teaspoon ground cinnamon
2 green chiles, seeded and minced	1 onion, sliced
1 teaspoon low-sodium beef bouillon	8 mushrooms, sliced
1 tablespoon paprika	2 bananas, peeled and sliced

1. In 9-inch-square ovenproof casserole, combine first 9 ingredients. Cover and refrigerate at least 4 hours.
2. Preheat oven to 350°.
3. Scatter onion and mushrooms around chicken. Cover and bake 40 minutes.
4. Add bananas. Bake, uncovered, 20 minutes more.

Per serving: 216.4 calories; 61.3 mg. sodium; 26.4 gm. carbohydrates; 4.8 gm. fat.

Chicken and Chorizo

SERVES 8

A traditional Mexican dish, this hearty and flavorful fare is a sumptuous complete meal. Wonderful with steamed broccoli.

3 cups hot water	1 teaspoon dried oregano
1 3-pound chicken, cut into large serving pieces	1⁄8 teaspoon ground nutmeg
2 onions, sliced	1 teaspoon paprika
2 tablespoons low-sodium chicken bouillon	1 tablespoon lemon juice
	2 teaspoons olive oil
Black pepper to taste	4 potatoes, boiled,* peeled, and sliced
2 tablespoons dried parsley	
2 cloves garlic, minced	2 green chiles, seeded and minced
2 tomatoes, chopped	1 leek, chopped, including greens
1⁄8 teaspoon ground cinnamon	4 ounces Chorizo (page 158)
	½ teaspoon dried basil

1. In Dutch oven, combine first 6 ingredients. Turn heat to medium and bring to a slow boil. Continue boiling 10 minutes.

2. Reduce heat to medium-low. Add garlic, tomatoes, cinnamon, oregano, nutmeg, paprika, and lemon juice. Cook 20 minutes, stirring occasionally.
3. While chicken is cooking, in skillet, heat oil over low heat. Add potatoes, chiles, and leek. Sauté 10 minutes, or until potatoes are lightly browned, stirring often. Transfer mixture to Dutch oven.
4. To skillet, add chorizo. Raise heat to medium and fry until chorizo is browned all over, stirring constantly. Transfer to Dutch oven.
5. Stir in basil. Cook 20 minutes more, stirring occasionally.

Per serving: 284.2 calories; 86.7 mg. sodium; 25.0 gm. carbohydrates; 9.7 gm. fat.

* Do not add salt to water.

Chicken and Spiced Fruit
SERVES 8

Sweet, hot, spicy, and quite simply marvelous. Mixed Salad San Miguel (page 101) is all the accompaniment you need.

1 orange, peeled and sectioned	1 teaspoon dried basil
1 can (8 ounces) dietetic peaches, including juice	¼ teaspoon ground cinnamon
½ pineapple, peeled, cored, and cut into chunks	1 tablespoon honey
	2 3-pound chickens, cut into serving pieces
¼ cup lime juice	Black pepper to taste
2 cups water	1 tablespoon paprika
2 cans (16 ounces) low-sodium tomato sauce	¼ cup cider vinegar
2 teaspoons Chili Powder (page 210)	½ cup pineapple juice
1 teaspoon dried mint	½ teaspoon ground cumin

1. In bowl, combine first 4 ingredients. Cover and chill at least 2 hours to allow flavors to blend.
2. In Dutch oven, combine water, tomato sauce, chili powder, mint, basil, cinnamon, and honey. Turn heat to low and cook 10 minutes, stirring often.
3. Add chicken, pepper, paprika, vinegar, pineapple juice, and cumin. Cover and cook 10 minutes.
4. Add fruit mixture. Cover and cook ½ hour, stirring occasionally. Uncover and cook ½ hour more.

Per serving: 338.6 calories; 130.6 mg. sodium; 19.8 gm. carbohydrates; 10.9 gm. fat.

Chicken and Squash   SERVES 4

Squash is very popular in Mexico. Most common are zucchini, yellow squash, or chayote, but for this dish, we have chosen the sweet goodness of butternut squash. We think you will be pleased because this dish is truly spectacular. Serve with any rice or noodle dish.

2 teaspoons unsalted margarine
2 leeks, chopped, including greens
1/4 teaspoon aniseed
2 tomatoes, chopped
4 chicken legs
1/4 teaspoon cayenne pepper
1/2 tablespoon dried oregano
1/4 teaspoon dried marjoram
1 teaspoon dried thyme

2 tablespoons low-sodium beef
  bouillon
1 cup water
1 small butternut squash, cut in
  chunks
1/2 cup dry red wine
1/4 teaspoon ground cinnamon
1/2 teaspoon orange peel powder

1. In large skillet, heat margarine over low heat. Add leeks, aniseed, and tomatoes, pushing mixture to sides of skillet.
2. In well created in center, place chicken. Season with cayenne pepper, oregano, marjoram, thyme, and bouillon. Cook 1/2 hour, or until chicken is lightly browned all over, turning chicken occasionally.
3. Pour water around chicken. Cover and cook 20 minutes.
4. Add remaining ingredients. Cover and cook 20 minutes more, or until squash is fork tender.

Per serving: 304.6 calories; 90.6 mg. sodium; 31.6 gm. carbohydrates; 8.7 gm. fat.

Chicken Colombian SERVES 4

A tantalizing medley of Mexican flavors makes this dish special indeed. Simple Beans (page 174) is an excellent companion.

4 chicken legs
3 cloves garlic, sliced
2 onions, chopped
1 small eggplant, cubed
½ cup white wine
1 can (8 ounces) low-sodium tomato sauce
2 cups water
4 tablespoons low-sodium beef bouillon

½ teaspoon ground black peppercorns
1 tablespoon dried tarragon
1½ tablespoons dried parsley
2 teaspoons paprika
2 poblano chiles (or 2 green peppers), seeded and chopped
1 large tomato, chopped
6 mushrooms, chopped

1. Preheat oven to 325°.
2. Gash chicken legs and insert garlic slices into gashes.
3. In 9-inch-square ovenproof casserole, place chicken. Add onions, eggplant, wine, tomato sauce, water, bouillon, green peppercorns, tarragon, parsley, and paprika. Stir to blend. Bake ½ hour.
4. Add remaining ingredients. Cover and bake 20 minutes more.

Per serving with poblano chiles: 306.5 calories; 118.6 mg. sodium; 35.7 gm. carbohydrates; 8.5 gm. fat.
Per serving with green peppers: 325.9 calories; 131.6 mg. sodium; 39.8 gm. carbohydrates; 8.7 gm. fat.

Chicken in Mustard Sauce   SERVES 8

The best of Mexican and German culinary styles are tastefully served up in this unique dish. Salad of Colors (page 102) is a marvelous accent.

1 4-pound chicken, cut into serving pieces	½ cup cider vinegar
	⅓ cup low-sodium Dijon mustard
1½ cups water	4 capers*
1 bay leaf	2 teaspoons paprika
1 teaspoon dried oregano	4 tomatoes, sliced
Black pepper to taste	2 onions, sliced
¼ cup dry sherry	1 green pepper, sliced

1. In large skillet, combine first 6 ingredients. Turn heat to low. Cover and simmer 15 minutes.
2. Add vinegar, mustard, capers, and paprika. Stir to blend.
3. Add remaining ingredients. Cover and cook 1 hour more, stirring occasionally and adding more water if necessary to prevent sticking.

Per serving: 216.1 calories; 89.1 mg. sodium; 10.6 gm. carbohydrates; 7.4 gm. fat.

* Preserved in vinegar only.

Chicken in Orange-Mint Sauce   SERVES 4

Mint—that marvelous herb which probably found its way into Mexico after the Spanish Conquest—is an often-used ingredient in Mexican cooking. Its sweet, delicate flavor certainly makes this dish very special. Creamed Cauliflower and Sweet Peppers (page 204) is a delightful side dish.

4 half chicken breasts	½ teaspoon dried sage
⅓ cup red wine vinegar	2 teaspoons low-sodium beef bouillon
3 onions, sliced	
8 cloves garlic, sliced	1 orange, peeled and sectioned, rind chopped fine
1 bay leaf	
1 teaspoon aniseed	2 tablespoons dried mint
1 cup hot water	1 tablespoon brandy
Black pepper to taste	3 tablespoons orange marmalade*

1. In 9 x 13-inch ovenproof casserole, combine first 6 ingredients. Cover and refrigerate at least 4 hours, turning chicken occasionally.

2. Preheat oven to 350°.
3. To casserole, add all but last 2 ingredients. Cover and bake ½ hour, turning chicken occasionally.
4. Stir in brandy. Then spread marmalade over chicken. Bake, uncovered, 20 minutes more.

Per serving: 236.4 calories; 57.2 mg. sodium; 35.0 gm. carbohydrates; 3.2 gm. fat.

* Preserved without pectin or sodium.

Chicken in Chile-Nut Sauce   SERVES 8

The special, piquant poblano chile coupled with pine nuts so enhances chicken that this dish is sure to become a favorite in your Mexican repertoire. Spicy Potato Casserole (page 180) adds the finishing touch.

4 half chicken breasts, cut into 2-inch pieces
4 chicken legs, cut into 2-inch pieces
4 cups boiling water
2 tablespoons dried parsley
Black pepper to taste
¼ cup unsalted pine nuts
¼ cup unsalted almonds
1 onion, chopped
1 clove garlic, chopped
2 tablespoons low-sodium chicken bouillon

6 poblano chiles (or 4 red peppers), seeded and chopped
2 tablespoons white vinegar
1 can (14 ounces) low-sodium tomatoes, chopped, including liquid
¼ cup dry red wine
1 tablespoon olive oil

1. In Dutch oven, combine first 5 ingredients. Turn heat to medium and bring to a slow boil. Reduce heat to low. Cover and simmer 1 hour.
2. While chicken is cooking, in blender, combine pine nuts, almonds, onion, and garlic. Grind to a paste. Set aside.
3. Drain chicken, reserving 2 cups stock.
4. Return reserved stock to Dutch oven. Stir in puree, bouillon, chiles, vinegar, tomatoes, and wine, blending thoroughly. Cook 10 minutes, stirring often.
5. Stir in oil. Add chicken. Cover and simmer 15 minutes more.

Per serving with poblano chiles: 226.1 calories; 67.6 mg. sodium; 9.8 gm. carbohydrates; 10.9 gm. fat.
Per serving with red peppers: 253.1 calories; 92.6 mg. sodium; 15.9 gm. carbohydrates; 11.2 gm. fat.

Chicken Mole

SERVES 8

Mole is an ancient Aztec word which means concoction. This dish, traditionally made with turkey and reserved for very special occasions, is the most famous of all the Mexican moles. It is truly an elaborate concoction whose base is a sauce made of many chiles. The use of chocolate is off-putting to some, but, in truth, it only adds a rich, bittersweet flavor to the whole spectacular and mouth-watering effect. Well worth the time and effort required, Chicken Mole will be the dish you serve when you want to delight your family and friends.

3 tablespoons vegetable oil, divided
2 ancho chiles (or ⅟₁₆ teaspoon hot pepper flakes)
2 pasilla chiles (or ⅟₁₆ teaspoon hot pepper flakes)
2 mulato chiles (or ⅟₁₆ teaspoon hot pepper flakes)
⅟₁₆ teaspoon cayenne pepper
2 quarts water, divided
2 3-pound chickens, cut into serving pieces
2 onions, chopped
1 carrot, sliced
10 black peppercorns
1 bay leaf
2 tablespoons unsalted almonds

2 tablespoons unsalted peanuts
1 tablespoon unsalted sesame seeds
1 slice low-sodium bread
2 cloves garlic, chopped
¼ teaspoon aniseed
¼ teaspoon ground cinnamon
⅛ teaspoon clove powder
4 tomatoes, chopped
1½ ounces low-sodium bittersweet chocolate
1 teaspoon sugar
2 tablespoons dark raisins*
Dash of vanilla extract
2 tablespoons dried parsley
1 tablespoon low-sodium chicken bouillon

1. In skillet, heat 1 tablespoon oil over low heat. Add all chiles and sauté 5 minutes, stirring often. Drain on paper towels.
2. In blender, combine chiles, cayenne pepper, and 1 cup water. **Puree.** Transfer to bowl.
3. In Dutch oven, combine remaining water, chicken pieces, half the onions, carrot, peppercorns, and bay leaf. Turn heat to high and bring to a boil. Reduce heat to low. Cover and simmer 1 hour.
4. With slotted spoon, transfer chicken to warm platter. Set aside.
5. Strain chicken broth, reserving 4 cups. Set aside.
6. In skillet, heat 1 tablespoon oil over medium-low heat. Add remaining onions, almonds, peanuts, sesame seeds, bread, garlic, aniseed, cinnamon, and clove powder. Sauté 2 minutes, or until bread is browned on both sides.
7. In blender, combine bread mixture and tomatoes. Puree.

8. In skillet, heat remaining tablespoon oil over low heat. Add chile puree and tomato puree. Cook 10 minutes, stirring often.
9. Add the 4 cups of reserved chicken broth. Stir to blend.
10. Add chocolate and sugar. Cook 5 minutes, or until sugar is dissolved, stirring often.
11. Stir in raisins, vanilla, and parsley. Cover and simmer 1½ hours. Uncover and cook 15 minutes more, or until sauce starts to thicken.
12. Add chicken. Stir in bouillon. Cook, uncovered, ½ hour more, stirring occasionally.

Note: If you wish, substitute an 8-pound turkey, cut into serving pieces, for the chicken.

Per serving with chicken: 459.3 calories; 140.0 mg. sodium; 21.1 gm. carbohydrates; 24.1 gm. fat.
Per serving with turkey: 476.2 calories; 164.3 mg. sodium; 21.1 gm. carbohydrates; 19.2 gm. fat.

* Preserved in non-sodium ingredient.

Chicken with Figs and Lemons   SERVES 4

Mexican Potato Salad (page 178) is a wonderful and zesty accompaniment to this exotically tasty dish.

1 tablespoon unsalted margarine
4 half chicken breasts, skinned
1 onion, minced
2 cloves garlic, minced
Black pepper to taste
2 tomatoes, chopped
1⁄16 teaspoon ground nutmeg
4 raw figs, chopped
2 lemons, chopped, including rind

2 cups boiling water
1⁄16 teaspoon hot pepper flakes
2 teaspoons low-sodium beef bouillon
1⁄8 teaspoon ground cumin
1⁄4 cup dry sherry
1 tablespoon dried parsley
2 teaspoons low-sodium chicken bouillon

1. In large skillet, heat margarine over low heat. Add chicken, onion, and garlic. Sauté 20 minutes, or until chicken is white all over, turning chicken often.
2. Season chicken with black pepper.
3. Add tomatoes, nutmeg, figs, lemons, water, and hot pepper flakes. Cover and simmer 40 minutes.
4. Add remaining ingredients. Cook, uncovered, 15 minutes more, stirring occasionally.

Per serving: 294.4 calories; 58.4 mg. sodium; 37.4 gm. carbohydrates; 6.9 gm. fat.

Festival Chicken in Wine SERVES 8

The name tells all. This dish is sure to bring you joy. Serve with Yellow Rice (page 190).

8 half chicken breasts
3 cloves garlic, minced
2 onions, chopped
Black pepper to taste
½ teaspoon celery seed*
½ teaspoon dried thyme
1 small eggplant (about 8 ounces), peeled and cubed
1½ cups boiling water
1 can (6 ounces) low-sodium tomato paste

2 tomatoes, chopped
1 bay leaf
2 apples, peeled, cored, and diced
½ cup dry red wine
⅛ teaspoon ground cinnamon
1 teaspoon paprika
2 zucchini, chopped
¼ teaspoon ground cumin
1½ tablespoons low-sodium beef bouillon

1. In Dutch oven, place chicken skin side down. Scatter garlic and onions all around. Season with black pepper. Turn heat to medium-low and cook 15 minutes.
2. Turn chicken and cook 15 minutes more.
3. Reduce heat to low. Add celery seed, thyme, and eggplant. Cover and simmer 20 minutes.
4. Add water, tomato paste, tomatoes, bay leaf, and apples. Cover and cook 20 minutes more, stirring occasionally.
5. Add remaining ingredients, stirring to blend thoroughly. Cook, uncovered, 15 minutes more, stirring occasionally.

Per serving: 218.8 calories; 64.5 mg. sodium; 23.4 gm. carbohydrates; 3.6 gm. fat.

* Do not use celery flakes, which contain salt.

Mint Chicken

In this dish, the spicy heat of chile powder and the sweet tingle of mint will do a provocative and very satisfying dance on your tongue. Baked Eggplant with Raisins (page 197) is a lovely companion along with Yellow Rice (page 190).

8 half chicken breasts
10 cups water
1 onion, minced
2 cloves garlic, sliced
Black pepper to taste
¼ cup lemon juice

1 tablespoon Chili Powder (page 210)
2 tablespoons dried parsley
4 tablespoons dried mint
1 tablespoon tequila

1. In Dutch oven, combine first 2 ingredients. Turn heat to high and bring to a boil. Continue boiling 20 minutes. Drain, reserving 1½ cups broth.
2. Return chicken and reserved broth to Dutch oven. Add onion, garlic, and pepper. Reduce heat to low. Cover and simmer 10 minutes.
3. Add all remaining ingredients, except tequila. Cover and simmer 20 minutes more.
4. Stir in tequila, just before serving.

Per serving: 133.2 calories; 62.3 mg. sodium; 5.3 gm. carbohydrates; 2.7 gm. fat.

Parsley Chicken

SERVES 4

Parsley (or cilantro) is the herb found in almost every Mexican dish. Used sometimes as a garnish, sometimes as a sauce base (as in this recipe), parsley reaches sublime heights in Mexican cuisine. This excellent dish goes well with any salad or vegetable of your choice.

4 tablespoons dried parsley
1 onion, chopped
2 cloves garlic, chopped
4 tomatoes, chopped
2 tablespoons cider vinegar
Cayenne pepper to taste
2 teaspoons low-sodium beef
   bouillon

⅛ teaspoon ground cumin
1 tablespoon dried mint
4 chicken legs
½ cup water
1 cup apple juice

1. In blender, combine first 9 ingredients. Puree. Transfer to skillet.
2. Place chicken on top of puree. Add water and apple juice. Turn heat to low. Cover and simmer 1 hour, adding more juice if necessary to prevent sticking.

Per serving: 211.8 calories; 87.3 mg. sodium; 21.7 gm. carbohydrates; 5.8 gm. fat.

Poached Chicken in Chile Cream Sauce

SERVES 4

The cream tempers and cools the hot chiles in this recipe to perfection. Peas and Almonds (page 206) is an elegant and delectable side dish.

4 half chicken breasts
2 green chiles, seeded and minced
1 onion, sliced
2 cloves garlic, sliced
Black pepper to taste
⅔ cup dry white wine

8 mushrooms, sliced
1 teaspoon low-sodium beef bouillon
⅛ teaspoon ground nutmeg
1 teaspoon dried oregano
1 teaspoon lemon peel powder
¼ cup heavy cream

1. In large skillet, place chicken breasts skin side down. Surround with chiles, onion, and garlic. Season with black pepper. Turn heat to low and cook ½ hour, or until skin is golden brown.

2. Turn chicken and cook 10 minutes more.
3. Add all remaining ingredients, except cream. Cover and cook ½ hour, stirring occasionally.
4. Stir in cream. Cook, uncovered, 5 minutes more.

Per serving: 223.7 calories; 66.8 mg. sodium; 10.5 gm. carbohydrates; 8.1 gm. fat.

Pineapple Chicken with Zucchini

SERVES 8

Bringing fruit and vegetables together is a favorite Mexican culinary device nowhere better displayed than in this mingling of sweet and hot flavors. A tossed salad vinaigrette and Beans with Cheese (page 175) are perfect accompaniments.

4 chicken breasts, cut into 2-inch pieces
2 leeks, chopped, including greens
⅛ teaspoon hot pepper flakes
1 cup boiling water
1 cup pineapple juice
2 bay leaves
1 teaspoon green peppercorns*
4 slices low-sodium sweet peppers, chopped

½ cup dry white wine
1 teaspoon paprika
8 fresh mushrooms, chopped
2 tablespoons low-sodium chicken bouillon
3 zucchini, chopped

1. In large skillet, place chicken. Turn heat to medium-low and cook 20 minutes, stirring often.
2. Add leeks and hot pepper flakes. Cook 5 minutes more.
3. Add water and cook 10 minutes more, stirring occasionally.
4. Reduce heat to low. Add juice, bay leaves, green peppercorns, sweet peppers, and wine, stirring to blend. Cover and cook 20 minutes.
5. Add remaining ingredients. Cover and cook 15 minutes more, stirring occasionally.

Per serving: 190.6 calories; 62.5 mg. sodium; 14.2 gm. carbohydrates; 3.4 gm. fat.

* Preserved in vinegar only.

Pueblo Chicken SERVES 4

Rice with Mushrooms and Cheese (page 188) will complete a most savory meal.

4 chicken legs
6 cloves garlic, sliced
2 onions, sliced
1 tablespoon low-sodium beef
 bouillon
1 teaspoon celery seed*
1½ tablespoons dried parsley
2 cups boiling water

1 lemon, sliced
4 carrots, cut in 1-inch rounds
1/16 teaspoon ground nutmeg
1/8 teaspoon ground cumin
2/3 cup dry white wine
4 tablespoons sour cream
1 green pepper, chopped

1. In large skillet, place chicken, garlic, and onions. Turn heat to medium-low and sauté 10 minutes, or until chicken is browned all over, turning often.
2. Add all but last 2 ingredients. Reduce heat to low. Cover and cook ½ hour, stirring occasionally.
3. Stir in sour cream. Then add pepper. Cover and cook 20 minutes more.

Per serving: 317.3 calories; 142.1 mg. sodium; 31.7 gm. carbohydrates; 11.4 gm. fat.

* Do not use celery flakes, which contain salt.

Red and Green Chicken with Cheese

SERVES 8

One bite and you will know the true meaning of the word *scrumptious.* Serve with Mexican Macaroni Salad (page 184).

4 chicken breasts, cut in bite-size
pieces
½ teaspoon achiote (or 1 strand
saffron)
4 cups boiling water
2 onions, minced
2 leeks, chopped, including greens
2 cloves garlic, minced
3 tomatoes, chopped
1 tablespoon dried parsley

1 teaspoon dried basil
1/16 teaspoon clove powder
⅛ teaspoon ground cinnamon
2 dried chiles
2 tablespoons low-sodium chicken
bouillon
2 ounces low-sodium Cheddar
cheese, grated

1. In Dutch oven, combine first 4 ingredients. Turn heat to medium-low. Cover and cook 45 minutes. Drain, reserving half the stock. Set aside.
2. In blender, combine leeks, garlic, tomatoes, parsley, basil, clove powder, cinnamon, and chiles. Puree.
3. In Dutch oven, combine reserved stock and puree, stirring to blend. Cook 10 minutes, stirring often.
4. Stir in bouillon and cheese. Return chicken to Dutch oven. Simmer 15 minutes more.

Per serving: 204.0 calories; 116.0 mg. sodium; 30.2 gm. carbohydrates; 8.4 gm. fat.

Spiced Chicken and Vegetable Stew

SERVES 8

Stewing is a fine art in Mexico, as a multitude of flavors slowly simmer and blend into a delicious, magical completion. This dish is one sublime example and needs only a boiled potato or some boiled white rice to soak up its juicy goodness.

4 chicken breasts
1 onion, minced
2 cloves garlic, minced
2 tablespoons red wine vinegar
1 2-inch cinnamon stick
3 carrots, cut in 1-inch rounds
1¼ cups boiling water
8 prunes, chopped
1 tablespoon Chili Powder (page 210)
½ cup orange juice

2 tomatoes, chopped
1 teaspoon dried oregano
2 cups cauliflowerettes
½ pound green beans, chopped in 2-inch pieces
½ cup dry red wine
⅛ teaspoon ground nutmeg
2 tablespoons low-sodium beef bouillon

1. In Dutch oven, place chicken skin side down. Surround with onion and garlic. Turn heat to low and cook ½ hour, or until skin is lightly browned.
2. Turn chicken and cook 15 minutes more.
3. Add vinegar, cinnamon, carrots, water, prunes, and chili powder. Cover and cook 20 minutes.
4. Add orange juice and tomatoes. Cover and cook 10 minutes more.
5. Add remaining ingredients. Cover and cook 15 minutes more. Discard cinnamon.

Per serving: 223.3 calories; 104.3 mg. sodium; 25.5 gm. carbohydrates; 3.9 gm. fat.

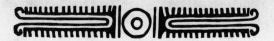

Meat

Ingenuity and ingenuousness best describe the Mexican cook's approach to meat. Heaped with a mixture of vegetables, fruit, spices, herbs, nuts, juice, cream, and wine, meat dishes have a festive look and a heady aroma. Mouth-watering temptations all, they reflect the potpourri of Mexico's culinary heritage.

For example, Mexican Pot Roast (page 153) has a distinctly Germanic quality. Baked Lamb in Drunken Sauce (page 156) has a Spanish flavor. But what matters to the Mexicans, and to us, are not the origins but the final results, which are excellent indeed.

In Mexican hands, meat of every kind is prepared with care, and the end product is invariably delicious. Goat and kid (called *cabrito*) are favorites, but are not featured in this book because they do not appeal to our palates. Lamb and veal are also enjoyed although they are not as widely available as other meats. Often, however, they are included in meatball mixtures, which are extraordinary. In Mexico, meatballs are rarely sautéed. Instead, they are simmered in wonderfully tasty sauces and infused with their flavors. For one of these fabulous treats, sample Saucy Meat Balls (page 171).

Beef is very popular here, and steak is the favorite cut. Cattle are home-grown in the northern part of the country, and their diet includes wild oregano, which Mexicans will swear is responsible for the rich, juicy flavor of the beef. We think the preparation may have something to do with it. See if you do not agree when you savor Steak with Chile Strips (page 156) and Boiled Beef (page 151).

But, of course, pork is the most popular meat on the Mexican menu, dating back to the wild pig of the Aztec era, and later replaced with its domestic cousin brought into Mexico after the Spanish Conquest. Indescribably tasty, as you will discover when you enjoy Roast Pork Loin (page 162), pork nevertheless is higher in fat, calories, and sodium than lean beef or veal. So, in this chapter, pork is given an equal but no more important role than other meats.

But whether you choose pork, lamb, veal, or beef, once you try meat with a Mexican flair, you may never want it any other way.

Beef Chile SERVES 12

A classic, Beef Chile, or Chile Con Carne, is one of the dishes of which northern Mexico is justly proud. Unlike the Texas variation, which includes kidney beans, real Mexican beef chile is a simple, pure stew whose two principal ingredients, meat and chiles, are accented only with herbs and spices. As a concession to our palates, we have added tomato puree and a touch of red wine. Whether you prefer your chile with beef or pork, this recipe will be a staple in your Mexican repertoire. Serve with Beans with Cheese (page 175) or Simple Beans (page 174) plus Basil-Tomato Sauce (page 212).

½ cup paprika
6 dried chiles, seeded and crushed
1 tablespoon low-sodium beef
  bouillon
1½ teaspoons ground cumin, divided
2 pounds stewing beef (or pork
  shoulder), cubed
3 tablespoons vegetable oil, divided

2 onions, chopped
4 cloves garlic, minced
4 cups water
2 cans (58 ounces) low-sodium
  tomato puree
1 tablespoon Chili Powder (page 210)
2 teaspoons dried oregano
2 tablespoons dry red wine

1. In bowl, combine paprika, chiles, bouillon, and ½ teaspoon cumin, blending thoroughly.
2. Roll beef in paprika mixture, coating all over. Set aside.
3. In Dutch oven, heat 2 tablespoons oil over medium heat. Add beef and sauté 5 minutes, or until beef is browned all over. With slotted spoon, remove beef to platter.
4. Reduce heat to low. Add remaining tablespoon oil plus onions and garlic. Cook 10 minutes, or until onions are lightly browned.
5. Return beef to Dutch oven. Add water. Cover and simmer 1 hour.
6. Stir in remaining ingredients. Cover and simmer 45 minutes more.

Per serving with beef: 339.9 calories; 73.2 mg. sodium; 20.7 gm. carbohydrates;
    20.3 gm. fat.
Per serving with pork: 315.5 calories; 90.7 mg. sodium; 20.7 gm. carbohydrates;
    15.7 gm. fat.

Boiled Beef

Simple, delicious, and fabulous when shredded and stuffed into Tortillas (pages 48, 49) along with shredded lettuce, minced cheese, and topped with your favorite sauce.

1½ pounds stewing beef
2½ cups water
2 onions, chopped
2 cloves garlic, minced
3 tomatoes, chopped
2 teaspoons vegetable oil
2 dried chiles
2 green peppers, chopped
Black pepper to taste

1½ teaspoons dried oregano
4 teaspoons low-sodium beef
  bouillon
2½ teaspoons low-sodium Dijon
  mustard
1 can (6 ounces) low-sodium tomato
  paste

1. In Dutch oven, combine first 2 ingredients. Turn heat to high and bring to a boil. Reduce heat to low. Cover and simmer 1½ hours. Remove from heat. Let stand ½ hour.
2. Transfer beef to platter and shred. Set aside.
3. In blender, combine onions, garlic, and tomatoes. Puree. Set aside.
4. In skillet, heat oil over low heat. Add chiles and tomato puree. Cook 5 minutes, stirring often.
5. Add meat, stewing liquid, and all remaining ingredients. Stir to blend. Cover and simmer 15 minutes, stirring occasionally.

Per serving: 327.9 calories; 67.6 mg. sodium; 16.9 gm. carbohydrates; 19.7 gm. fat.

Citrus Steak

SERVES 4

A puckery adaptation of a Yucatan recipe. What citrus does to beef—or 1 pound of pork or veal shoulder for that matter—is unbelievably wonderful. Serve with soothing Cucumber Salad La Jolla (page 100) or Broiled Tomatoes with Avocado (page 200) and Yellow Rice (page 190).

1 pound bottom round, 1½ inches thick
½ cup grapefruit juice
¼ cup lemon juice
1 tablespoon vegetable oil
2 onions, sliced

2 cloves garlic, minced
1 tablespoon low-sodium beef bouillon
½ teaspoon dried thyme
1/16 teaspoon cayenne pepper

1. In 9 x 13-inch ovenproof casserole, combine first 3 ingredients. Cover and chill overnight, turning meat occasionally.
2. In skillet, heat oil over low heat. Add onions and garlic and cook 5 minutes, or until onions are golden.
3. Preheat oven to broil.
4. Spoon onion mixture around meat. Broil 4 inches from heat 5 minutes, or until browned on top.
5. Stir in remaining ingredients.
6. Turn meat and broil 6 minutes more.

Per serving with beef: 413.7 calories; 68.0 mg. sodium; 16.6 gm. carbohydrates; 27.8 gm. fat.
Per serving with pork: 377.2 calories; 94.3 mg. sodium; 16.6 gm. carbohydrates; 20.8 gm. fat.
Per serving with veal: 361.2 calories; 117.2 mg. sodium; 16.6 gm. carbohydrates; 25.2 gm. fat.

Mexican Pot Roast

SERVES 8

This dish has a distinctly German flavor, tastefully enhanced in a decidedly Mexican way. Delicious with Mixed Salad San Miguel (page 101) and Chessy Hot Noodles (page 182).

1½ pounds bottom round
2 tablespoons paprika
3 onions, chopped
4 cloves garlic, minced
4 cups water, divided
2 tablespoons all-purpose flour
¼ teaspoon clove powder
2 teaspoons dried oregano

⅛ teaspoon cayenne pepper
4 apples, peeled, cored, and
 quartered
½ cup dry red wine
1 tablespoon low-sodium beef
 bouillon

1. Sprinkle meat with paprika. In Dutch oven, place meat. Turn heat to high and sear on all sides.
2. Reduce heat to medium-low. Add onions, garlic, and ½ cup water. Cover and cook 20 minutes.
3. Stir in flour, blending thoroughly.
4. Add remaining water. Reduce heat to low. Cover and simmer 1 hour, turning meat occasionally.
5. Stir in clove powder, oregano, cayenne pepper, apples, and wine. Cover and simmer ½ hour more, or until meat is fork tender, stirring occasionally.
6. Stir in bouillon. Cook, uncovered, 5 minutes more.
7. Transfer meat and apples to serving platter. Let stand 15 minutes to cool before carving.
8. While meat is cooling, cover Dutch oven and continue to simmer sauce 10 minutes.
9. Slice meat. Spoon 1 cup sauce over meat. Serve remaining sauce on the side.

Per serving: 356.3 calories; 50.8 mg. sodium; 27.1 gm. carbohydrates; 18.5 gm. fat.

Steak and Tomatoes

SERVES 8

Clove powder and nutmeg do wonderfully tasty magic on beef in this very Mexican dish. Fabulous with Spicy Potato Casserole (page 180) and Zucchini in Cheese Sauce (page 207).

1½ pounds bottom round, sliced thin
2 onions, sliced in rounds, divided
2 cups water
½ teaspoon garlic powder
1 tablespoon capers*
1/16 teaspoon clove powder
1/8 teaspoon ground nutmeg

4 tomatoes, chopped
¼ cup dry red wine
1 tablespoon low-sodium chicken bouillon
Black pepper to taste
1 bay leaf

1. In skillet, lay meat slices and half the onion slices. Add water. Bring to a boil. Reduce heat. Cover and simmer 1 hour.
2. While meat is cooking, in blender, combine remaining onion, garlic powder, capers, clove powder, nutmeg, and tomatoes. Puree. Set aside.
3. Pour wine over meat. Season with bouillon and pepper.
4. Spoon tomato puree over meat. Add bay leaf. Cover and simmer 1 hour more, or until meat is fork tender.
5. Discard bay leaf.

Per serving: 287.7 calories; 47.5 mg. sodium; 9.4 gm. carbohydrates; 18.2 gm. fat.

* Preserved in vinegar only.

Steak Guacamole with Dates

SERVES 8

The imaginative and lavish combination of ingredients rises to new heights in this sumptuous dish. Serve with Cauliflower Salad (page 99) and boiled white rice.

1½ pounds bottom round
¼ cup lime juice
¼ cup cider vinegar
1 cup orange juice
2 teaspoons dried oregano
1 tablespoon vegetable oil
2 onions, minced
4 cloves garlic, minced

2 dried chiles, seeded and crushed
1½ cups boiling water
2 tablespoons low-sodium beef
   bouillon
¼ cup rum
¼ cup dates, pitted and chopped
1 cup Guacamole (page 34), if
   desired

1. In 9 x 13-inch ovenproof casserole, place meat. Add lime juice, vinegar, and orange juice. Season meat with oregano. Cover and refrigerate overnight, turning meat occasionally.
2. Preheat oven to 375°.
3. In skillet, heat oil over low heat. Add onions, garlic, and chiles. Cook 5 minutes, or until onions are golden.
4. Add onion mixture to meat in casserole. Cover and bake 15 minutes.
5. Reduce oven to 350°.
6. To casserole, add water, bouillon, rum, and dates. Cover and bake 1 hour more, or until meat is fork tender.
7. Spoon Guacamole over meat and bake, uncovered, 15 minutes more.

Note: For plain Steak with Dates, omit Step 7.

Per serving with guacamole: 392.2 calories; 64.0 mg. sodium; 21.0 gm. carbohydrates; 24.0 gm. fat.
Per serving plain: 351.7 calories; 61.2 mg. sodium; 18.5 gm. carbohydrates; 20.4 gm. fat.

Steak with Chile Strips   SERVES 8

The rich flavors of the marinade soak into the beef, resulting in an absolutely sublime dish that works well with any accompaniment.

1½ pounds London broil, 2 inches thick
1 cup Garlic Dressing (page 228)
4 poblano chiles, seeded and halved lengthwise (or 1 teaspoon hot pepper flakes)

2 ounces low-sodium Cheddar cheese, shredded
2 limes, cut in wedges

1. In 9 x 13-inch casserole, place meat. Cover with garlic dressing and chiles. Cover and refrigerate overnight, turning meat occasionally. Transfer meat to baking sheet. Reserve marinade.
2. Preheat oven to broil.
3. Broil meat 4 inches from heat 10 minutes.
4. Turn meat and broil 10 minutes more. Transfer to platter.
5. While meat is cooking, in saucepan, over low heat, cook marinade 20 minutes, stirring occasionally.
6. Slice meat very thin. Sprinkle cheese over all. Pour marinade over all.
7. Garnish with lime wedges.

Per serving: 253.9 calories; 58.1 mg. sodium; 4.6 gm. carbohydrates; 12.8 gm. fat.

Baked Lamb in Drunken Sauce   SERVES 8

Green Beans and Corn (page 202) is the perfect companion for this delightful, flavorful, meltingly tender specialty.

4 pounds lamb shanks
1¾ cups Drunken Sauce (page 220)
½ teaspoon ground cumin
1 tablespoon dried oregano

1 bay leaf
¼ cup dry red wine
1 tablespoon low-sodium chicken bouillon

1. In 9 x 13-inch ovenproof casserole, combine all ingredients, except bouillon. Cover and refrigerate overnight, turning lamb occasionally.
2. Preheat oven to 300°.
3. Cover lamb and bake ½ hour.

4. Raise oven to 350°. Bake lamb 2 hours more, or until fork tender, turning occasionally. Stir in bouillon.
5. Remove lamb from oven and let stand 20 minutes. Then transfer to serving platter.
6. Discard bay leaf and skim fat from sauce, then serve on the side.

Per serving: 258.9 calories; 71.1 mg. sodium; 8.9 gm. carbohydrates; 11.6 gm. fat.

Leg of Lamb Condata   SERVES 8

Richly flavorful and festive, this dish should be saved for extra-special occasions. Serve with either Sherried Carrots in Rum Cream (page 203) or Asparagus and Mushrooms (page 196) and boiled new potatoes.

4 cloves garlic, sliced
4-pound leg of lamb, gashed
¾ cup Honey-Lime Dressing
  (page 229), including the oil
2 onions, chopped

3 tomatoes, chopped
2 cups Meat Stock (page 78), divided
¼ cup golden raisins*

1. Preheat oven to 350°.
2. Insert garlic in gashes in lamb and place in 9 x 13-inch ovenproof casserole.
3. Spoon dressing over all. Set aside.
4. In blender, combine onions, tomatoes, and ½ cup stock. Puree. Spoon over lamb.
5. Pour remaining stock around lamb.
6. Scatter raisins around lamb. Then cover and bake 2½ hours. Uncover and bake ½ hour more, or until lamb is fork tender.
7. Remove lamb from oven. Let stand 20 minutes. Then transfer to platter and slice thin.
8. Skim fat from sauce and serve on the side.

Per serving: 296.4 calories; 93.9 mg. sodium; 20.5 gm. carbohydrates; 11.6 gm. fat.

* Preserved in non-sodium ingredient.

Mint Lamb Chops with Peanuts   SERVES 4

An exquisite dish by any taste standards. A mixed green salad and Rice with Tomatoes (page 188) will complete your savory meal.

1 tablespoon unsalted margarine	1 cup Meat Stock (page 78), divided
¼ cup unsalted peanuts, crushed	4 rib lamb chops
4 cloves garlic, minced	1 tablespoon dried mint
2 leeks, chopped, including greens	1 lime, cut into wedges
2 dried chiles, crushed	

1. Preheat oven to broil.
2. In skillet, heat margarine over low heat. Add peanuts, garlic, leeks, and chiles. Cook 10 minutes, or until garlic is lightly browned, stirring often.
3. Stir in half the stock. Simmer 5 minutes. Set aside.
4. On baking sheet, place lamb chops. Pour remaining stock over all. Broil 6 inches from heat 7 minutes.
5. Turn lamb. Sprinkle mint over all. Then pour peanut mixture over all and broil 10 minutes more.
6. Garnish with lime wedges.

Per serving: 324.0 calories; 86.1 mg. sodium; 18.3 gm. carbohydrates; 20.0 gm. fat.

Chorizo   MAKES 1½ POUNDS

Chorizo is the very highly seasoned and spicy ground pork blend we know as Mexican sausage. Although it is available in links or canned in Mexican, Spanish, and Puerto Rican food stores, commercially sold chorizo often contains salt. Thus we offer our own version below.

Chorizo adds its tangy spark to many Mexican dishes. We think you will love it.

1½ pounds boneless pork shoulder	1 teaspoon paprika
1 onion, chopped	⅛ teaspoon ground cumin
4 cloves garlic, chopped	3 tablespoons cider vinegar
2 tablespoons Chili Powder (page 195)	½ teaspoon sugar
2 tablespoons dried basil	Black pepper to taste
1½ tablespoons low-sodium beef bouillon	

1. In blender, grind pork to coarse consistency. Transfer to bowl.
2. In blender, combine remaining ingredients. Grind.

3. Add onion mixture to pork and blend thoroughly. Cover and chill overnight to allow flavors to blend.
4. Before use, form into small patties or into 2-inch sausage rolls and wrap individually.
5. May be refrigerated in tightly closed container up to 3 days, or frozen in tightly closed container up to 2 months.

Per recipe: 2,042.9 calories; 687.0 mg. sodium; 65.3 gm. carbohydrates; 105.7 gm. fat.

Cinnamon-Chile Pork Chops
SERVES 4

Pork or lamb can be transformed with this flavorful spice blend. Green Bean and Sweet Pepper Salad (page 100) and Rice with Mushrooms and Cheese (page 188) are two tempting accompaniments.

4 pork (or lamb) chops
1/4 teaspoon garlic powder, divided
Black pepper to taste
2 dried chiles, crushed and divided
1/4 teaspoon ground cinnamon, divided

2 tablespoons red wine vinegar
2 tomatoes, chopped
1 1/2 teaspoons low-sodium beef bouillon

1. Preheat oven to broil.
2. On baking sheet, place pork chops. Season with half the garlic powder, black pepper, chiles, and cinnamon. Broil 6 inches from heat 7 minutes, or until chops are browned.
3. Turn chops. Season with remaining garlic powder, black pepper, chiles, and cinnamon. Broil 7 minutes more.
4. While chops are broiling, in blender, combine remaining ingredients. Puree.
5. Top pork with puree and broil 3 minutes more.

Per serving with pork: 329.0 calories; 104.2 mg. sodium; 7.4 gm. carbohydrates; 17.2 gm. fat.
Per serving with lamb: 263.9 calories; 109.9 mg. sodium; 7.4 gm. carbohydrates; 10.8 gm. fat.

Pork and Pecans

SERVES 8

Nuts are often used in Mexican cooking with fabulous results. This dish is a notable example. Lovely and elegant with Cabbage and Apples in Piquant Sour Cream Sauce (page 224).

6 pasilla chiles (or 6 dried chiles)
1½ pounds pork loin, cubed
4 cups water
1 onion
4 cloves
2 cloves garlic
4 tomatoes, chopped
¼ cup cider vinegar
1 teaspoon dried basil

½ teaspoon ground cumin
1½ teaspoons Chili Powder
  (page 210)
1 teaspoon sugar
2 tablespoons dry sherry
1 tablespoon low-sodium beef
  bouillon
1 tablespoon unsalted margarine
¼ cup unsalted pecans, crushed

1. In Dutch oven, combine first 3 ingredients. Turn heat to high and bring to a boil.
2. Stud onion with cloves. Add to Dutch oven. Reduce heat to medium-low. Cover and cook 1 hour.
3. While pork is cooking, in blender, combine garlic, tomatoes, vinegar, basil, cumin, chili powder, and sugar. Puree.
4. Stir puree into pork mixture. Cover and cook 10 minutes more.
5. Stir in sherry and bouillon. Cover and cook 10 minutes more.
6. While pork is cooking, in skillet, heat margarine over low heat. Add pecans and sauté 10 minutes, stirring often.
7. Stir pecans into pork mixture. Cook, uncovered, 20 minutes more, stirring often.

Per serving with pork:
  With fresh chiles: 305.7 calories; 73.6 mg. sodium; 11.0 gm. carbohydrates;
    17.1 gm. fat.
  With dried chiles: 324.7 calories; 100.2 mg. sodium; 14.3 gm. carbohydrates;
    18.2 gm. fat.
Per serving with beef:
  With fresh chiles: 333.2 calories; 53.9 mg. sodium; 11.0 gm. carbohydrates;
    22.7 gm. fat.
  With dried chiles: 352.1 calories; 80.5 mg. sodium; 14.3 gm. carbohydrates;
    23.4 gm. fat.

Pork Stew

SERVES 8

This is one of the easiest, most temptingly delicious meals you will ever make or enjoy. For variety, substitute an equal amount of veal for the pork. Either way, Refried Beans (page 177) is a must.

1½ pounds pork loin, cubed
3 cups water
¼ pound Chorizo (page 158)
1 onion, chopped
1½ tablespoons low-sodium beef
　bouillon
Black pepper to taste
2 teaspoons dried oregano

2 tomatoes, chopped
6 carrots, cut in 1-inch rounds
1 teaspoon sugar
¼ cup dry white wine
3 potatoes, parboiled,* peeled, and
　cubed
1 bay leaf

1. In large skillet, place pork. Turn heat to high and sear on all sides.
2. Transfer pork to saucepan. Add water. Turn heat to low. Cover and simmer 1½ hours.
3. While pork is cooking, in skillet, combine chorizo and onion. Turn heat to medium-low and sauté 5 minutes, or until chorizo is browned all over, stirring often.
4. Stir in bouillon, pepper, oregano, and tomatoes.
5. Add tomato mixture and all remaining ingredients to pork. Cover and simmer ½ hour more, stirring occasionally.
6. Raise heat to medium-high. Cook, uncovered, 15 minutes more. Discard bay leaf.

Per serving with pork: 364.3 calories; 103.8 mg. sodium; 24.0 gm. carbohydrates;
　　15.2 gm. fat.
Per serving with veal: 352.3 calories; 120.9 mg. sodium; 24.0 gm. carbohydrates;
　　18.5 gm. fat.

* Do not add salt to water.

Roast Pork Loin

SERVES 8

If you like roast beef, you will also love this Mexican-style pork roast. A mixed green salad vinaigrette and Yellow Rice (page 190) are the perfect subtle and tasty accompaniments.

2 ancho chiles, seeded
2 cloves garlic
1 onion, chopped
2 cups Meat Stock (page 78), divided
1½ pounds pork loin
1 teaspoon black pepper
¼ cup molasses

¼ cup dry sherry
2 teaspoons dried oregano
½ teaspoon dried thyme
4 raw figs, chopped
1 tablespoon low-sodium beef
   bouillon

1. Preheat oven to 350°.
2. In blender, combine first 3 ingredients plus ½ cup stock. Puree. Set aside.
3. Sprinkle pork with black pepper. In skillet, over medium-high heat, sear pork until browned all over. Transfer to roasting pan.
4. Pour molasses and sherry over pork. Then season with oregano and thyme.
5. Spread chile mixture over pork.
6. Pour remaining stock in pan. Then add figs and bouillon. Roast 2 hours, or until meat is fork tender, basting often.
7. Let pork stand 20 minutes before slicing.
8. Skim fat from sauce and serve on the side.

Per serving: 307.2 calories; 80.5 mg. sodium; 17.3 gm. carbohydrates; 14.6 gm. fat.

Shredded Pork

This traditional dish makes a great filling for tacos, enchiladas, etc. Or combine it with some Basic Salsa (page 210) for Mexican-style sloppy Joe sandwiches.

1½ pounds pork shoulder
4 cups water
2 onions
2 cloves garlic, chopped
2 teaspoons low-sodium beef
  bouillon

½ teaspoon Chili Powder (page 210)
⅛ teaspoon ground cinnamon
½ cup low-sodium chili ketchup

1. In Dutch oven, combine first 4 ingredients. Turn heat to high and bring to a boil. Reduce heat to low. Cover and simmer 2 hours. Drain, reserving 1 cup broth.
2. Preheat oven to 350°.
3. In roasting pan, place pork. Season with bouillon, chili powder, and cinnamon.
4. Spoon chili ketchup over pork.
5. Pour reserved pork broth in pan. Bake ½ hour, or until pork is fork tender. Transfer pork to warm platter.
6. Shred pork with 2 forks (texture will be coarse).

Per serving: 244.8 calories; 71.5 mg. sodium; 6.4 gm. carbohydrates; 12.5 gm. fat.
Per cup: 489.7 calories; 142.9 mg. sodium; 12.8 gm. carbohydrates; 25.0 gm. fat.

Sweetly Hot Pork Stew

SERVES 8

Deliciously spicy and oh-so-good. For an exciting flavor contrast, serve with Salad of Colors (page 102).

1½ pounds pork shoulder, cubed
4 poblano chiles, seeded and halved
   diagonally (or 4 dried chiles)
1 onion, sliced
4 cloves
1 stick cinnamon
3 cups water
⅓ cup golden raisins*
4 tomatoes, chopped

1 teaspoon vegetable (or peanut) oil
¼ cup unsalted chopped walnuts
1 teaspoon dried basil
1 teaspoon dried parsley
1 tablespoon paprika
2 teaspoons low-sodium chicken
   bouillon

1. In Dutch oven, combine first 2 ingredients.
2. Stud onion with cloves and add to Dutch oven along with cinnamon and water. Turn heat to high and bring to a boil. Reduce heat to low. Cover and simmer 1 hour.
3. While pork is cooking, in blender, combine raisins and tomatoes. Puree. Set aside.
4. In skillet, heat oil over low heat. Add walnuts and cook 5 minutes, stirring often.
5. Add tomato puree and cook 3 minutes more, stirring often.
6. To Dutch oven, add tomato puree and walnuts plus remaining ingredients. Cover and simmer ½ hour more, or until veal is fork tender, stirring occasionally. Discard cinnamon before serving.

Per serving with fresh chiles: 323.9 calories; 67.9 mg. sodium; 15.5 gm. carbohydrates; 17.5 gm. fat.
Per serving with dried chiles: 336.6 calories; 85.6 mg. sodium; 17.7 gm. carbohydrates; 18.0 gm. fat.

* Preserved in non-sodium ingredient.

Sherry Veal Chops

SERVES 4

Creamy Carrot Soup (page 83), a mixed green salad, and Beans with Pork in Lime Sauce (page 176) provide a superb variety of flavors to embellish this truly delicious dish. Twelve chopped dried apricots is a good alternate to the prunes.

½ cup boiling water
1½ teaspoons low-sodium chicken
   bouillon
1 teaspoon low-sodium Dijon
   mustard
¼ cup dry sherry
1 tablespoon unsalted margarine
2 large veal chops (bone in, 12
   ounces each)

Black pepper to taste
6 prunes, pitted and chopped
1 Granny Smith apple, peeled, cored,
   and chopped
1 lemon, sliced thin

1. In bowl, combine first 3 ingredients, stirring to dissolve mustard.
2. Stir in sherry. Set aside.
3. Preheat oven to 350°.
4. In skillet, heat margarine over low heat. Add veal chops and cook 20 minutes, or until chops are lightly browned on bottom.
5. Turn chops. Raise heat to medium and cook 10 minutes more. Season with pepper. Transfer to 9-inch-square ovenproof casserole.
6. Pour sherry mixture over all.
7. Scatter prunes and apple around chops.
8. Top veal chops with lemon slices. Cover and bake 20 minutes, or until chops are fork tender.

Per serving with prunes: 255.0 calories; 57.6 mg. sodium; 20.6 gm. carbohydrates;
   14.0 gm. fat.
Per serving with apricots: 240.8 calories; 58.7 mg. sodium; 16.7 gm. carbohydrates;
   14.0 gm. fat.

Veal and Apples in Green Sauce   SERVES 8

Veal takes on a tart sweetness thanks to the mix of Granny Smith apples and cinnamon in this dish. For variety, substitute 1½ pounds of bottom round for the veal. Either way, it is, quite simply, marvelous. Serve with Sweet Rice with Green Beans (page 189).

1½ pounds stewing veal, cubed
2 tablespoons paprika
2 cups Meat Stock (page 78)
3 Granny Smith apples, peeled,
  cored, and chopped

1 cup Green Sauce I (page 216)
¼ teaspoon ground cumin
¼ teaspoon ground cinnamon

1. In Dutch oven, over high heat, sear veal.
2. Reduce heat to low. Add paprika and stock. Cover and simmer 45 minutes.
3. Add remaining ingredients. Cover and simmer 1 hour more, or until veal is fork tender, stirring occasionally.

Per serving with veal: 307.0 calories; 97.9 mg. sodium; 17.3 gm. carbohydrates;
    20.3 gm. fat.
Per serving with beef: 346.5 calories; 48.9 mg. sodium; 17.3 gm. carbohydrates;
    22.2 gm. fat.

Veal Balls in Sour Cream Sauce   SERVES 8

A like amount of beef or pork can be substituted for the veal in this lip-smacking dish. Enjoy it with boiled noodles and Glazed Carrots with Minced Shrimp (page 202). If you like, this dish also makes a wonderful appetizer.

1½ pounds ground veal
1 teaspoon dried parsley
½ teaspoon dried oregano
⅛ teaspoon ground cumin
1/16 teaspoon clove powder
2 teaspoons low-sodium beef
  bouillon
1 tablespoon unsalted margarine

2 onions, chopped
2 cloves garlic, minced
2 cups water
2 tomatoes, chopped
½ cup dry red wine
8 mushrooms, sliced
1 green pepper, chopped
¼ cup sour cream

1. In bowl, combine first 6 ingredients, blending thoroughly. Shape into tiny balls. Set aside.

2. In Dutch oven, over medium heat, sauté veal balls until browned all over.
3. Add margarine, onions, and garlic. Cook 10 minutes, or until onions are golden, stirring occasionally.
4. Add water and cook 15 minutes.
5. Add remaining ingredients, except sour cream. Cook ½ hour more.
6. Stir in sour cream and cook 15 minutes more.

Per serving with veal: 291.3 calories; 91.6 mg. sodium; 10.4 gm. carbohydrates; 20.0 gm. fat.
Per serving with beef: 330.8 calories; 54.7 mg. sodium; 10.4 gm. carbohydrates; 22.0 gm. fat.
Per serving with pork: 303.3 calories; 74.4 mg. sodium; 10.4 gm. carbohydrates; 16.8 gm. fat.

Veal Loaf
SERVES 8

Start your meal with heart-warming, savory Lentil and Okra Soup (page 90). Then, a lettuce and tomato salad is all you need to complement the moist goodness of this flavorful dish. But for a special treat, try Tomato Sauce with Cayenne (page 212) over hot Veal Loaf; Piquant Sour Cream Sauce (page 224), over cold.

1½ pounds ground veal
1 tablespoon low-sodium beef bouillon
2 teaspoons dried basil
1 teaspoon low-sodium Dijon mustard
1 egg, lightly beaten
1 onion, minced
⅛ teaspoon cayenne pepper

⅛ teaspoon ground cinnamon
¼ teaspoon orange peel powder
1 tablespoon dried parsley
1 teaspoon dried mint
⅛ teaspoon aniseed
¼ cup low-sodium bread crumbs
½ red pepper, diced

1. Preheat oven to 350°.
2. In bowl, combine first 5 ingredients, blending thoroughly.
3. Add remaining ingredients, blending thoroughly.
4. In 5 x 9-inch baking pan, form veal mixture into loaf and bake 1 hour.

Per serving: 251.5 calories; 95.6 mg. sodium; 7.9 gm. carbohydrates; 16.6 gm. fat.

Sweet-and-Spicy Veal Stew
SERVES 8

The combination of spicy herbs and succulent pineapple (or an 8-ounce can of dietetic peaches) will delight your senses. Bean Salad (page 98) is a flavorful accompaniment.

1 tablespoon paprika
1½ pounds veal shoulder, cut in
   1-inch chunks
2 onions, sliced
3 dried chiles, crushed
¼ cup rum
1½ cups Chicken Stock (page 76)
3 carrots, cut into 1-inch rounds
4 halves low-sodium sweet peppers,
   chopped

Black pepper to taste
1 tablespoon dried mint
1 can (8 ounces) dietetic pineapple
   chunks, including juice
⅛ teaspoon ground cumin
2 green peppers, chopped

1. Sprinkle paprika all over veal.
2. In Dutch oven, over high heat, sear veal.
3. Reduce heat to low. Add all remaining ingredients, except green peppers. Cover and simmer 1 hour.
4. Add green peppers. Cover and simmer ½ hour more, or until veal is fork tender.

Per serving with pineapple: 310.3 calories; 134.4 mg. sodium; 20.8 gm. carbohydrates;
   16.4 gm. fat.
Per serving with peaches: 308.0 calories; 134.8 mg. sodium; 20.2 gm. carbohydrates;
   16.4 gm. fat.

Picadillo with Vegetables

SERVES 8
MAKES 6 CUPS

Every Mexican region, indeed, every Latin country, has its own favorite version of this marvelous dish: one made with fruit; another more like Indian chutney; yet another featuring vegetables (like the recipe below). Picadillo in any form can be a flavorful dip, a meal in itself, or a popular stuffing for tortillas, burritos, and other Mexican baked goods. Try it. It is wonderful.

½ pound ground beef
½ pound ground pork
4 new potatoes, diced
1 onion, chopped
2 cloves garlic
2 carrots, diced
1 cucumber, peeled, seeded, and
    chopped
3 tomatoes, chopped

¼ cup dark raisins*
4 cups water
2 tablespoons low-sodium beef
    bouillon
Cayenne pepper to taste
2 teaspoons dried oregano
1 tablespoon paprika
⅛ teaspoon ground cinnamon

1. In skillet, combine first 5 ingredients. Turn heat to medium and sauté 5 minutes, or until meat is browned all over.
2. Add carrots, cucumber, tomatoes, raisins, and water. Stir to blend.
3. Reduce heat to low. Cover and simmer 45 minutes, stirring occasionally.
4. Stir in remaining ingredients. Cook, uncovered, ½ hour more, stirring often.

Per serving: 286.6 calories; 65.0 mg. sodium; 31.0 gm. carbohydrates; 10.9 gm. fat.
Per cup: 382.1 calories; 86.7 mg. sodium; 41.3 gm. carbohydrates; 14.5 gm. fat.

* Preserved in non-sodium ingredient.

Minced Meats with Fruit
SERVES 8

Along with Picadillo with Vegetables (page 169), this dish is exceedingly popular in Mexico, most especially for stuffing tortillas. But it is equally wonderful as a main meal accompanied by Cauliflower Salad (page 99) or Vegetable-Stuffed Chiles (page 195) and your favorite bean, potato, or rice dish.

1 pound ground pork
1/4 pound ground beef
1/4 pound ground veal
4 cloves garlic, minced
1/4 teaspoon dried thyme
1/4 teaspoon dried marjoram
1/2 teaspoon dried oregano
2 onions, chopped
1 1/2 tablespoons low-sodium beef bouillon
1/16 teaspoon cayenne pepper

2 cups Basic Salsa (page 210)
1 can (8 ounces) dietetic pineapple chunks, including juice
2 pears, cored and diced
2 bananas, peeled and cubed
1/8 teaspoon ground cinnamon
1/8 teaspoon ground nutmeg
1/16 teaspoon clove powder
2 teaspoons paprika

1. In skillet, combine first 4 ingredients. Turn heat to medium-high and sauté until meats lose all pink color, stirring often.
2. Stir in thyme, marjoram, and oregano. Then push meat mixture to sides of skillet.
3. To well created in center, add onions. Sauté 3 minutes more, or until onions are lightly browned. Stir into meat mixture.
4. Stir in bouillon and cayenne pepper.
5. Stir in salsa. Cook 15 minutes, stirring often.
6. Reduce heat to low. Add remaining ingredients and cook 20 minutes more, stirring occasionally.

Per serving: 338.5 calories; 75.5 mg. sodium; 30.5 gm. carbohydrates; 14.8 gm. fat.

Saucy Meat Balls

SERVES 8

An exotic and fabulous appetizer and a marvelous main dish, these meat balls will become one of your favorite Mexican recipes. In its company, any side dish you choose will taste all the better.

2 slices low-sodium bread, cubed
⅓ cup low-fat milk
½ pound ground beef
½ pound ground pork
½ pound ground veal
1 egg
1 onion, minced
1 teaspoon dried parsley
1 teaspoon dried oregano
¼ teaspoon garlic powder
¼ teaspoon celery seed*

⅛ teaspoon ground cinnamon
1 teaspoon low-sodium beef bouillon
1 teaspoon low-sodium chicken
  bouillon
3 cups Chicken Stock (page 76)
2 dried chiles
1 can (6 ounces) low-sodium tomato
  paste
Black pepper to taste
¼ cup dry red wine

1. In bowl, combine first 2 ingredients. Let stand 15 minutes. Chop.
2. In second bowl, combine soaked bread cubes, beef, pork, veal, egg, onion, parsley, oregano, garlic powder, celery seed, cinnamon, and beef and chicken bouillons. Blend thoroughly and form into small meat balls. Set aside.
3. In Dutch oven, combine stock, chiles, tomato paste, pepper, and wine. Turn heat to high and bring to a boil.
4. Add meat balls. Reduce heat to low and simmer 1 hour.

Per serving: 320.9 calories; 99.7 mg. sodium; 15.3 gm. carbohydrates; 17.0 gm. fat.

* Do not use celery flakes, which contain salt.

South-of-the-Border Meat Loaf SERVES 8

This dish proves that meat loaf can be as tasty and as special as the most elegant fare. If you want to be casual, serve it with Mexican Macaroni Salad (page 184) or Mexican Potato Salad (page 178). For more formal dining, Cheddar Cheese Soup (page 85), Salad of Colors (page 102), and Spicy Potato Casserole (page 180) make an excellent combination.

2 slices low-sodium bread
⅓ cup low-fat milk
¾ pound ground beef
¾ pound ground pork
2 teaspoons low-sodium Dijon
  mustard
1 egg
1 onion, minced
2 teaspoons low-sodium chicken
  bouillon

¼ teaspoon garlic powder
½ teaspoon dried basil
⅛ teaspoon dried thyme
¼ teaspoon ground cumin
2 halves low-sodium sweet peppers,
  sliced
2 cups Basil-Tomato Sauce (page 212)
1 teaspoon paprika

1. In bowl, combine first 2 ingredients. Let stand ½ hour. Chop.
2. In second bowl, combine beef, pork, mustard, egg, and onion. Blend thoroughly.
3. Add bouillon, garlic powder, basil, thyme, cumin, and bread. Blend thoroughly.
4. Preheat oven to 350°.
5. In 5 x 9-inch baking pan, shape meat mixture into a loaf.
6. On top of meat loaf, lay sweet pepper strips.
7. Pour tomato sauce over all. Season with paprika and bake 1 hour.

Per serving: 315.8 calories; 79.1 mg. sodium; 16.4 gm. carbohydrates; 16.7 gm. fat.

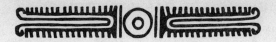

Beans, Potatoes, Pasta, and Rice

Red and yellow and pink and brown and, we might add, black and purple and green. We are talking about beans, a Mexican rainbow of beans. They are a constant at every Mexican meal.

Although bits of cheese, pork, and tomato are sometimes added to the pot, beans are most often cooked in their own broth with nothing more than a little onion, lard, and seasoning. Simple Beans (page 174) is one example of this basic dish. Even the famous Refried Beans (page 177) are fried in their own juices, so that not even one teaspoon of their own flavor is lost.

With beans, the rule of thumb is the simpler, the better; and they are always simply delicious.

In contrast, potatoes and pasta suffer from neglect in the Mexican home. It is odd, since potatoes, for one, are indigenous to Mexico, but they have never sparked the local palate, and few dishes feature them. It is a shame, for potatoes—baked, mashed, boiled, fried—have a sweet, full, meaty flavor which blends so well with the distinctive herbs, spices, and other seasonings of the Mexican kitchen. Spicy Potato Casserole (page 180) is a prime example.

With regard to pasta, you cannot really say that Mexicans dislike it. In fact, their Aztec ancestors readily adapted to this food, which had journeyed to Spain via China. But in modern Mexican cuisine, these delicious wheat-based strands and twists and twirls are virtually unknown. More's the pity, because chorizo, any Mexican tomato sauce, and all the heady seasonings would be taste-magic coupled with pasta. This is why in this chapter we have included some Mexican-style pasta dishes like Mexican Macaroni Salad (page 184) and Cheesy Hot Noodles (page 182) which we think you will enjoy.

Rice is another story. Introduced to Mexico at the same time as pasta, rice immediately became part of the Aztec cuisine and is today almost as popular as beans in the Mexican diet. The more famous rice dishes, like Rice with Chicken (page 187), frequently feature rice in combination with a potpourri of foods. But, in Mexico, rice is just as often served as a dry soup, first sautéed in oil, then simmered in a flavorful, seasoned stock, as in Yellow Rice (page 190).

Mexicans love beans, rice, and the like, and they are a substantial part of their daily menu. Happily, these foods also provide the complex carbohydrates that should be the bulk of any diet. Once you sample the recipes in this chapter, you will want them to be your mainstay, too.

Simple Beans   SERVES 8

In Mexico, every bean recipe starts with this most basic and delicious preparation.

1½ cups dried beans (pinto, kidney, or black)
6 cups water
1 onion, minced
⅛ teaspoon garlic powder
1 tablespoon low-sodium beef bouillon

Black pepper to taste
½ tablespoon vegetable oil
2 tablespoons low-sodium chicken bouillon

1. In saucepan, combine first 4 ingredients. Turn heat to high and bring to a boil.
2. Reduce heat to low. Cover and simmer 1½ hours.
3. Add beef bouillon, pepper, and oil. Cover and simmer 1½ hours more.
4. Add chicken bouillon. Cover and cook ½ hour more, or until beans are tender.

Note: You may serve this dish at once, but the beans will be tastier if refrigerated overnight and reheated the next day. They will keep up to 1 week, but should not be frozen because their flavor will be lost.

Per serving: 143.8 calories; 12.1 mg. sodium; 24.6 gm. carbohydrates; 2.6 gm. fat.

Beans with Cheese

SERVES 8

A wonderfully zesty side dish, especially tasty with pork, but thoroughly enjoyable with any main dish.

1 recipe Simple Beans (page 174)
4 scallions, chopped, including greens
½ teaspoon ground cumin
1 can (8 ounces) low-sodium tomato
  sauce

3 ounces low-sodium Cheddar
  cheese, minced

1. In saucepan, combine all ingredients, except cheese. Turn heat to high and bring to a boil.
2. Reduce heat to medium-low. Add cheese and cook 10 minutes, or until cheese starts to melt.

Per serving: 200.2 calories; 15.5 mg. sodium; 28.0 gm. carbohydrates; 6.1 gm. fat.

Beans with Chorizo and Salsa

SERVES 8

Cauliflower Salad (page 99) is all you need to complete this terrific meal.

½ tablespoon olive oil
½ pound Chorizo (page 158)
1 recipe Simple Beans (page 174)

2 cups Basic Salsa (page 210)
1 teaspoon paprika

1. In saucepan, heat oil over medium-low heat. Add chorizo and sauté 5 minutes, or until chorizo loses all pink color, stirring often.
2. Add beans. Reduce heat to low and cook 10 minutes, stirring occasionally.
3. Stir in remaining ingredients. Cook 20 minutes more, stirring occasionally.

Per serving: 256.6 calories; 45.9 mg. sodium; 32.2 gm. carbohydrates; 8.2 gm. fat.

Beans with Pork in Lime Sauce   SERVES 8

A surprising taste experience that you will definitely love. Just as good with the cubed meat from one chicken breast. Either way, add a tasty finishing touch with Chile-Vegetable Sauce (page 214).

1 teaspoon unsalted margarine	¼ cup lime juice
½ pound pork, cut in ½-inch strips	¹⁄₁₆ teaspoon cayenne pepper
1 leek, chopped, including greens	1 recipe Simple Beans (page 174)
2 red chiles, seeded and minced	1 tablespoon dried parsley

1. In saucepan, heat margarine over medium-low heat. Add pork, leek, and chiles and sauté 3 minutes, or until pork loses all pink color, stirring often.
2. Raise heat to medium. Stir in lime juice and cayenne pepper. Cook 2 minutes more, stirring often.
3. Stir in remaining ingredients. Reduce heat to low. Cover and simmer 20 minutes, stirring occasionally.

Per serving with pork: 234.9 calories; 34.9 mg. sodium; 28.0 gm. carbohydrates; 7.2 gm. fat.
Per serving with chicken: 184.0 calories; 24.8 mg. sodium; 28.0 gm. carbohydrates; 4.0 gm. fat.

Mexican Baked Beans   SERVES 12

If you like baked beans, you will love this version. And if you feel extravagant, add ½ pound minced pork to Step 8. With pork or without, Mexican baked beans are a rich, tangy accompaniment to any dish.

12 ounces dried pinto beans	¼ teaspoon clove powder
6 cups water	¼ cup white vinegar
6 cups Meat Stock (page 78)	3 tablespoons low-sodium mustard
2 tablespoons low-sodium beef bouillon	¼ teaspoon cayenne pepper
4 tomatoes, chopped	1 can (6 ounces) low-sodium tomato paste
1 onion, chopped	3 tablespoons honey
½ teaspoon ground cinnamon	

1. In Dutch oven, combine first 3 ingredients. Turn heat to high and bring to a boil.

2. Reduce heat to low. Cover and simmer 2 hours.
3. Add bouillon. Cover and cook 1 hour more.
4. While beans are cooking, in blender, combine tomatoes, onion, cinnamon, and clove powder. Puree.
5. In bowl, combine tomato puree, vinegar, and mustard, blending thoroughly.
6. Preheat oven to 350°.
7. Transfer beans, including liquid, to 9 x 13-inch ovenproof casserole.
8. Stir in tomato mixture. Then stir in remaining ingredients. Cover and bake 1½ hours. Uncover and bake 15 minutes more.

Per serving plain: 195.3 calories; 34.9 mg. sodium; 32.6 gm. carbohydrates; 5.0 gm. fat.
Per serving with pork: 243.7 calories; 48.2 mg. sodium; 32.6 gm. carbohydrates;
   7.7 gm. fat.

Refried Beans SERVES 8

This classic Mexican dish is as much a constant at the Mexican table as the tortilla. Although traditionally fried in a considerable amount of lard, we have taken the liberty of using oil, and very little at that. Nevertheless, we think you will enjoy our version and find it worthy of its true Mexican name: well-fried beans.

1 tablespoon vegetable oil   ½ cup hot water, divided
1 recipe Simple Beans (page 174)
½ tablespoon Chili Powder (page
   210, optional)

1. In skillet, heat oil over medium-low heat. Add beans, chili powder, if desired, and half the water. Simmer 10 minutes, stirring often.
2. Add remaining water. Simmer 10 minutes more, or until liquid is absorbed, stirring often.

Per serving: 167.2 calories; 21.0 mg. sodium; 26.1 gm. carbohydrates; 4.6 gm. fat.

Mexican Potato Salad

SERVES 12

A worthy rival to its American and German counterparts, this potato salad adds a tangy spark to any meal.

3 tablespoons low-sodium
  mayonnaise
4 tablespoons white vinegar
1 teaspoon lemon juice
1 small onion, minced
2 green chiles, seeded and minced
2 halves low-sodium sweet peppers,
  chopped

6 tablespoons juice from low-sodium
  sweet peppers
6 potatoes, parboiled,* peeled, and
  cubed
4 ounces low-sodium Cheddar
  cheese, grated

1. In bowl, combine all but last 2 ingredients, blending thoroughly.
2. Stir in potatoes and cheese, blending thoroughly. Cover and chill at least 4 hours to allow flavors to blend.

Per serving: 127.5 calories; 10.0 mg. sodium; 15.7 gm. carbohydrates; 5.9 gm. fat.

* Do not add salt to water.

Potato Fritters

SERVES 8

These fritters lie lightly on the tongue and their spicy goodness is just as tempting cold or hot. Fabulous with Sweet Hot Apple Relish (page 45) or Sour Cream Dip (page 37).

4 potatoes, parboiled,* peeled, and
  mashed
⅛ teaspoon garlic powder
1½ teaspoons low-sodium chicken
  bouillon
1/16 teaspoon cayenne pepper

1 egg, lightly beaten
¼ cup low-fat milk
¼ cup low-sodium cottage cheese
1 teaspoon dried basil
2 cups vegetable oil

1. In bowl, mash together first 4 ingredients, blending thoroughly.
2. Beat in egg, milk, and cheese, blending thoroughly.
3. Stir in basil. Divide mixture into 16 small cakes.
4. In skillet, heat oil over medium heat. Add potato cakes and fry 3 minutes, or until bottoms are browned.

5. Turn cakes and fry 3 minutes more, or until second sides are browned.
6. Drain cakes on paper towels.

Per serving: 170.0 calories; 15.7 mg. sodium; 13.2 gm. carbohydrates; 11.9 gm. fat.

* Do not add salt to water.

Baked Stuffed Potatoes

SERVES 8

Potatoes stuffed with all sorts of goodies are very popular in the United States. This absolutely scrumptious Mexican version should make them even more so.

2 tablespoons unsalted margarine
2 onions, chopped
1 clove garlic, chopped
¼ pound ground beef (or ground
  pork or 1 half chicken breast,
  skinned, boned, and diced)
2 green chiles, seeded and minced
¹⁄₁₆ teaspoon ground nutmeg
1 teaspoon Chili Powder (page 210)

2 teaspoons dried parsley
4 potatoes, baked
¼ cup low-fat milk
3 ounces low-sodium Swiss cheese,
  minced
1½ teaspoons low-sodium chicken
  bouillon

1. In skillet, heat margarine over low heat. Add onion, garlic, beef, and chiles. Cook 10 minutes, or until beef loses all pink color, stirring often.
2. Stir in nutmeg, chili powder, and parsley. Set aside.
3. Preheat oven to 325°.
4. In bowl, scoop potatoes from shells. Reserve shells. Mash potatoes with milk.
5. Stir in beef mixture, blending thoroughly.
6. Stir in remaining ingredients.
7. Stuff potato shells with potato mixture.
8. On aluminum foil, place stuffed potatoes. Bake ½ hour, or until lightly browned on top.

Per serving with beef: 183.0 calories; 21.9 mg. sodium; 19.3 gm. carbohydrates;
    9.2 gm. fat.
Per serving with pork: 178.4 calories; 25.1 mg. sodium; 19.3 gm. carbohydrates;
    8.3 gm. fat.
Per serving with chicken: 155.9 calories; 21.4 mg. sodium; 19.3 gm. carbohydrates;
    6.6 gm. fat.

Potatoes with Chiles   SERVES 8

The tasty magic of poblano chiles is put to savory use in this marvelous recipe. It is a wonderful accompaniment to any dish. Steak and Tomatoes (page 154) and Fish-Stuffed Eggplant (page 114) are two suggestions.

3 tablespoons olive oil, divided
2 onions, chopped
1 clove garlic, minced
3 poblano chiles, seeded and
  chopped (or 3 green chiles)
4 potatoes, parboiled,* peeled, and
  sliced

Black pepper to taste
1/16 teaspoon ground nutmeg
1 1/2 teaspoons low-sodium chicken
  bouillon

1. In skillet, heat 1 tablespoon oil over medium-low heat. Add onions, garlic, and chiles and cook 5 minutes, or until onions are golden.
2. Push onion mixture to sides of skillet. To well created in center, add 1 tablespoon oil and potatoes. Season with black pepper, nutmeg, and bouillon. Fry 10 minutes, or until bottoms are lightly browned.
3. Turn potatoes. Add remaining oil and cook 5 minutes more, or until second sides are browned.

Per serving: 119.0 calories; 6.1 mg. sodium; 18.3 gm. carbohydrates; 5.9 gm. fat.

* Do not add salt to water.

Spicy Potato Casserole   SERVES 8

An elegant way to enjoy the versatile potato. Lovely with Chicken in Mustard Sauce (page 138). Or for variety, top with Tomato Sauce with Cayenne (page 212).

6 potatoes, boiled,* peeled, and
  mashed
1/4 cup low-fat milk
1/4 cup plain yogurt
1 1/2 teaspoons low-sodium baking
  powder

2 leeks, chopped, including greens
1/16 teaspoon ground cinnamon
1/4 teaspoon ground cumin
1 teaspoon dried basil
2 teaspoons paprika

1. Preheat oven to 350°.
2. In bowl, combine first 4 ingredients, blending thoroughly.

3. Stir in all remaining ingredients, except paprika, blending thoroughly. Transfer mixture to 9-inch-square ovenproof casserole.
4. Sprinkle paprika over all and bake ½ hour, or until potatoes are browned on top.

Per serving: 107.8 calories; 12.4 mg. sodium; 23.2 gm. carbohydrates; 0.4 gm. fat.

* Do not add salt to water.

Spaghetti and Chorizo SERVES 8

This dish is so fabulous it needs no improving. But if you want to be lavish, add either ¼ pound green beans or 1 cup fresh peas* to Step 3.

1 tablespoon unsalted margarine
1 onion, minced
2 cloves garlic, minced
¼ pound Chorizo (page 158)
3 tomatoes, chopped
1 cup Chicken Stock (page 76)
Dash of clove powder

1 teaspoon dried parsley
2 ounces low-sodium Swiss cheese, minced
¾ pound spaghetti, boiled al dente†
3 tablespoons heavy cream
Dash of ground nutmeg

1. In saucepan, heat margarine over medium-low heat. Add onion, garlic, and chorizo and cook 10 minutes, or until chorizo loses all pink color, stirring often.
2. Stir in tomatoes, blending thoroughly.
3. Add stock, clove powder, parsley, and cheese. Cook 10 minutes, stirring often.
4. Add spaghetti. Raise heat to medium and cook 5 minutes more, stirring often.
5. Reduce heat to low. Stir in remaining ingredients and cook 5 minutes more, stirring often.

Per serving plain: 307.4 calories; 32.6 mg. sodium; 41.0 gm. carbohydrates; 9.6 gm. fat.
Per serving with green beans: 312.0 calories; 33.6 mg. sodium; 42.0 gm. carbohydrates; 9.6 gm. fat.
Per serving with peas: 325.4 calories; 33.0 mg. sodium; 44.1 gm. carbohydrates; 9.7 gm. fat.

* Do not use frozen, which contain salt. If fresh are not available, substitute 1 can (8 ounces) low-sodium peas.
† Do not add salt to water.

Noodles with Minced Meats SERVES 8

A delectable meal. Choose either Zucchini, Tomatoes, and Corn Casserole (page 208) or Lima Beans and Tomatoes in Butter Sauce (page 199) as a side dish.

1 recipe Minced Meats with Fruit
  (page 170)
4 scallions, chopped, including greens

½ pound noodles, boiled al dente*
1 tablespoon unsalted margarine
1 teaspoon dried parsley

1. In saucepan, combine first 2 ingredients. Turn heat to medium-low and cook 15 minutes, stirring often.
2. Stir in remaining ingredients, blending thoroughly. Cook 10 minutes more, stirring occasionally.

Per serving: 465.0 calories; 77.8 mg. sodium; 51.8 gm. carbohydrates; 17.6 gm. fat.

* Do not add salt to water.

Cheesy Hot Noodles SERVES 8

As its name suggests, this is a delectable combination of flavors and textures. Great with Mint Chicken (page 143).

1 cup Tomato Sauce with Cayenne
  (page 212)
1 teaspoon red wine vinegar
1 cup low-sodium cottage cheese

2 teaspoons dried parsley
2 teaspoons low-sodium beef
  bouillon
½ pound noodles, boiled al dente*

1. In saucepan, combine all ingredients, except noodles. Stir to blend.
2. Turn heat to medium-low and cook 10 minutes, or until mixture bubbles around the edges, stirring often.
3. Stir in noodles and cook 5 minutes more, stirring occasionally.

Per serving: 149.1 calories; 14.3 mg. sodium; 24.5 gm. carbohydrates; 2.3 gm. fat.

* Do not add salt to water.

Mexican Lasagna

SERVES 18

A uniquely tasty adaptation of the Italian favorite. Serve with the salad of your choice.

1 pound lasagna, boiled al dente,*
  divided
1 recipe Picadillo with Vegetables
  (page 169), divided
1 recipe Shredded Pork (page 163) or
  ¾ pound Chorizo (page 158),
  divided

3 ounces low-sodium mozzarella
  cheese, shredded
1 can (29 ounces) low-sodium
  tomato puree
2 ounces low-sodium Cheddar
  cheese, shredded

1. Preheat oven to 350°.
2. In 9 x 13-inch ovenproof casserole, place ⅓ of the lasagna. Spoon ⅓ of the picadillo over lasagna. Then add ⅓ of the pork.
3. Repeat Step 2 until lasagna, picadillo, and pork are gone.
4. Top with mozzarella cheese.
5. Pour tomato puree over all.
6. Sprinkle Cheddar cheese on top.
7. Cover and bake 40 minutes. Uncover and bake 10 minutes more.

Per serving with pork: 402.6 calories; 74.5 mg. sodium; 39.2 gm. carbohydrates;
   14.7 gm. fat.
Per serving with chorizo: 318.3 calories; 53.0 mg. sodium; 38.1 gm. carbohydrates;
   10.3 gm. fat.

* Do not add salt to water.

Mexican Macaroni Salad   SERVES 12

A little bit German, a lot Mexican, and thoroughly delicious. Wonderful
with the simplest as well as the most elegant dishes.

4 tablespoons low-sodium
  mayonnaise
½ cup plain yogurt
¼ cup lemon juice
2 low-sodium hot cherry peppers,
  seeded and minced
6 low-sodium cucumber pickles,
  diced

1½ teaspoons sugar
6 scallions, chopped, including greens
1⁄16 teaspoon cayenne pepper
½ teaspoon low-sodium Dijon
  mustard
¾ pound elbow macaroni, boiled
  al dente*

In bowl combine all ingredients, blending thoroughly. Cover and chill at
least 4 hours to allow flavors to blend.

Per serving: 158.8 calories; 7.8 mg. sodium; 25.5 gm. carbohydrates; 4.4 gm. fat.

* Do not add salt to boiling water.

Chile Rice
with Shrimp and Cheese   SERVES 4

To paraphrase an old saying, one taste is better than a thousand words.

1 onion, chopped
1 clove garlic, chopped
2 tomatoes, chopped
2 teaspoons vegetable oil
1 cup white rice
2 green chiles, seeded and chopped
2 cups boiling water

1½ tablespoons low-sodium chicken
  bouillon
1 teaspoon dried basil
2 ounces low-sodium Gouda cheese
¼ pound fresh shrimp, shelled,
  deveined, and halved diagonally

1. In blender, combine first 3 ingredients. Puree. Set aside.
2. In saucepan, heat oil over low heat. Add rice and chiles and cook 5
   minutes, or until rice is golden, stirring often.
3. Add tomato puree and cook 3 minutes more, stirring occasionally.

4. Add water, bouillon, basil, and cheese. Stir to blend. Cover and cook 10 minutes.
5. Add shrimp. Cover and cook 5 minutes more, or until liquid is absorbed.
6. Remove from heat. Let stand, covered, 5 minutes more.
7. Stir to blend before serving.

Per serving: 311.3 calories; 54.9 mg. sodium; 47.0 gm. carbohydrates; 8.8 gm. fat.

Baked Rice
with Chicken and Chorizo SERVES 8

Rice—that perennial Mexican favorite—was never so tasty as in this dish, which requires only Green Bean and Sweet Pepper Salad (page 100) to make a perfect meal.

3 tablespoons unsalted margarine, divided
2 onions, chopped
½ pound Chorizo (page 158)
1½ cups white rice
1 can (8 ounces) low-sodium tomato sauce
3 half chicken breasts, cut in 2-inch pieces
1 teaspoon dried parsley
½ teaspoon dried basil
Black pepper to taste
3 cups boiling water
1 tablespoon low-sodium beef bouillon
2 tablespoons low-sodium chicken bouillon
¼ pound fresh peas*

1. In saucepan, heat 1 tablespoon margarine over medium-low heat. Add onions and chorizo and cook 10 minutes, or until chorizo loses all pink color, stirring often.
2. Push onion mixture to sides of saucepan. To well created in center, add rice and cook 5 minutes more, stirring often.
3. Add tomato sauce, chicken, parsley, basil, and pepper. Reduce heat to low. Cover and cook 10 minutes.
4. Add remaining ingredients, except peas. Raise heat to medium and bring to a slow boil. Continue boiling 5 minutes, stirring occasionally.
5. Reduce heat to low. Cover and cook 15 minutes.
6. Sprinkle peas on top. Cover and cook 10 minutes more, or until liquid is absorbed.

Per serving: 336.2 calories; 62.4 mg. sodium; 40.5 gm. carbohydrates; 11.1 gm. fat.

* Do not use frozen, which contain salt. If fresh are not available, substitute 1 can (8 ounces) low-sodium peas.

Green Rice

SERVES 4

A beautiful representative of Mexico's best. For the deluxe version, add one ounce of shredded low-sodium Cheddar cheese to Step 3.

2 cups boiling water
1½ tablespoons low-sodium chicken bouillon

½ cup Green Sauce (page 216)
1¼ cups white rice

1. In saucepan, combine first 2 ingredients, stirring until bouillon is dissolved.
2. Stir in sauce. Turn heat to medium and bring to slow boil.
3. Add rice. Reduce to low. Cover and cook 20 minutes, or until liquid is absorbed.

Per serving plain: 247.7 calories; 17.0 mg. sodium; 49.6 gm. carbohydrates; 3.5 gm. fat.
Per serving with Cheddar cheese: 276.1 calories; 17.9 mg. sodium; 49.8 gm. carbohydrates; 5.8 gm. fat.

Mexican White Rice

SERVES 4

The modest name does not begin to describe the savory charms of this dish. Serve with any main dish. You cannot go wrong.

1 tablespoon vegetable oil
1 onion, minced
2 cloves garlic, minced

1 cup white rice
2 cups Chicken Stock (page 76)

1. In saucepan, heat oil over low heat. Add onion and garlic and cook 5 minutes, or until onion is golden, stirring occasionally.
2. Add rice and cook 3 minutes more, stirring often.
3. Add stock. Cover and simmer 15 minutes, or until liquid is absorbed.

Per serving: 232.4 calories; 20.8 mg. sodium; 43.8 gm. carbohydrates; 4.8 gm. fat.

Rice with Chicken

SERVES 8

This international dish, known by its Mexican name, Arroz con Pollo, is an unbeatable meal. If you want to try new variations of perfection, replace the chicken with any one of the following: ½ pound cubed pork, added to Step 3; or ¼ pound fresh shrimp, shelled, deveined, and minced, or 2 pints shucked oysters, liquid included, added to Step 5.

4 half chicken breasts, chopped into
   2-inch pieces
1 teaspoon low-sodium beef bouillon
Black pepper to taste
1 tablespoon olive oil
2 onions, chopped
2 cloves garlic, minced
2 red chiles, seeded and minced
1½ cups white rice
4 tomatoes, chopped

¼ teaspoon ground cumin
1 teaspoon dried oregano
3 carrots, cut in ½-inch rounds
4 cups Chicken Stock (page 76)
1 can (8 ounces) low-sodium
   tomato sauce
1 teaspoon paprika
2 green peppers, chopped

1. In bowl, place chicken. Season with bouillon and pepper. Set aside.
2. In Dutch oven, heat oil over low heat. Add onions, garlic, and chiles and cook 5 minutes, or until onions are golden, stirring often.
3. Add chicken and cook 20 minutes more, or until skin turns golden brown, stirring often.
4. Add all remaining ingredients, except paprika and green peppers. Cover and cook 45 minutes.
5. Stir in paprika and green peppers. Cover and cook 15 minutes more, or until liquid is absorbed.

Per serving with chicken: 288.5 calories; 73.5 mg. sodium; 47.4 gm. carbohydrates;
   4.6 gm. fat.
Per serving with pork: 246.5 calories; 68.5 mg. sodium; 47.6 gm. carbohydrates;
   3.5 gm. fat.
Per serving with shrimp: 290.1 calories; 110.1 mg. sodium; 50.3 gm. carbohydrates;
   4.9 gm. fat.
Per serving with oysters: 306.0 calories; 68.5 mg. sodium; 47.4 gm. carbohydrates;
   7.5 gm. fat.

Rice with Mushrooms and Cheese

SERVES 4

This combination is irresistible. Serve with any number of dishes, including Flounder with Walnut-Orange Sauce (page 111).

1 teaspoon unsalted margarine
12 mushrooms, chopped
1 tablespoon dried parsley
¼ teaspoon dried marjoram
1 tablespoon dry sherry
1 cup white rice

2 cups Meat Stock (page 78)
¹⁄₁₆ teaspoon hot pepper flakes
2 ounces low-sodium mozzarella
  cheese, shredded

1. In saucepan, heat margarine over low heat. Add mushrooms and cook 3 minutes, stirring often.
2. Stir in parsley, marjoram, and sherry.
3. Stir in rice. Cook 5 minutes more, stirring often.
4. Add stock and hot pepper flakes. Cover and cook 10 minutes.
5. Sprinkle cheese on top. Cover and cook 5 minutes more, or until liquid is absorbed.

Per serving: 245.7 calories; 32.4 mg. sodium; 41.0 gm. carbohydrates; 5.8 gm. fat.

Rice with Tomatoes

SERVES 8

Nobody makes rice as delicious as does a Mexican cook and this dish is a perfect example. If you wish, you can substitute one-half pound of chopped eggplant for the tomatoes. Any way you make it, this dish is a winner. Two serving suggestions are Festival Chicken in Wine (page 142) and Steak with Chile Strips (page 156).

2 tomatoes, chopped
1 onion, chopped
1 clove garlic, chopped
2 teaspoons dried parsley
1 tablespoon vegetable oil
2 cups white rice

3 cups Chicken Stock (page 76)
1 tablespoon low-sodium chicken
  bouillon
1 can (8 ounces) low-sodium tomato
  sauce

1. In blender, combine first 4 ingredients. Puree. Set aside.
2. In saucepan, heat oil over low heat. Add rice and cook 5 minutes, or until rice turns golden, stirring often.

3. Add tomato puree. Raise heat to medium and cook 3 minutes, stirring constantly.
4. Stir in remaining ingredients. Reduce heat to low. Cover and cook 20 minutes, or until liquid is absorbed.

Per serving with tomatoes; 226.4 calories; 20.3 mg. sodium; 44.7 gm. carbohydrates;
  3.2 gm. fat.
Per serving with eggplant: 225.7 calories; 25.0 mg. sodium; 44.6 gm. carbohydrates;
  3.2 gm. fat.

Sweet Rice with Green Beans   SERVES 8

The contrast of flavors (pungent garlic, sweet cinnamon, and piquant mint) adds up to a deliciously different dish. Excellent with Sherry Veal Chops (page 165).

2 tablespoons vegetable oil	Dash of ground nutmeg
1 onion, minced	1 teaspoon dried parsley
2 cloves garlic, minced	1 teaspoon dry sherry
1½ cups white rice	½ pound green beans, cut in 1-inch
1 teaspoon paprika	pieces
4½ cups Chicken Stock (page 76)	½ teaspoon dried mint
⅛ teaspoon ground cinnamon	

1. In saucepan, heat oil over low heat. Add onion, garlic, and rice. Cook 10 minutes, or until rice is golden, stirring often.
2. Stir in paprika, blending thoroughly.
3. Add stock, cinnamon, nutmeg, parsley, and sherry. Cover and cook 5 minutes.
4. Sprinkle green beans and mint on top. Cover and cook 10 minutes more, or until liquid is absorbed.
5. Remove from heat. Let stand, covered, 5 minutes more.

Per serving: 199.3 calories; 22.6 mg. sodium; 34.6 gm. carbohydrates; 4.9 gm. fat.

Yellow Rice
SERVES 8

The tomatoes and cayenne pepper actually color this rice red. But just as Mexicans stubbornly refer to limes as lemons, so do they whimsically persist in calling this dish Yellow Rice. Whatever the name, it is special. Try it with Mixed Seafood in Lime Sauce (page 128).

2 onions, chopped
2 cloves garlic, chopped
3½ cups boiling water, divided
1 tablespoon olive oil
1½ cups white rice
4 tomatoes, chopped

⅛ teaspoon cayenne pepper
2 tablespoons low-sodium chicken bouillon
1 teaspoon turmeric
1 tablespoon unsalted margarine

1. In blender, combine onions, garlic, and ½ cup water. Grind to a paste. Set aside.
2. In saucepan, heat oil over low heat. Add onion paste and sauté 2 minutes, stirring often.
3. Add rice. Cook 5 minutes more, stirring often.
4. Stir in tomatoes and cayenne pepper.
5. Add remaining water, bouillon, and turmeric. Raise heat to high and bring to a boil.
6. Reduce heat to low. Cover and cook ½ hour, or until liquid is absorbed.
7. Add margarine. Let melt before serving.

Per serving: 187.8 calories; 11.0 mg. sodium; 36.2 gm. carbohydrates; 4.4 gm. fat.

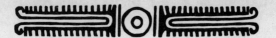

Vegetables

Small, dark, hazelnut-flavored avocados; lovely green zucchini trailing on the ground; sweet peas in flower; white and yellow stalks of corn swaying against the sky; sun-drenched rosy tomatoes bursting on the vine—a cornucopia of vegetables colors the Mexican landscape with even greater and more riotous abundance than do the flowers.

Indeed, vegetables are so important to the Mexican diet that they dominate every scene, and every family, rich and poor alike, has a little vegetable plot of their own to guarantee the freshest possible flavor for the day's meals.

Vegetables are part of almost every main dish in the Mexican kitchen. But they are so relished that they are often served as special courses before the main meal as well. Take your pick: Creamed Chile Corn (page 204); Broiled Tomatoes with Avocado (page 200); Cabbage, Walnuts, and Pears (page 201); or any of the other sumptuous offerings in this chapter. They will make vegetable devotees of you all.

Bean-Stuffed Chiles

SERVES 8

For a true Mexican feast, serve this dish with Sour Cream-Chicken Enchiladas (page 60).

4 poblano chiles (or 4 green peppers)
2 cups Refried Beans (page 177)
1 egg, separated
¼ cup low-fat milk
⅓ cup all-purpose flour
⅓ cup vegetable oil
1 cup Chicken Stock (page 76)

Black pepper to taste
¼ teaspoon onion powder
2 ounces low-sodium Cheddar
   cheese, chopped
2 tablespoons heavy cream
1⁄16 teaspoon ground cinnamon

1. Preheat oven to broil.
2. Cut ½-inch caps from tops of chiles. Remove seeds.
3. On baking sheet, place chiles and broil 4 inches from heat until skins start to blacken, turn often. Transfer to platter.
4. Reduce oven to 350°.
5. Stuff chiles with refried beans. Set aside.
6. In bowl, beat egg yolk.
7. In second bowl, beat egg white until stiff. Fold into egg yolk.
8. Stir in milk. Set aside.
9. Sprinkle flour over chiles. Then dip chiles in egg mixture.
10. In skillet, heat oil over medium-low heat. Add chiles and sauté until golden brown, turning once. Transfer to 9-inch-square ovenproof casserole.
11. Pour stock over chiles. Season with black pepper and onion powder. Sprinkle cheese over all and bake 15 minutes.
12. Add cream and cinnamon. Bake 5 minutes more, or until cheese is melted.
13. Cut each chile in half and serve immediately.

Per serving with poblano chiles: 197.5 calories; 27.0 mg. sodium; 22.3 gm. carbohydrates; 8.7 gm. fat.
Per serving with green peppers: 216.9 calories; 40.0 mg. sodium; 26.5 gm. carbohydrates; 8.9 gm. fat.

Chiles with
Cream Sauce and Nut Sauce

SERVES 16

This is an adaptation of a renowned Mexican dish called Chiles en Nogada, which means chiles in walnut sauce. Folklore tells us the dish was created in Puebla to honor General Iturbide who led the final revolution that freed Mexico from Spanish rule. The colors—red, white, and green—represent the Mexican flag. We have substituted almonds and peanuts for the walnuts.

8 poblano chiles (or 8 green peppers)
2 cups Picadillo with Vegetables
   (page 169)
¼ cup unsalted, slivered almonds
¼ cup unsalted peanuts
1⅔ cups Cream Cheese Sauce
   (page 222)

¹⁄₁₆ teaspoon clove powder
1 pomegranate, peeled, seeds
   separated and reserved

1. Preheat oven to broil.
2. Cut ½-inch caps from tops of chiles. Remove seeds.
3. On baking sheet, place chiles and broil 4 inches from heat until skins start to blacken, turning often. Transfer to platter.
4. Stuff chiles with picadillo. Set aside.
5. In bowl, combine almonds, peanuts, cheese sauce, and clove powder, blending thoroughly. Spoon sauce over chiles.
6. Cut each chile in half and garnish with pomegranate seeds.

Per serving with poblano chiles: 144.7 calories; 20.7 mg. sodium; 13.3 gm. carbohydrates; 8.8 gm. fat.
Per serving with green peppers: 164.0 calories; 33.7 mg. sodium; 17.5 gm. carbohydrates; 8.9 gm. fat.

Meat-Stuffed Chiles

SERVES 8

Simply fabulous and one of the most popular chile dishes in Mexico. Serve with Mexican Vegetable Soup (page 87) and Simple Beans (page 174) or with Cucumber Salad La Jolla (page 100) and Rice with Eggplant (page 188).

8 poblano chiles (or 8 green peppers)
2 cups Picadillo with Vegetables
   (page 169)
2 eggs, separated
¼ cup water

⅔ cup all-purpose flour
⅔ cup vegetable oil
3 cups Basil-Tomato Sauce (page 212)

1. Preheat oven to broil.
2. Cut ½-inch caps from tops of chiles. Remove seeds.
3. On baking sheet, place chiles and broil 4 inches from heat until skins start to blacken, turning often. Transfer to platter. Let stand 5 minutes.
4. Spoon picadillo with vegetables into chiles. Set aside.
5. Reduce oven to 350°.
6. In bowl, beat egg yolks.
7. In second bowl, beat egg whites until stiff. Fold into egg yolks.
8. Stir in water. Set aside.
9. Sprinkle flour over chiles. Then dip chiles in egg mixture.
10. In skillet, heat oil over medium-low heat. Add chiles and fry until golden brown, turning once. Transfer to 9 x 13-inch ovenproof casserole.
11. Pour tomato sauce over chiles and bake ½ hour, or until sauce is bubbly.

Per serving: 265.9 calories; 44.3 mg. sodium; 35.8 gm. carbohydrates; 9.8 gm. fat.

Vegetable-Stuffed Chiles

SERVES 16

Another favorite chile recipe in Mexico. Great with anything you choose.

8 poblano chiles (or 8 green peppers)
1 tablespoon vegetable oil, divided
2 cloves garlic, chopped
2 onions, chopped
2 tomatoes, chopped
1 zucchini, chopped
1 can (8 ounces) low-sodium corn
 niblets, drained
Cayenne pepper to taste
1/16 teaspoon ground nutmeg

2 cups Chile-Avocado Sauce
 (page 214)
1/2 cup sour cream
2 ounces low-sodium Gouda cheese,
 minced
3/4 cup boiling water
1 teaspoon low-sodium chicken
 bouillon

1. Preheat oven to broil.
2. Cut 1/2-inch caps from tops of chiles. Remove seeds.
3. On baking sheet, place chiles and broil 4 inches from heat until skins start to blacken, turning often. Transfer to platter.
4. Reduce oven to 350°.
5. In skillet, heat oil over low heat. Add garlic and onions and cook 5 minutes, or until garlic is lightly browned.
6. Add tomatoes, zucchini, and corn. Stir to blend. Cook 5 minutes more, stirring often.
7. Stir in cayenne pepper and nutmeg, blending thoroughly.
8. Stuff chiles with vegetable mixture. Transfer to 9 x 13-inch ovenproof casserole.
9. In bowl, combine Chile-Avocado Sauce and sour cream, blending thoroughly. Spoon over chiles.
10. Sprinkle cheese over all.
11. In second bowl, combine water and bouillon, stirring until bouillon is dissolved. Pour around chiles.
12. Bake chiles 20 minutes, or until cheese is melted.
13. Cut chiles in half and serve immediately.

Per serving with poblano chiles: 134.3 calories; 9.3 mg. sodium; 10.4 gm. carbohydrates; 10.6 gm. fat.
Per serving with green peppers: 142.7 calories; 12.5 mg. sodium; 11.2 gm. carbohydrates; 10.7 gm. fat.

Asparagus and Mushrooms SERVES 4

The delicate sweetness of asparagus takes on a new dimension with the flavorings in this dish. Mint Lamb Chops with Peanuts (page 158) and Cheesy Hot Noodles (page 182) combine to make a lovely main course.

1 tablespoon unsalted margarine	Dash of ground cinnamon
8 mushrooms, chopped	12 stalks asparagus, steamed* al dente
1 dried chile, seeded and crushed	1/16 teaspoon ground nutmeg
1 cup boiling water	1 orange, peeled and chopped
1 teaspoon low-sodium chicken bouillon	

1. In skillet, heat margarine over low heat. Add mushrooms and chile and cook 3 minutes, stirring often.
2. Add water, bouillon, and cinnamon. Raise heat to medium and cook 5 minutes, stirring often.
3. Divide asparagus among 4 plates. Pour bouillon mixture over all.
4. Sprinkle nutmeg over all. Garnish with orange.

Per serving: 100.1 calories; 17.7 mg. sodium; 15.0 gm. carbohydrates; 3.8 gm. fat.

* Do not add salt to water.

Asparagus in Crumb Sauce SERVES 4

Mint and asparagus and cream, too—a heavenly combination that is so special you will want to serve it with your favorite dish.

1 tablespoon unsalted margarine	1 teaspoon low-sodium chicken bouillon
3 tablespoons low-sodium bread crumbs	2 tablespoons heavy cream
1/16 teaspoon cayenne pepper	16 stalks asparagus, steamed* al dente
1 teaspoon dried mint (or 1 1/2 tablespoons fresh mint) minced	

1. In skillet, heat margarine over low heat. Add bread crumbs, cayenne pepper, and mint and cook 3 minutes, stirring often.

2. Stir in bouillon and cream and cook 3 minutes more.
3. Divide asparagus among 4 plates. Spoon bread crumb mixture over all.

Per serving: 116.6 calories; 10.5 mg. sodium; 12.3 gm. carbohydrates; 6.8 gm. fat.

* Do not add salt to water.

Baked Green Peppers with Raisins

SERVES 4

An unbeatable blend of flavors to tease the tongue. Equally delicious when one medium eggplant, sliced, or 2 yellow squash, halved diagonally, replace the green peppers. Try serving with Sea Bass and Tomatoes (page 119), Chicken in Orange-Mint Sauce (page 138), or Veal Balls in Sour Cream Sauce (page 166).

2 large green peppers, halved
  lengthwise
1½ cups Tomato Sauce with Cayenne
  (page 212)
⅛ teaspoon ground cinnamon

¼ cup dark raisins*
½ cup orange juice
2 ounces low-sodium mozzarella
  cheese, sliced in thin strips

1. Preheat oven to 400°.
2. Place peppers, cut side down, in 9-inch-square ovenproof casserole. Add tomato sauce, cinnamon, raisins, and juice. Cover and bake 10 minutes.
3. Add cheese. Bake, uncovered, 10 minutes more.

Per serving with peppers: 134.9 calories; 30.7 mg. sodium; 28.6 gm. carbohydrates;
  2.4 gm. fat.
Per serving with eggplant: 130.5 calories; 13.5 mg. sodium; 27.8 gm. carbohydrates;
  2.3 gm. fat.
Per serving with squash: 121.9 calories; 12.2 mg. sodium; 25.7 gm. carbohydrates;
  2.3 gm. fat.

* Preserved in non-sodium ingredient.

Green Peppers and Avocado SERVES 4

This refreshingly flavorful dish is especially delightful with Scrod in Pecan Sauce (page 118).

1 teaspoon unsalted margarine
1 onion, chopped
1 avocado, peeled, pitted, and
   chopped
⅛ teaspoon ground cumin
¹⁄₁₆ teaspoon ground nutmeg

1 teaspoon dried parsley
1 teaspoon low-sodium chicken
   bouillon
1 tablespoon sour cream
2 green peppers, halved lengthwise

1. Preheat oven to broil.
2. In skillet, heat margarine over low heat. Add onion and sauté 5 minutes, or until onion is golden.
3. In blender, combine onion and all remaining ingredients, except green peppers. Puree.
4. Stuff green peppers with avocado mixture. Broil 6 inches from heat 6 minutes, or until peppers are tender.

Per serving: 202.2 calories; 22.4 mg. sodium; 15.9 gm. carbohydrates; 16.9 gm. fat.

Lime Eggplant with Tomatoes SERVES 4

Wonderfully spicy and pungent. Truly fabulous with the simplest or the most elegant fare: Burritos II (page 51) or Sea Bass in Red Wine Sauce (page 118), for example.

1 eggplant, cut into ½-inch rounds
¼ cup lime juice
2 teaspoons low-sodium beef
   bouillon
Black pepper to taste

¼ teaspoon ground cumin
2 tablespoons dried parsley
½ teaspoon ground cinnamon
3 tomatoes, chopped

1. Preheat oven to 350°.
2. In 9 x 13-inch ovenproof casserole, place eggplant. Add remaining ingredients, stirring to blend. Cover and bake 20 minutes.
3. Uncover and bake 5 minutes more.

Per serving: 68.0 calories; 13.8 mg. sodium; 14.4 gm. carbohydrates; 1.0 gm. fat.

Lima Beans and
Tomatoes in Butter Sauce

SERVES 8

Whether you choose the lima beans or an equal amount of peas or cauliflower (chopped), this dish is a flavorful delight that enhances any meal.
South-of-the-Border Meat Loaf (page 172) and Spicy Potato Casserole
(page 180) are just two of many possible serving options.

2 tablespoons unsalted margarine,
  divided
1 onion, chopped
½ pound lima beans, steamed*
  al dente
Black pepper to taste

3 tomatoes, chopped
1/16 teaspoon ground cinnamon
1 cup Chicken Stock (page 76)
½ teaspoon paprika
⅛ teaspoon garlic powder

1. In skillet, heat 1 tablespoon margarine over low heat. Add onion and
   cook 5 minutes, or until onion is golden, stirring occasionally.
2. Add remaining margarine, lima beans, and pepper. Stir to blend.
3. Add remaining ingredients, blending thoroughly. Raise heat to medium
   and cook 10 minutes, stirring occasionally.

Per serving with lima beans: 85.5 calories; 7.9 mg. sodium; 12.1 carbohydrates; 3.4 gm.
   fat.
Per serving with peas: 74.3 calories; 7.9 mg. sodium; 9.9 gm. carbohydrates; 3.4 gm. fat.
Per serving with cauliflower: 58.0 calories; 11.0 mg. sodium; 7.3 gm. carbohydrates;
   3.3 gm. fat.

* Do not add salt to water.

Broccoli and Mushrooms with Pork
SERVES 8

Flounder in Chile-Corn Sauce (page 110) and a simple tossed salad will guarantee you a lovely meal.

2 tablespoons olive oil, divided
10 cloves garlic, minced
1 onion, minced
1 head broccoli, broken into
    flowerettes, stalks cut in ½-inch
    rounds

2 green chiles, seeded and minced
¼ pound pork, shredded
8 mushrooms, sliced

1. In skillet, heat 1 tablespoon oil over low heat. Add garlic and onion and cook 10 minutes, or until garlic is lightly browned, stirring often.
2. Add broccoli and chiles and stir to blend.
3. Add pork and remaining oil. Raise heat to medium-low and sauté 2 minutes, or until pork loses all pink color.
4. Add mushrooms and sauté 1 minute more, stirring constantly.

Per serving: 109.1 calories; 23.9 mg. sodium; 9.6 gm. carbohydrates; 6.0 gm. fat.

Broiled Tomatoes with Avocado
SERVES 8

This very Mexican dish will enhance any meal.

4 tomatoes
1 avocado, peeled, pitted, and
    chopped
1 green chile, seeded and minced
1 leek, chopped, including greens

Black pepper to taste
1 tablespoon dried parsley
⅛ teaspoon ground cumin
1½ teaspoons paprika

1. Preheat oven to broil.
2. Cut ½ inch from tops of tomatoes. Remove pulp and chop.
3. In blender, combine tomato pulp and remaining ingredients, except tomato shells. Puree.
4. Stuff tomato shells with avocado mixture. Broil 6 inches from heat 10 minutes, or until tomatoes start to brown.

Per serving: 98.0 calories; 5.6 mg. sodium; 8.4 gm. carbohydrates; 7.2 gm. fat.

Cabbage and Apples in Piquant Sour Cream Sauce
SERVES 8

Very German in origin, very delicious at any time. You might try this dish with Spaghetti and Chorizo (page 158).

1 head cabbage, shredded
3 apples, peeled, cored, and chopped
1½ cups water
1 cup apple juice

½ cup Piquant Sour Cream Sauce
(page 224)

1. In Dutch oven, combine first 3 ingredients. Turn heat to low. Cover and simmer 45 minutes, adding more water if necessary to prevent sticking, stirring occasionally.
2. Add apple juice. Cover and simmer 15 minutes more.
3. Stir in sour cream sauce. Cover and simmer 15 minutes more, stirring occasionally.

Per serving: 98.9 calories; 13.4 mg. sodium; 18.3 gm. carbohydrates; 3.2 gm. fat.

Cabbage, Walnuts, and Pears
SERVES 8

An elegant, unusual medley. Try it with Saucy Meat Balls (page 171).

2 tablespoons unsalted margarine
1 head cabbage, shredded
1 onion, chopped
2 pears, cored and chopped
½ teaspoon ground cinnamon

⅟₁₆ teaspoon clove powder
2 cups water
¼ cup dry red wine

1. In Dutch oven, heat margarine over low heat. Add cabbage and onion. Cover and simmer 15 minutes, stirring often.
2. Add all remaining ingredients, except wine. Cover and simmer 20 minutes.
3. Add wine, stirring to blend. Raise heat to medium and cook, uncovered, 20 minutes more, stirring occasionally.

Per serving: 82.0 calories; 14.7 mg. sodium; 13.5 gm. carbohydrates; 3.2 gm. fat.

Glazed Carrots with Minced Shrimp

SERVES 8

An unusual and highly satisfying combination. Chicken with Figs and Lemons (page 141) and boiled white rice are great companions.

4 carrots, cut in 2-inch pieces
1½ cups water
¼ cup sugar
2 tablespoons dark raisins*
1 orange, chopped, including rind
1 tablespoon unsalted margarine

1 leek, chopped, including greens
¼ pound fresh shrimp, shelled, deveined, and minced
1/16 teaspoon ground nutmeg

1. In saucepan, combine first 5 ingredients. Turn heat to high and bring to a boil. Reduce heat to medium-low and cook 20 minutes, or until carrots are fork tender.
2. While carrots are cooking, in skillet, heat margarine over medium-low heat. Add leek and shrimp and sauté 5 minutes, or until shrimp are pink all over, stirring often.
3. Combine shrimp mixture with carrots. Add nutmeg. Stir to blend. Cook 5 minutes more, stirring often.

Per serving: 106.2 calories; 43.9 mg. sodium; 20.0 gm. carbohydrates; 1.8 gm. fat.

* Preserved in non-sodium ingredient.

Green Beans and Corn

SERVES 8

Shrimp Salad Mazatlan (page 106) and Chicken Salad Cozumel (page 104) are two refreshing options to accompany this tasty, tangy treat.

1½ cups Basic Salsa (page 210)
1/16 teaspoon ground nutmeg
6 dried apricots, chopped
1 teaspoon dry sherry

1½ pounds green beans, steamed* al dente
2 cans (16 ounces) low-sodium corn niblets, including liquid

In saucepan, combine all ingredients. Turn heat to medium and bring to a slow boil. Reduce heat to medium-low and cook 5 minutes, stirring occasionally.

Per serving: 86.5 calories; 12.1 mg. sodium; 20.4 gm. carbohydrates; 0.7 gm. fat.

* Do not add salt to water.

Sherried Carrots in Rum Cream   SERVES 8

Any main course will taste better when accompanied by this delectable and distinctly Mexican dish.

6 carrots, sliced and parboiled*
¼ cup dry sherry
1 cup boiling water
2 teaspoons low-sodium chicken
    bouillon

¼ cup lime juice
1 tablespoon rum
¼ cup heavy cream
1/16 teaspoon clove powder

1. In saucepan, combine first 5 ingredients. Turn heat to medium and bring to a slow boil. Continue boiling 5 minutes.
2. Reduce heat to low. Stir in remaining ingredients. Cook 5 minutes more.

Per serving: 73.6 calories; 36.2 mg. sodium; 8.9 gm. carbohydrates; 3.1 gm. fat.

* Do not add salt to water.

Green Beans, Mushrooms, and Sweet Peppers   SERVES 8

Baked Lamb in Drunken Sauce (page 156) is a terrific main course with this superbly tasty dish.

1 tablespoon unsalted margarine
12 mushrooms, sliced
4 halves low-sodium sweet peppers,
    chopped
1/16 teaspoon cayenne pepper
¾ teaspoon low-sodium chicken
    bouillon

1½ pounds green beans, steamed*
    al dente
½ cup sour cream
4 ounces low-sodium Cheddar
    cheese, grated

1. In skillet, heat margarine over low heat. Add mushrooms and sauté 2 minutes, stirring often.
2. Stir in remaining ingredients. Raise heat to medium-low. Cook 10 minutes more, stirring often.

Per serving: 174.0 calories; 29.7 mg. sodium; 11.9 gm. carbohydrates; 12.1 gm. fat.

* Do not add salt to water.

Creamed Cauliflower and Sweet Peppers

SERVES 8

Whether you serve this dish with meat, fish, or poultry, the inventive blend of flavors and textures is sure to meet with your approval.

1 head cauliflower, chopped
3 cups boiling water
2 tablespoons low-sodium beef
   bouillon
½ teaspoon dried parsley

⅟₁₆ teaspoon cayenne pepper
⅟₁₆ teaspoon ground nutmeg
2 halves low-sodium sweet peppers,
   sliced
⅓ cup heavy cream

1. In saucepan, combine first 2 ingredients. Cook 5 minutes, or until cauliflower is tender crisp. Drain, reserving half the liquid.
2. In blender, combine ⅓ cup cauliflower and ½ cup reserved liquid. Puree.
3. Return puree to saucepan. Add remaining cauliflower, remaining reserved liquid, bouillon, parsley, cayenne pepper, nutmeg, and sweet peppers. Turn heat to medium-low and cook 10 minutes, stirring occasionally.
4. Stir in cream and cook 5 minutes more, stirring often.

Per serving: 66.5 calories: 22.5 mg. sodium; 5.8 gm. carbohydrates; 4.5 gm. fat.

Creamed Chile Corn

SERVES 4

A fabulous, spicy way to enjoy corn. Flounder in Green Garlic Sauce (page 110) sets off this dish.

2 cans (16 ounces) low-sodium corn,
   niblets, including liquid
2 green chiles, seeded and minced
⅟₁₆ teaspoon ground cinnamon
1 teaspoon low-sodium chicken
   bouillon

1 tablespoon dry sherry
1 teaspoon dried parsley
¼ cup heavy cream

1. In saucepan, combine all ingredients, except cream. Stir to blend. Turn heat to medium-low. Cook 10 minutes, stirring often.
2. Stir in cream. Cook 5 minutes more, stirring often.

Per serving: 126.2 calories; 10.0 mg. sodium; 17.4 gm. carbohydrates; 6.2 gm. fat.

Creamed Corn, Eggplant, and Chicken

SERVES 8

Sweet yet spicy, as only Mexican food can be. This dish makes a lovely light lunch when accompanied by Mixed Salad San Miguel (page 101). For a slightly different taste experience, omit the eggplant and add one head of broccoli, chopped, to Step 3.

1 tablespoon olive oil
2 leeks, chopped, including greens
1 clove garlic, minced
1 teaspoon paprika
1 cup cooked chicken, diced
1 eggplant, peeled and diced
2 cans (16 ounces) low-sodium
   creamed corn

Dash of clover powder
½ teaspoon dried basil
1 teaspoon low-sodium chicken
   bouillon
1 teaspoon dry sherry
3 tablespoons heavy cream

1. In skillet, heat oil over low heat. Add leeks and garlic and cook 5 minutes, stirring often.
2. Stir in paprika and chicken, blending thoroughly. Add eggplant. Cover and simmer 20 minutes.
3. Stir in remaining ingredients, blending thoroughly. Cover and cook 20 minutes more, stirring occasionally.

Per serving with eggplant: 136.3 calories; 14.9 mg. sodium; 18.5 gm. carbohydrates; 5.6 gm. fat.
Per serving with broccoli: 140.3 calories; 22.4 mg. sodium; 18.7 gm. carbohydrates; 5.7 gm. fat.

Peas and Almonds

SERVES 8

The sophisticated touch of French culinary artistry is the influencing factor here. Red and Green Chicken with Cheese (page 147) and Rice with Oysters (page 187) are equally elegant and flavorful companions.

⅓ cup unsalted slivered almonds
1 tablespoon unsalted margarine
1 pound peas, steamed* al dente

½ teaspoon sugar
Dash of ground nutmeg

1. Preheat oven to 350°.
2. On baking sheet, place almonds. Toast 5 minutes. Set aside.
3. In saucepan, heat margarine over low heat. Add peas, sugar, and nutmeg. Stir to blend. Cook 5 minutes, stirring often.
4. Stir in almonds.

Per serving: 97.6 calories; 1.6 mg. sodium; 9.7 gm. carbohydrates; 4.9 gm. fat.

* Do not add salt to water.

Peas in Cream Cheese Sauce

SERVES 4

As deliciously Mexican as you could possibly want. For variety, steam three cups of broccoli flowerettes or ½ pound of green beans instead of the peas. Serve any of these options with Jicama and Chorizo Salad (page 105) and Rice with Chicken (page 187) for a truly sensational meal.

½ pound peas, steamed* al dente
½ cup Cream Cheese Sauce
   (page 222)

1 orange, peeled and sectioned

In bowl, combine all ingredients, blending thoroughly.

Per serving with peas: 140.5 calories; 12.6 mg. sodium; 18.7 gm. carbohydrates;
   5.8 gm. fat.
Per serving with broccoli: 110.8 calories; 12.3 mg. sodium; 13.9 gm. carbohydrates;
   5.7 gm. fat.
Per serving with green beans: 110.8 calories; 15.4 mg. sodium; 14.6 gm. carbohydrates;
   5.7 gm. fat.

* Do not add salt to water.

Spinach in
Almond-Cream Sauce
SERVES 4

Absolutely lip-smacking. Chicken with Figs and Lemons (page 141) and Potatoes with Chiles (page 180) provide an unforgettable taste combination.

1½ tablespoons unsalted margarine	Black pepper to taste
1 onion, minced	1 pound spinach, chopped
2 tablespoons unsalted, slivered	¼ cup water
almonds	¼ cup sour cream
1⁄16 teaspoon ground nutmeg	1 teaspoon low-sodium beef bouillon

1. In saucepan, heat margarine over medium-low heat. Add onion and almonds. Season with nutmeg and pepper. Cook 10 minutes, or until onion is lightly browned, stirring often.
2. Stir in spinach. Add water. Cover and cook 5 minutes.
3. Stir in sour cream and bouillon. Cover and cook 5 minutes more, stirring occasionally.

Per serving: 160.7 calories; 92.0 mg. sodium; 11.7 gm. carbohydrates; 12.8 gm. fat.

Zucchini in Cheese Sauce
SERVES 4

The prickly combination of chili powder and Swiss cheese works wonders with zucchini. The sweet cream is a bonus. This dish is especially wonderful with swordfish and flounder.

2 zucchini, halved lengthwise	½ teaspoon Chili Powder (page 210)
⅔ cup boiling water	1 teaspoon dried basil
1 teaspoon low-sodium beef bouillon	2 ounces low-sodium Swiss cheese
⅓ cup heavy cream	

1. Preheat oven to 350°.
2. In 9-inch-square ovenproof casserole, place zucchini, cut side down.
3. Add remaining ingredients. Cover and bake 20 minutes, or until zucchini are fork tender.

Per serving: 149.1 calories; 20.2 mg. sodium; 6.4 gm. carbohydrates; 11.7 gm. fat.

Zucchini, Tomatoes, and Corn Casserole

SERVES 8

Not only colorful, but bursting with flavor. Almond-Sherry Chicken (page 132) and boiled white rice go beautifully with this dish.

1 tablespoon unsalted margarine
1 onion, minced
2 cloves garlic, minced
¼ cup low-sodium bread crumbs
1 teaspoon low-sodium chicken bouillon
1 teaspoon dried basil
2 red chiles, seeded and minced
3 zucchini, cut in 1-inch rounds

3 tomatoes, cut in wedges
2 cans (16 ounces) low-sodium corn niblets, including liquid
½ cup water
1/16 teaspoon cayenne pepper
1 teaspoon paprika
⅛ teaspoon ground cinnamon
1 tablespoon vegetable oil

1. Preheat oven to 350°.
2. In skillet, heat margarine over low heat. Add onion, garlic, and bread crumbs and cook 5 minutes, stirring often.
3. Stir in bouillon, basil, and chiles. Set aside.
4. In 9 x 13-inch ovenproof casserole, place zucchini, cut side down.
5. Layer tomato wedges on top.
6. Pour corn, including liquid, over all.
7. Add water, cayenne pepper, paprika, cinnamon, and oil. Then add onion mixture. Cover and bake ½ hour.

Per serving: 117.4 calories; 9.6 mg. sodium; 20.5 gm. carbohydrates; 4.2 gm. fat.

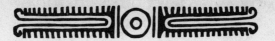

Sauces

Every Mexican meal features at least one sauce, Basic Salsa (page 210), which is used as a seasoning as well as a condiment. But the real truth is that every dish at every meal is either prepared or served with one or more of the excellent sauces that highlight the cuisine.

This penchant for sauces dates back to the pre-Columbian era, and the variety is endless, ranging from mild, like Onion Sauce (page 219), to sweet, such as Cream Cheese Sauce (page 222), to pungent, like Hot-and-Sweet Dressing (page 228), to the very spicy, like Tomato Sauce with Cayenne (page 212).

Sauces are spooned over everything: tortillas, eggs, fish, poultry, meat, beans, and vegetables. They are even added to soups.

However and whenever you use them, Mexican sauces are sure to tantalize your tongue and enhance any dish they touch.

Chili Powder

MAKES ⅝ CUP

A traditional blend of ground spices, chief among which are dried chiles. For a lively change of pace, use a little Chili Powder where you might normally use black pepper.

20 dried chiles
3 tablespoons paprika
2½ teaspoons ground cumin

¾ teaspoon garlic powder
2½ teaspoons dried oregano
¼ teaspoon cayenne pepper

1. In blender, combine all ingredients. Grind to a fine powder. Transfer to jar.
2. Will keep indefinitely if stored in tightly closed jar in cool, dry place.

Per recipe: 612.0 calories; 710.0 mg. sodium; 114.0 gm. carbohydrates; 18.0 gm. fat.
Per tablespoon: 61.2 calories; 71.0 mg. sodium; 11.4 gm. carbohydrates; 1.8 gm. fat.

Basic Salsa

MAKES 3 CUPS

Salsa is a staple in Mexican homes, served with every meal and used on every conceivable kind of dish. It is the one condiment no home is ever without. After tasting it, you will know why. For a milder version, see Basil-Tomato Sauce (page 212).

4 tomatoes, chopped and pureed
1 onion, minced
2 serrano chiles, seeded and minced
   (or ⅛ teaspoon hot pepper flakes)
1 bay leaf

½ teaspoon sugar
2 teaspoons low-sodium beef
   bouillon
2 tablespoons dried parsley
¾ cup water

1. In saucepan, combine all ingredients. Turn heat to low. Cover and simmer ½ hour, stirring occasionally.
2. Transfer mixture to blender. Puree.
3. Return mixture to saucepan and simmer, uncovered, ½ hour more.
4. May be refrigerated up to 3 weeks in tightly closed jars, or frozen indefinitely in plastic containers.

Per recipe: 237.5 calories; 61.3 mg. sodium; 58.2 gm. carbohydrates; 3.6 gm. fat.
Per cup: 79.2 calories; 20.4 mg. sodium; 19.4 gm. carbohydrates; 1.2 gm. fat.
Per tablespoon: 4.9 calories; 1.3 mg. sodium; 1.2 gm. carbohydrates; 0.07 gm. fat.

Sweet Tomato Sauce   MAKES 5 CUPS

Every Mexican cook has several tomato sauce recipes in his or her repertoire, not because they are used differently, but just for variety. The sauce
below is one you will want to call your own. The sweet spices it contains
make it especially appealing for pork, veal, and poultry.

1 tablespoon salad oil	¼ teaspoon ground cinnamon
1 onion, chopped	⅛ teaspoon clove powder
2 cloves garlic, minced	¹⁄₁₆ teaspoon ground nutmeg
8 tomatoes, chopped	
Cayenne pepper to taste	
1 can (8 ounces) low-sodium tomato sauce	

1. In skillet, heat oil over low heat. Add onion and garlic. Cook 5 minutes, stirring often.
2. Add tomatoes and cayenne pepper. Cook 10 minutes more, stirring
   often.
3. Transfer tomato mixture to blender. Puree.
4. Return tomato mixture to skillet. Stir in remaining ingredients. Cook
   10 minutes more, or until mixture bubbles around the edges.
5. May be refrigerated in tightly closed jars up to 3 weeks, or frozen in
   plastic containers indefinitely.

Per recipe: 529.3 calories; 62.3 mg. sodium; 98.2 gm. carbohydrates; 17.9 gm. fat.
Per cup: 105.9 calories; 12.5 mg. sodium; 19.6 gm. carbohydrates; 3.6 gm. fat.
Per tablespoon: 6.6 calories; 0.8 mg. sodium; 1.2 gm. carbohydrates; 0.2 gm. fat.

Basil-Tomato Sauce

MAKES 5 CUPS

Very similar to an Italian tomato sauce, this delicious blend is a flavorful and milder alternative to Basic Salsa (page 210).

2 teaspoons olive oil, divided
2 cloves garlic, minced
2 onions, chopped
1 bay leaf
4 tomatoes, chopped
Black pepper to taste

1 can (29 ounces) low-sodium
   tomato puree
1 tablespoon dry sherry
1½ tablespoons dried basil
2 teaspoons low-sodium beef
   bouillon

1. In skillet, heat 1 teaspoon oil over low heat. Add garlic and cook 1 minute, stirring often.
2. Add remaining oil and onions. Cover and cook 5 minutes more, or until onions are golden. Transfer mixture to saucepan.
3. Add remaining ingredients. Cover and simmer ½ hour, stirring occasionally. Uncover and cook 15 minutes more.
4. May be refrigerated in tightly closed jars up to 2 weeks, or frozen in plastic containers indefinitely.

Per recipe: 687.3 calories; 113.2 mg. sodium; 149.3 gm. carbohydrates; 15.2 gm. fat.
Per cup: 137.5 calories; 22.6 mg. sodium; 29.8 gm. carbohydrates; 3.0 gm. fat.
Per tablespoon: 8.6 calories; 1.4 mg. sodium; 1.9 gm. carbohydrates; 0.2 gm. fat.

Tomato Sauce
with Cayenne

MAKES 2½ CUPS

When you feel like having a tomato sauce with a little "oomph," try this one. Superb for beef or poultry, and surprisingly good with fish.

1 pound tomatoes
1 teaspoon vegetable oil
1 onion, minced
1 teaspoon low-sodium chicken
   bouillon

1 green chile, seeded and minced
1 teaspoon dried parsley
1/16 teaspoon cayenne pepper
½ teaspoon paprika

1. In blender, puree tomatoes. Set aside.
2. In skillet, heat oil over low heat. Add onion and cook 5 minutes, or until onion is lightly browned, stirring occasionally.

3. Add tomato puree and cook 2 minutes, stirring frequently.
4. Add remaining ingredients, stirring to blend. Cover and simmer 20 minutes.
5. May be refrigerated in tightly closed jars up to 3 weeks, or frozen in plastic containers indefinitely.

Per recipe: 211.4 calories; 35.8 mg. sodium; 45.1 gm. carbohydrates; 9.6 gm. fat.
Per cup: 84.6 calories; 14.3 mg. sodium; 18.0 gm. carbohydrates; 3.8 gm. fat.
Per tablespoon: 5.3 calories; 0.9 mg. sodium; 1.1 gm. carbohydrates; 1.2 gm. fat.

Chile-Tomato Sauce

MAKES 2½ CUPS

A very snappy tomato sauce, indeed. Wonderful to perk up leftovers or to enhance main dishes, such as Chicken Ancho (page 133).

4 tomatoes, chopped
3 serrano chiles (or 1 large pepper), seeded and toasted
2 cloves garlic, chopped
1 small onion, chopped
1 tablespoon vegetable oil
½ teaspoon sugar

½ teaspoon ground cumin
1 can (6 ounces) low-sodium tomato paste
1 teaspoon white vinegar
1 cup water
1 tablespoon dried parsley

1. In blender, combine first 4 ingredients. Grind to a coarse paste. Transfer to saucepan.
2. Stir in oil, sugar, and cumin. Turn heat to medium-low and cook 5 minutes, stirring occasionally.
3. Stir in remaining ingredients, except parsley. Reduce heat to low. Cover and simmer ½ hour, or until mixture bubbles around the edges, stirring occasionally.
4. Stir in parsley. Cover and simmer 5 minutes more.
5. May be refrigerated in tightly closed jars up to 3 weeks, or frozen in plastic containers indefinitely.

With chiles:
Per recipe: 397.2 calories; 54.9 mg. sodium; 66.6 gm. carbohydrates; 16.6 gm. fat.
Per cup: 158.9 calories; 22.0 mg. sodium; 26.6 gm. carbohydrates; 6.6 gm. fat.
Per tablespoon: 9.9 calories; 1.4 mg. sodium; 1.7 gm. carbohydrates; 0.4 gm. fat.

With red pepper:
Per recipe: 487.6 calories; 129.8 mg. sodium; 87.0 gm. carbohydrates; 17.5 gm. fat.
Per cup: 195.0 calories; 51.9 mg. sodium; 34.8 gm. carbohydrates; 7.0 gm. fat.
Per tablespoon: 12.2 calories; 3.2 mg. sodium; 2.2 gm. carbohydrates; 0.4 gm. fat.

Chile-Vegetable Sauce

MAKES 4 CUPS

This sauce makes a wonderful cold dip for tacos, crudités, cold meat, fish, or poultry. For variety, try it as a basting sauce when broiling or barbecuing.

6 green chiles, seeded and minced
1 cucumber, peeled, seeded, and
  diced
1 green pepper, diced
6 tomatoes, chopped

1 onion, grated
1/16 teaspoon clove powder
1/8 teaspoon garlic powder
1 teaspoon dried oregano
1 tablespoon lime juice

1. In blender, combine first 4 ingredients. Blend briefly. Transfer to bowl.
2. Stir in remaining ingredients. Cover and chill at least 2 hours before serving to allow flavors to blend.
3. May be refrigerated in tightly closed jars up to 1 week. If you wish to freeze, prepare initially without cucumber. Sauce may then be frozen indefinitely in plastic containers. Before serving, stir in cucumber.

Per recipe: 421.0 calories; 132.0 mg. sodium; 86.6 gm. carbohydrates; 2.8 gm. fat.
Per cup: 105.3 calories; 33.0 mg. sodium; 21.7 gm. carbohydrates; 0.7 gm. fat.
Per tablespoon: 6.6 calories; 2.1 mg. sodium; 1.4 gm. carbohydrates; 0.04 gm. fat.

Chile-Avocado Sauce

MAKES 2½ CUPS

If there are a thousand ways to enjoy the sweet, nutty flavor of the avocado, Mexican cooks will know them all. This sauce is one beautiful example. Serve it as a dip or use it to perk up leftover fish or poultry; any way at all, it will delight.

1 onion, minced
½ green pepper, minced
1 red chile, seeded and minced
2 large, ripe avocados, peeled, pitted,
  and cut in chunks

3 tablespoons low-sodium chili
  ketchup
1/16 teaspoon cayenne pepper
1/16 teaspoon ground nutmeg
2½ teaspoons dried parsley

1. In blender, combine first 3 ingredients. Grind to a coarse blend.
2. Add avocados and puree. Transfer mixture to bowl.

3. Stir in ketchup, cayenne pepper, and nutmeg, blending thoroughly.
4. Stir in parsley. Cover and refrigerate at least 1 hour to allow flavors to blend.
5. May be refrigerated in tightly closed jars up to 3 weeks, or frozen in plastic containers indefinitely.

Per recipe: 1,249.0 calories; 73.6 mg. sodium; 71.6 gm. carbohydrates; 112.9 gm. fat.
Per cup: 499.6 calories; 29.4 mg. sodium; 28.7 gm. carbohydrates; 45.2 gm. fat.
Per tablespoon: 31.2 calories; 1.8 mg. sodium; 1.8 gm. carbohydrates; 2.8 gm. fat.

Sweet-and-Hot Chile Sauce   MAKES 2 CUPS

Be careful. Once you taste the sweet, hot blend of this richly seasoned sauce, you might not be able to stop until it is gone. Fabulous on meat, fish, or poultry, it is sure to become a standard item in your kitchen.

4 green chiles, seeded and chopped	1/16 teaspoon ground nutmeg
1 onion, minced	Dash of allspice
1 1/2 cups Meat Stock (page 78)	1/2 tablespoon vegetable oil
1/8 teaspoon ground cinnamon	1/4 cup dark raisins*

1. In saucepan, combine first 6 ingredients. Turn heat to medium-low and cook 15 minutes, stirring occasionally.
2. Add remaining ingredients. Cover and cook 1/2 hour more, stirring occasionally.
3. May be refrigerated in tightly closed jars up to 1 week, or frozen in plastic containers indefinitely.

Per recipe: 442.0 calories; 109.5 mg. sodium; 81.8 gm. carbohydrates; 19.6 gm. fat.
Per cup: 221.1 calories; 54.8 gm. sodium; 40.9 gm. carbohydrates; 9.8 gm. fat.
Per tablespoon: 13.8 calories; 3.4 mg. sodium; 2.6 gm. carbohydrates; 0.6 gm. fat.

* Preserved in non-sodium ingredient.

Green Sauce I

MAKES 1¾ CUPS

Green sauce gets its name from the herbs it contains, the primary and most essential being parsley. Spanish in origin, it has been adapted by Mexican chefs to suit their spicier tastes. Delicious on plain broiled fish or poultry, it is also a special treat on salads.

2 tablespoons olive oil
2 onions, chopped
1 clove garlic, minced
2 dried chiles
1 cup boiling water
2 teaspoons low-sodium chicken
  bouillon

2½ tablespoons dried parsley
1 teaspoon dried basil
⅛ teaspoon dried thyme

1. In skillet, heat oil over medium-low heat. Add onions and garlic and cook 3 minutes, or until onions are lightly browned, stirring often.
2. Add chiles and cook 2 minutes more, stirring often.
3. Add water and bouillon, stirring to blend thoroughly. Cook 5 minutes, stirring occasionally.
4. Stir in remaining ingredients. Reduce heat to low. Simmer 10 minutes, or until mixture bubbles around the edges, stirring occasionally.
5. May be refrigerated in tightly closed jars up to 3 weeks.

Per recipe: 461.6 calories; 121.2 mg. sodium; 60.4 gm. carbohydrates; 34.1 gm. fat.
Per cup: 263.8 calories; 69.3 mg. sodium; 34.5 gm. carbohydrates; 19.5 gm. fat.
Per tablespoon: 16.5 calories; 4.3 mg. sodium; 2.2 gm. carbohydrates; 1.2 gm. fat.

Green Sauce II

MAKES 2 CUPS

An absolutely scrumptious topping for fish or chilled vegetables. For something unusual and terrific, mix this dressing with pasta and fresh-cooked shrimp. Absolutely superb.

1¾ cups Green Sauce I (page 216) divided
½ cup low-sodium mayonnaise

1 cucumber, seeded and chopped

1. In blender, combine ½ cup of green sauce with mayonnaise and cucumber. Grind. Transfer to bowl.
2. Stir in remaining sauce, blending thoroughly. Cover and chill at least 1 hour to allow flavors to blend.
3. May be refrigerated in tightly closed jars up to 2 weeks.

Per recipe: 1,371.3 calories; 200.3 mg. sodium; 68.2 gm. carbohydrates; 122.2 gm. fat.
Per cup: 685.7 calories; 100.2 mg. sodium; 34.1 gm. carbohydrates; 61.1 gm. fat.
Per tablespoon: 42.9 calories; 6.3 mg. sodium; 2.1 gm. carbohydrates; 3.8 gm. fat.

Lime Sauce

MAKES ¾ CUP

When you want a sauce that is very Mexican, very easy, and totally wonderful, try this one. Goes with everything.

12 dried chiles
1 onion, minced
Dash of ground cinnamon

1 tablespoon dried parsley
⅔ cup lime juice

1. In blender, combine first 3 ingredients. Grind to blend. Transfer to bowl.
2. Stir in remaining ingredients. Cover and refrigerate at least ½ hour to allow flavors to blend.
3. May be refrigerated in tightly closed containers up to 1 week.

Per recipe: 456.5 calories; 445.8 mg. sodium; 103.2 gm. carbohydrates; 11.3 gm. fat.
Per tablespoon: 38.0 calories; 37.2 mg. sodium; 8.6 gm. carbohydrates; 0.9 gm. fat.

Almond Sauce

MAKES 2½ CUPS

Nuts are very popular in Mexican cuisine for the subtle, rich, meaty flavor they impart to any dish. This sauce is just one example. Use it on meat, fish, poultry, or vegetables when you want to add elegance to the simplest meal. For variety, substitute any nuts you prefer for the almonds.

1 tablespoon olive oil
1 onion, chopped
2 cloves garlic, halved
¼ cup unsalted slivered almonds
1 potato, boiled,* peeled, and
   chopped
1 tomato, chopped

2 cups Chicken Stock (page 76)
   divided
½ teaspoon dried basil
1/16 teaspoon hot pepper flakes
¼ teaspoon sugar

1. In saucepan, heat oil over low heat. Add onion, garlic, and almonds and cook until onion is golden. Transfer mixture to blender. Grind to a coarse paste.
2. To blender, add potato, tomato, and ½ cup stock. Puree. Return mixture to saucepan.
3. Add remaining stock and all remaining ingredients. Over low heat, simmer 20 minutes, or until sauce thickens.
4. May be refrigerated in tightly closed jars up to 1 week, or frozen in plastic containers up to 1 month.

Per recipe: 670.2 calories; 84.4 mg. sodium; 77.8 gm. carbohydrates; 38.2 gm. fat.
Per cup: 268.0 calories; 33.8 mg. sodium; 31.1 gm. carbohydrates; 15.3 gm. fat.
Per tablespoon: 16.8 calories; 2.1 mg. sodium; 1.9 gm. carbohydrates; 1.0 gm. fat.

* Do not add salt to water.

Onion Sauce

MAKES 3 CUPS

Most unusual. Especially good on fish, poultry, peas, carrots, and asparagus.

2 tablespoons olive oil
2 onions, chopped
3 cloves garlic, minced
1 slice low-sodium bread
4 tablespoons cider vinegar
2 cups Chicken Stock (page 76),
   divided

¼ teaspoon dried thyme
1½ tablespoons dried parsley
Black pepper to taste

1. In saucepan, heat oil over low heat. Add onions and garlic and cook 10 minutes, or until onion is golden. Set aside.
2. While onion and garlic are cooking, in bowl, combine bread and vinegar. Let stand 10 minutes.
3. In blender, combine onion mixture, bread, and ½ cup stock. Puree. Transfer mixture to saucepan.
4. Add remaining stock and all remaining ingredients. Turn heat to medium-low and cook 15 minutes, or until mixture thickens, stirring occasionally.

Per recipe: 581.0 calories; 110.8 mg. sodium; 78.8 gm. carbohydrates; 34.5 gm. fat.
Per cup: 193.7 calories; 36.9 mg. sodium; 26.3 gm. carbohydrates; 11.5 gm. fat.
Per tablespoon: 12.1 calories; 2.3 mg. sodium; 1.6 gm. carbohydrates; 0.7 gm. fat.

Drunken Sauce

MAKES 1¾ CUPS

A little tequila packs a powerful punch as this sauce will prove. It is simply wonderful on meat, fish, or poultry.

2 tablespoons peanut oil, divided
6 pasilla chiles (or 10 dried chiles), seeded
1¼ cups orange juice
½ tablespoon lime juice

1 onion, chopped
Cayenne pepper to taste
½ teaspoon sugar
¼ cup tequila

1. In skillet, heat 1 tablespoon oil over low heat. Add chiles and sauté 2 minutes, or until chiles are lightly browned, stirring constantly. Transfer to blender. Add orange and lime juices. Blend. Set aside.
2. In skillet, heat remaining oil over low heat. Add onion. Season with cayenne pepper. Cook 5 minutes, or until onion is golden.
3. Add juice mixture and sugar, stirring to blend thoroughly. Cook 10 minutes, stirring occasionally. Remove from heat. Let stand ½ hour.
4. Stir in tequila immediately before serving.

With fresh chiles:
  Per recipe: 617.7 calories; 36.6 mg. sodium; 62.7 gm. carbohydrates; 30.6 gm. fat.
  Per cup: 353.0 calories; 20.9 mg. sodium; 35.8 gm. carbohydrates; 17.5 gm. fat.
  Per tablespoon: 22.1 calories; 1.3 mg. sodium; 2.2 gm. carbohydrates; 1.1 gm. fat.

With dried chiles:
  Per recipe: 891.9 calories; 370.0 mg. sodium; 111.9 gm. carbohydrates; 39.4 gm. fat.
  Per cup: 509.7 calories; 211.4 mg. sodium; 63.9 gm. carbohydrates; 22.5 gm. fat.
  Per tablespoon: 31.9 calories; 13.2 mg. sodium; 36.5 gm. carbohydrates; 1.4 gm. fat.

Creamy Wine Sauce

MAKES 2 CUPS

Hot or cold, this sauce lends an elegant air to any dish. Veal Loaf (page 167), Honey Fish (page 113), and Broccoli and Mushrooms with Pork (page 200) are just a few examples.

1 teaspoon peanut (or vegetable) oil
2 dried chiles, crushed
1 onion, chopped
1 clove garlic, minced
⅓ cup olive oil
1 cup hot water

1 teaspoon low-sodium beef bouillon
1 teaspoon dried oregano
⅓ cup dry red wine
¼ cup heavy cream

1. In skillet, heat peanut oil over low heat. Add chiles and sauté 1 minute, stirring constantly.
2. Add onion and garlic and cook 3 minutes more, or until onion and garlic are slightly browned, stirring occasionally.
3. While onion mixture is cooking, in bowl, combine olive oil and water, stirring to blend thoroughly.
4. Stir in bouillon. Then add oregano and wine.
5. Add onion mixture.
6. Stir in cream, blending thoroughly.

Per recipe: 1,112.4 calories; 115.8 mg. sodium; 40.5 gm. carbohydrates; 108.2 gm. fat.
Per cup: 556.2 calories; 57.9 mg. sodium; 20.3 gm. carbohydrates; 54.1 gm. fat.
Per tablespoon: 34.8 calories; 3.6 mg. sodium; 1.3 gm. carbohydrates; 3.4 gm. fat.

Cream Cheese Sauce

MAKES 1⅔ CUPS

Talk about spine-tingling good, and you have described this sauce. Richly flavored but modest in calories, it will dress up any dish from the simplest salad to the most elegant roast or extravagant seafood combination. This is a "must try." But we warn you, it is definitely addictive.

1 red pepper
2 dried chiles
1 onion, diced
3 cloves garlic, minced
¼ teaspoon sugar
¼ cup olive oil
⅓ cup boiling water

½ cup red wine vinegar
Black pepper to taste
½ teaspoon dried oregano
2 tablespoons low-sodium cream
    cheese, diced

1. On broiler pan, place red pepper. Toast 6 inches from heat, turning constantly to prevent burning. Transfer to platter. Let cool. Seed and dice. Transfer to bowl.
2. Stir in dried chiles, onion, and garlic. Set aside.
3. In second bowl, combine oil and water, stirring to blend.
4. Stir in sugar, blending to dissolve.
5. Stir in vinegar, black pepper, and oregano.
6. Stir in onion-chile mixture. Let stand 1 hour to allow flavors to blend.
7. Add cream cheese immediately before serving.
8. May be refrigerated, without cream cheese, in tightly closed jars up to 2 weeks, or frozen in plastic containers up to 1 month.

Per recipe: 908.6 calories; 145.7 mg. sodium; 58.7 gm. carbohydrates; 72.6 gm. fat.
Per cup: 544.1 calories; 87.3 mg. sodium; 35.1 gm. carbohydrates; 43.5 gm. fat.
Per tablespoon: 34.0 calories; 5.5 mg. sodium; 2.2 gm. carbohydrates; 2.7 gm. fat.

Potato Sauce

MAKES 2½ CUPS

This hearty and zesty sauce will add a rich taste to any meat dish.

2 cups Fish Stock (page 77) or
  Meat Stock (page 78)
¹⁄₁₆ teaspoon cayenne pepper
2 potatoes, boiled,* peeled, and
  mashed
1 tablespoon olive oil

1 tablespoon red wine vinegar
1 teaspoon paprika
1 tablespoon low-sodium chicken
  bouillon

1. In saucepan, combine stock and cayenne pepper. Turn heat to medium-low and cook 10 minutes.
2. While stock is cooking, in bowl, combine potatoes, oil, and vinegar, blending thoroughly. Transfer mixture to saucepan.
3. Add paprika and bouillon. Cook 10 minutes more, stirring occasionally.

With fish stock:
  Per recipe: 522.6 calories; 64.3 mg. sodium; 69.1 gm. carbohydrates; 22.3 gm. fat.
  Per cup: 209.0 calories; 25.7 mg. sodium; 27.6 gm. carbohydrates; 8.9 gm. fat.
  Per tablespoon: 13.1 calories; 1.6 mg. sodium; 1.7 gm. carbohydrates; 0.5 gm. fat.

With meat stock:
  Per recipe: 598.4 calories; 115.6 mg. sodium; 72.2 gm. carbohydrates; 33.6 gm. fat.
  Per cup: 239.4 calories; 46.2 mg. sodium; 28.9 gm. carbohydrates; 13.4 gm. fat.
  Per tablespoon: 15.0 calories; 2.9 mg. sodium; 1.8 gm. carbohydrates; 0.8 gm. fat.

* Do not add salt to water.

Piquant Sour Cream Sauce   MAKES 2¼ CUPS

Nothing can beat the flavor of this puckery sauce on roast meats or fish. It has a most enticing taste that everyone will love, and a talent for making leftovers taste special all over again.

8 ancho chiles (or 6 dried chiles), seeded
1 onion, minced
1 clove garlic, minced
⅓ cup olive oil
¾ cup hot water

1 teaspoon low-sodium chicken bouillon
⅓ cup red wine vinegar
3 tablespoons sour cream
½ teaspoon sugar

1. In bowl, combine first 6 ingredients, stirring until bouillon is dissolved.
2. Stir in vinegar, blending thoroughly.
3. Stir in sour cream, blending thoroughly.
4. Stir in sugar, blending thoroughly. Cover and chill at least 2 hours to allow flavors to blend.

With fresh chiles:
    Per recipe: 1,012.0 calories; 35.4 mg. sodium; 41.3 gm. carbohydrates; 93.8 gm. fat.
    Per cup: 451.8 calories; 15.7 mg. sodium; 18.4 gm. carbohydrates; 41.7 gm. fat.
    Per tablespoon: 28.2 calories; 1.0 mg. sodium; 1.1 gm. carbohydrates; 2.6 gm. fat.

With dried chiles:
    Per recipe: 1,153.2 calories; 248.4 mg. sodium; 65.1 gm. carbohydrates; 99.9 gm. fat.
    Per cup: 512.5 calories; 110.4 mg. sodium; 28.9 gm. carbohydrates; 44.4 gm. fat.
    Per tablespoon: 32.0 calories; 6.9 mg. sodium; 1.8 gm. carbohydrates; 2.8 gm. fat.

Sour Cream Dressing

MAKES 1¾ CUPS

Much more festive and full of tasty surprises than its name suggests, this dressing is wonderful on salads and fish or with any chilled leftovers.

1 tablespoon olive oil
2 onions, minced
2 cloves garlic, minced
2 green chiles, seeded and minced
1 cup boiling water
1 tablespoon low-sodium chicken
  bouillon

1 tablespoon low-sodium
  Worcestershire sauce
1 teaspoon low-sodium Dijon
  mustard
½ cup sour cream

1. In skillet, heat oil over low heat. Add onions and garlic and cook until onions are wilted, stirring occasionally.
2. Add chiles and cook 2 minutes more, stirring often.
3. Raise heat to medium. Add water and bouillon, stirring to blend thoroughly.
4. Reduce heat to low. Stir in remaining ingredients. Cover and simmer 10 minutes, or until mixture bubbles around the edges, stirring occasionally.
5. May be refrigerated in tightly closed jars up to 2 weeks.

Per recipe: 742.8 calories; 84.9 mg. sodium; 68.2 gm. carbohydrates; 61.0 gm. fat.
Per cup: 424.5 calories; 48.5 mg. sodium; 39.0 gm. carbohydrates; 34.9 gm. fat.
Per tablespoon: 26.5 calories; 3.0 mg. sodium; 2.4 gm. carbohydrates; 2.2 gm. fat.

Lemon Dressing

MAKES 1⅓ CUPS

Perfect for basting chicken or veal; a surprising delight on pork or beef; an excellent salad dressing; extraordinary with seafood. What more is there to say.

⅓ cup olive oil
¾ cup hot water
1 tablespoon low-sodium beef
  bouillon

½ teaspoon Chili Powder (page 210)
¼ cup lemon juice

1. In bowl, combine all ingredients, blending thoroughly.
2. May be refrigerated in tightly closed jars indefinitely.

Per recipe: 750.8 calories; 42.4 mg. sodium; 12.3 gm. carbohydrates; 79.7 gm. fat.
Per cup: 563.1 calories; 24.2 mg. sodium; 7.0 gm. carbohydrates; 59.7 gm. fat.
Per tablespoon: 35.2 calories; 1.5 mg. sodium; 0.4 gm. carbohydrates; 3.7 gm. fat.

Fruit Juice Dressing

MAKES 1¾ CUPS

A delightfully refreshing and unusual salad dressing, this juicy concoction can be adapted to make a wonderful sauce for meats and poultry. Simply eliminate the vegetable oil and use the sauce for basting during cooking. Try Fruit Juice Chicken Wings (page 44) to see what we mean.

½ cup orange juice
¼ cup pineapple juice
¼ cup low-sodium chili ketchup
¼ cup vegetable oil
¼ cup hot water

1/16 teaspoon cayenne pepper
1/16 teaspoon ground cumin
¼ teaspoon paprika
¼ cup cold water
1 teaspoon mustard powder

1. In bowl, combine first 3 ingredients, blending thoroughly. Set aside.
2. In second bowl, combine oil, hot water, pepper, cumin, and paprika, blending thoroughly. Set aside.
3. In third bowl, combine water and mustard powder, stirring to dissolve mustard. Set aside.
4. Add juice mixture to oil mixture, stirring to blend.

5. Add mustard mixture, stirring to blend. Cover and chill ½ hour to allow flavors to blend. Stir well before serving.
6. May be refrigerated in tightly closed jars up to 3 weeks, or frozen in plastic containers indefinitely.

With oil:
Per recipe: 622.3 calories; 18.8 mg. sodium; 21.1 gm. carbohydrates; 59.5 gm. fat.
Per cup: 355.6 calories; 10.7 mg. sodium; 12.1 gm. carbohydrates; 34.0 gm. fat.
Per tablespoon: 22.2 calories; 0.7 mg. sodium; 0.8 gm. carbohydrates; 2.1 gm. fat.

Without oil:
Per recipe: 118.3 calories; 18.8 mg. sodium; 21.1 gm. carbohydrates; 0.3 gm. fat.
Per cup: 67.6 calories; 10.7 mg. sodium; 12.1 gm. carbohydrates; 0.2 gm. fat.
Per tablespoon: 4.2 calories; 0.7 mg. sodium; 0.8 gm. carbohydrates; 0.01 gm. fat.

Oil and Vinegar Dressing   MAKES 1½ CUPS

Everybody's standby dressing made special by the Dijon mustard and hot pepper flakes. Sometimes the familiar is the best.

⅓ cup olive oil
¾ cup hot water
1 teaspoon low-sodium Dijon
    mustard
1 tablespoon low-sodium chicken
    bouillon

Black pepper to taste
⅓ cup red wine vinegar
Dash of hot pepper flakes (optional)

1. In bowl, combine first 5 ingredients, stirring until mustard and bouillon are thoroughly blended.
2. Add remaining ingredients, stirring to blend.
3. Refrigerate in tightly closed jars at least 1 hour to allow flavors to blend. Stir well before serving.
4. May be refrigerated in tightly closed jars indefinitely.

Per recipe: 792.3 calories; 18.8 mg. sodium; 9.2 gm. carbohydrates; 79.2 gm. fat.
Per cup: 528.2 calories; 12.5 mg. sodium; 6.1 gm. carbohydrates; 52.8 gm. fat.
Per tablespoon: 33.0 calories; 0.8 mg. sodium; 0.4 gm. carbohydrates; 3.3 gm. fat.

Garlic Dressing

MAKES 1½ CUPS

The nutty garlic flavor permeates this Mexican-style vinaigrette. Do not just limit this dressing to salads. It is a fabulous marinade for meat, fish, and poultry as well.

¼ cup olive oil
¾ cup boiling water
½ cup cider vinegar
10 cloves garlic, chopped

2 teaspoons dried oregano
⅛ teaspoon black pepper
1 tablespoon dried parsley

1. In bowl, combine all ingredients. Transfer to jar.
2. Close jar tightly. Shake vigorously to blend.
3. May be refrigerated up to one month.

Per recipe: 625.3 calories; 21.5 mg. sodium; 29.9 gm. carbohydrates; 57.3 gm. fat.
Per cup: 416.9 calories; 8.6 mg. sodium; 12.0 gm. carbohydrates; 38.2 gm. fat.
Per tablespoon: 26.1 calories; 0.5 mg. sodium; 0.7 gm. carbohydrates; 2.4 gm. fat.

Hot-and-Sweet Dressing

MAKES 1½ CUPS

Add a Mexican touch to any meal with this tangy dressing.

⅓ cup olive oil
¾ cup hot water
½ teaspoon sugar
1 teaspoon low-sodium
   Worcestershire sauce

¼ teaspoon Chili Powder (page 210)
1/16 teaspoon ground cinnamon
⅓ cup red wine vinegar
½ teaspoon dried basil

1. In bowl, combine first 3 ingredients, stirring until sugar is dissolved.
2. Add remaining ingredients, stirring to blend thoroughly.
3. May be refrigerated in tightly closed jars indefinitely.

Per recipe: 767.1 calories; 9.9 mg. sodium; 6.6 gm. carbohydrates; 76.4 gm. fat.
Per cup: 511.4 calories; 6.6 mg. sodium; 4.4 gm. carbohydrates; 50.9 gm. fat.
Per tablespoon: 32.0 calories; 0.4 mg. sodium; 0.3 gm. carbohydrates; 3.2 gm. fat.

Honey-Lime Dressing

MAKES 1½ CUPS

A most unusual and delicious accent. For variety, and a different taste sensation, substitute 2 tablespoons low-sodium mayonnaise for the vegetable oil. Another option is to eliminate the oil altogether, and use the sauce to glaze pork, poultry, or vegetables.

⅔ cup boiling water
⅓ cup honey
2 tablespoons vegetable oil
¼ cup lime juice
⅛ teaspoon cayenne pepper

½ teaspoon celery seed*
1 teaspoon dried parsley
Dash of clove powder

1. In saucepan, combine first 3 ingredients. Turn heat to low and cook 10 minutes, or until mixture is completely blended, stirring often.
2. Stir in remaining ingredients and cook 5 minutes more.
3. May be refrigerated in tightly closed jars up to 1 month.

With oil:
   Per recipe: 501.2 calories; 6.5 mg. sodium; 68.2 gm. carbohydrates; 28.7 gm. fat.
   Per cup: 334.1 calories; 4.3 mg. sodium; 45.5 gm. carbohydrates; 19.1 gm. fat.
   Per tablespoon: 20.9 calories; 0.3 mg. sodium; 2.8 gm. carbohydrates; 1.2 gm. fat.

With mayonnaise:
   Per recipe: 448.6 calories; 14.5 mg. sodium; 68.2 gm. carbohydrates; 22.9 gm. fat.
   Per cup: 299.0 calories; 9.7 mg. sodium; 45.5 gm. carbohydrates; 15.3 gm. fat.
   Per tablespoon: 18.7 calories; 0.6 mg. sodium; 2.8 gm. carbohydrates; 1.0 gm. fat.

Without oil:
   Per recipe: 248.6 calories; 6.5 mg. sodium; 68.2 gm. carbohydrates; 0.1 gm. fat.
   Per cup: 165.7 calories; 4.3 mg. sodium; 45.5 gm. carbohydrates; 0.07 gm. fat.
   Per tablespoon: 10.4 calories; 0.3 mg. sodium; 2.8 gm. carbohydrates; trace of fat.

* Do not use celery flakes, which contain salt.

Sweet Dressing

MAKES 1¼ CUPS

Only a Mexican cook would be able to imagine the delicious result of the assorted ingredients below. And delicious it is on vegetables, salads, potatoes, fish, and anything else you please.

¾ cup red wine vinegar
⅛ teaspoon cayenne pepper
⅛ teaspoon ground cinnamon
2 teaspoons sugar

¼ cup low-sodium mayonnaise
¼ cup sour cream
1 tablespoon dried parsley

1. In blender, combine all ingredients. Whip briefly. Transfer mixture to jar. Cover tightly and chill at least 2 hours to allow flavors to blend.
2. May be refrigerated in tightly closed jar up to 2 weeks.

Per recipe: 668.1 calories; 42.4 mg. sodium; 22.5 gm. carbohydrates; 65.5 gm. fat.
Per cup: 534.5 calories; 33.9 mg. sodium; 18.0 gm. carbohydrates; 52.4 gm. fat.
Per tablespoon: 33.4 calories; 2.1 mg. sodium; 1.1 gm. carbohydrates; 3.3 gm. fat.

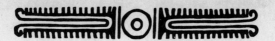

Eggs

Mexican breakfasts are prodigious affairs by American standards, consisting of fruit, tortillas, refried beans, and, of course, eggs. Huevos Rancheros (page 237) is perhaps the most famous and, like most Mexican egg dishes, makes a most filling and satisfying lunch when accompanied by soup, bread, salad, or a vegetable.

For those of you who prefer to or have to restrict egg consumption to two or three per week, beware. Once you taste Eggs and Chorizo (page 232), Scrambled Eggs Mexicana (page 238), and Spiced Eggs, Peppers, and Cheese (page 241), you will want to enjoy the sweet goodness of eggs in the Mexican fashion every single day.

Egg and Chicken Liver Casserole   SERVES 8

This is an adaptation of a national Mexican dish served as part of every wedding feast. It also makes a delicious brunch, lunch, or easy dinner. Wonderful topped with Chile-Vegetable Sauce (page 214) and served with Avocado, Tomato, and Cheese Salad (page 98) on the side.

3 cups water	Black pepper to taste
¼ pound chicken livers	⅟₁₆ teaspoon clove powder
1 teaspoon vegetable oil	½ teaspoon dried basil
1 onion, chopped	2 tomatoes, chopped
1 clove garlic, minced	1 cup Meat Stock (page 78)
⅛ teaspoon ground cumin	8 eggs, lightly beaten

1. In saucepan, combine first 2 ingredients. Turn heat to high and bring to a boil. Reduce heat to medium-low and cook ½ hour. Drain livers and chop fine. Set aside.
2. In skillet, heat oil over low heat. Add onion and garlic and cook 3 minutes, or until onion is golden, stirring often.
3. Stir in cumin, pepper, clove powder, basil, and tomatoes, blending thoroughly.
4. Add stock and continue cooking 20 minutes, stirring occasionally.
5. Slowly pour eggs around edges of skillet. Continue cooking until eggs are set.

Per serving: 128.6 calories; 73.4 mg. sodium; 6.3 gm. carbohydrates; 6.5 gm. fat.

Eggs and Chorizo   SERVES 4

This Mexican version of eggs and sausage is absolutely sensational.

1 tablespoon unsalted margarine, divided	4 eggs, lightly beaten
4 ounces Chorizo (page 158)	1 teaspoon cider vinegar
1 red chile, seeded and minced	1 teaspoon paprika
	½ cup Basil-Tomato Sauce (page 212)

1. In skillet, heat ½ teaspoon margarine over medium-low heat. Add chorizo and cook 2 minutes, or until chorizo is browned all over, stirring often.

2. Add remaining margarine. Add chile, eggs, vinegar, and paprika, stirring to blend. Cook 5 minutes, or until eggs are set.
3. Pour tomato sauce over all and cook 5 minutes more.

Per serving: 221.7 calories; 99.6 mg. sodium; 9.2 gm. carbohydrates; 12.1 gm. fat.

Eggs and Shrimp with Yogurt Sauce

SERVES 4

A mixed green salad or a juicy sliced tomato is just right for this heavenly blend of flavors. When you want to delight the senses, serve this dish accompanied by Tortillas (pages 48, 49).

½ pint plain yogurt
2 green chiles, seeded and minced
1 avocado, peeled, pitted, and diced
Dash of clove powder
⅟₁₆ teaspoon ground cinnamon
1 tablespoon unsalted margarine, divided
¼ pound fresh shrimp, shelled, deveined, and halved diagonally

2 tablespoons low-sodium seasoned bread crumbs
½ teaspoon dried parsley
3 eggs, lightly beaten
Cayenne pepper to taste
1½ teaspoons low-sodium chicken bouillon

1. In bowl, combine first 5 ingredients, stirring to blend thoroughly. Cover and chill ½ hour to allow flavors to blend.
2. In skillet, heat 1 teaspoon margarine over medium-low heat. Add shrimp, bread crumbs, and parsley. Sauté 2 minutes, or until shrimp are pink all over, stirring often.
3. While shrimp are cooking, in bowl, beat together eggs, cayenne pepper, and bouillon.
4. In skillet, heat remaining 2 teaspoons margarine. Add egg mixture and cook 3 minutes, or until eggs are set, stirring occasionally.
5. Divide egg mixture among 4 plates. Top each portion with 1 tablespoon of yogurt sauce. Serve remaining yogurt sauce on the side.

Per serving: 314.0 calories; 95.3 mg. sodium; 14.2 gm. carbohydrates; 22.8 gm. fat.

Eggs in a Nest
SERVES 8

That eggs are far more than breakfast fare is sublimely evident here. Serve with Asparagus in Crumb Sauce (page 196) for that final elegant touch.

2½ tablespoons unsalted margarine, divided
1 can (7½ ounces) low-sodium salmon, including liquid
2 onions, minced
1 teaspoon low-sodium chicken bouillon

1/16 teaspoon ground cumin
Black pepper to taste
1 large tomato, sliced thick
6 eggs, lightly beaten
2 teaspoons dried parsley

1. In skillet, heat 1 tablespoon margarine over medium-low heat. Add salmon and onions and cook 5 minutes, or until onions are golden, stirring often.
2. Season mixture with bouillon, cumin, and pepper, stirring to blend thoroughly. Push mixture to sides of skillet.
3. In well created in center, heat ½ tablespoon margarine. Add tomatoes and cook 2 minutes more.
4. Turn tomatoes. Add remaining tablespoon margarine. Pour eggs over tomatoes and cook 5 minutes, or until eggs are set.
5. Garnish with parsley.

Per serving: 151.0 calories; 65.8 mg. sodium; 7.3 gm. carbohydrates; 8.7 gm. fat.

Eggs, Potatoes, and Onion
SERVES 8

German in origin, this hearty meal is distinctly Mexican in flavor.

2 tablespoons unsalted margarine, divided
1 large onion, chopped
2 potatoes, parboiled,* peeled, and sliced
2 green chiles, seeded and minced
6 eggs, lightly beaten

½ teaspoon Chili Powder (page 210)
½ teaspoon low-sodium beef bouillon
¼ cup water
¼ cup heavy cream
1 teaspoon dried parsley

1. In skillet, heat 1 tablespoon margarine over low heat. Add onion and potatoes and cook 10 minutes, or until potatoes are lightly browned, stirring occasionally.

2. Add chiles and cook 1 minute more.
3. While onion mixture is cooking, in bowl, beat together remaining ingredients except parsley. Add to skillet and cook 10 minutes more, or until eggs are set.
4. Sprinkle parsley over all.

Per serving: 176.5 calories; 52.6 mg. sodium; 12.6 gm. carbohydrates; 11.7 gm. fat.

* Do not add salt to water.

Eggs, Sweet Pepper, and Cheddar Cheese

SERVES 4

A wonderful start to any day, especially with Comb Bread (page 67) as an accompaniment.

1 tablespoon unsalted margarine, divided
1 onion, minced
1 serrano chile (or 1 green pepper), seeded and julienned
4 eggs
Black pepper to taste
¼ teaspoon ground cumin

1 teaspoon low-sodium chicken bouillon
4 halves low-sodium sweet peppers
4 thin slices (½ ounce each) low-sodium Cheddar cheese
1 teaspoon paprika

1. In skillet, heat 1 teaspoon margarine over low heat. Add onion and chile and cook 5 minutes, or until onion is golden, stirring occasionally.
2. Heat remaining 2 teaspoons margarine. Add eggs. Season with black pepper, cumin, and bouillon. Cook 5 minutes, or until eggs are almost set.
3. Top eggs first with sweet pepper halves, then with cheese. Sprinkle paprika over all and cook 5 minutes more.

Per serving with chile: 208.3 calories; 86.4 mg. sodium; 13.6 gm. carbohydrates; 12.4 gm. fat.
Per serving with green pepper: 217.9 calories; 92.9 mg. sodium; 15.7 gm. carbohydrates; 12.5 gm. fat.

Eggs with Lemon-Pepper Chicken
SERVES 4

The perfect diet meal. It is delectable, tastes like a lot of food, yet is beautifully low in calories. Add Lime Eggplant with Tomatoes (page 198) as a side dish, and your day will be complete.

1 tablespoon unsalted margarine, divided
½ chicken breast, skinned, boned, and cubed
½ cup boiling water
1 teaspoon low-sodium chicken bouillon

1 tablespoon lemon juice
¹⁄₁₆ teaspoon black pepper
4 eggs, lightly beaten
1 teaspoon dry sherry
¼ teaspoon dried oregano

1. In skillet, heat 1 teaspoon margarine over low heat. Add chicken and cook 5 minutes, or until chicken is white all over, stirring often.
2. While chicken is cooking, in bowl, combine water, bouillon, lemon juice, and pepper. Add to skillet and cook 10 minutes more.
3. While chicken mixture is cooking, in second bowl, beat together remaining ingredients, except margarine. Set aside.
4. In skillet, heat 2 remaining teaspoons margarine. Add egg mixture. Raise heat to medium and cook 5 minutes, or until eggs are set.

Per serving: 137.6 calories; 69.4 mg. sodium; 1.2 gm. carbohydrates; 8.1 gm. fat.

Eggs Yucatan
SERVES 4

A spicier and heartier version of the universally popular Huevos Rancheros (page 237). You will love this dish with Crescent Rolls (page 70).

1 tablespoon unsalted margarine, divided
2 ounces pork, minced
1 carrot, steamed* and minced
½ teaspoon low-sodium beef bouillon

4 eggs
½ cup Tomato Sauce with Cayenne (page 212)
2 tablespoons low-sodium Swiss cheese, minced

1. In skillet, heat 1 teaspoon margarine over low heat. Add pork and sauté 5 minutes, or until pork loses its pink color.

2. Stir in carrot and bouillon. Move mixture to sides of skillet.
3. In well created in center, heat remaining margarine.
4. Add eggs and fry until eggs are set.
5. Pour sauce over all. Sprinkle with cheese and cook until cheese starts to melt.

Per serving: 181.6 calories; 80.9 mg. sodium; 5.5 gm. carbohydrates; 11.1 gm. fat.

* Do not add salt to water.

Huevos Rancheros   SERVES 4

The most famous of all Mexican egg dishes and deservedly so, Huevos Rancheros are, quite simply, fantastic, and are especially delicious when topped with grated low-sodium Cheddar cheese. Serve this classic with Refried Beans (page 177) as the Mexicans most often do. Or fry up a little Chorizo (page 158) if you prefer.

4 Corn Tortillas (page 48)   **1 cup Chile-Tomato Sauce (page 213)**
1 tablespoon unsalted margarine   **Black pepper to taste**
4 eggs

1. Preheat oven to 325°.
2. On baking tray, toast tortillas 3 minutes each side. Transfer to individual plates.
3. In skillet, heat margarine over low heat. Add eggs and fry until set.
4. While eggs are cooking, in saucepan, over medium-low heat, cook tomato sauce 10 minutes, or until mixture bubbles around the edges.
5. Top each tortilla with an egg. Season with pepper.
6. Spoon some sauce over each egg.

Per serving: 241.6 calories; 64.8 mg. sodium; 24.7 gm. carbohydrates; 10.3 gm. fat.

Scrambled Eggs Mexicana   SERVES 8

The Chile-Avocado Sauce raises simple scrambled eggs to new heights. Lovely with Orange-Banana Wheat Rolls (page 69).

1 tablespoon unsalted margarine,
  divided
1 onion, minced
6 eggs, beaten
2 tablespoons low-sodium cottage
  cheese
1 tablespoon sour cream

Black pepper to taste
1 teaspoon low-sodium chicken
  bouillon
½ cup Chile-Avocado Sauce
  (page 214)

1. Preheat oven to broil.
2. In skillet, heat 1 teaspoon margarine over low heat. Add onion and cook 5 minutes, or until onion is golden, stirring occasionally.
3. While onion is cooking, in bowl, beat together eggs, cottage cheese, sour cream, pepper, and bouillon. Set aside.
4. In skillet, heat remaining 2 teaspoons margarine. Add egg mixture. Raise heat to medium-low and cook 3 minutes, or until eggs are almost set.
5. Spoon sauce over eggs. Slide skillet under broiler and cook 2 minutes more.

Per serving: 126.5 calories; 47.2 mg. sodium; 5.3 gm. carbohydrates; 9.1 gm. fat.

Scrambled Eggs with Asparagus   SERVES 4

Elegant, delectable asparagus in a marvelous, tasty setting. Turn this dish into a main course by serving Rice with Tomatoes (page 188) on the side.

4 eggs, lightly beaten
4 tablespoons sour cream, divided
Cayenne pepper to taste
1 teaspoon dried parsley
Dash of ground nutmeg
1 teaspoon low-sodium beef bouillon

1 tablespoon unsalted margarine,
  divided
8 stalks asparagus, halved diagonally
  and blanched
1 slice (1 ounce) low-sodium
  Muenster cheese

1. In bowl, beat together eggs, 2 tablespoons sour cream, cayenne pepper, parsley, nutmeg, and bouillon. Set aside.

2. In skillet, heat 1 teaspoon margarine over low heat. Add asparagus and cook 5 minutes, stirring often.
3. To skillet, add remaining 2 teaspoons margarine. Add egg mixture and cook 10 minutes.
4. Raise heat to medium-low. Add remaining sour cream. Top with cheese and cook 2 minutes more.

Per serving: 203.5 calories; 65.5 mg. sodium; 5.4 gm. carbohydrates; 15.0 gm. fat.

Scrambled Eggs with Green Sauce

SERVES 4

There is nothing we can say about this dish, except try it. It eloquently speaks for itself.

1 tablespoon unsalted margarine, divided
1 onion, chopped
1 tomato, chopped
4 eggs
¼ cup water

½ teaspoon low-sodium chicken bouillon
Black pepper to taste
Dash of hot pepper flakes
½ cup Green Sauce II (page 217)

1. In skillet, heat 1 teaspoon margarine over low heat. Add onion and cook 5 minutes, or until onion turns golden, stirring occasionally.
2. Add tomato and cook 1 minute more.
3. While tomato is cooking, in bowl, beat together eggs, water, bouillon, black pepper, pepper flakes, and green sauce. Set aside.
4. In skillet, heat remaining 2 teaspoons margarine. Add egg mixture. Raise heat to medium-low and cook eggs 3 minutes, or until they are set, stirring constantly.

Per serving: 253.2 calories; 85.7 mg. sodium; 15.9 mg. carbohydrates; 37.9 mg. fat.

Mexican Deviled Eggs

SERVES 12

Stuffed hard-cooked eggs are often last-minute appetizers because they are so easy to make. Unfortunately, they are also usually boring, mayonnaise and pepper being the primary ingredients. But not this time. These deviled eggs are a wonderful surprise, imaginatively teasing the tongue with sparks of hot and sweet, creamy and crunchy. A great dish to add to your list of cocktail foods.

1 teaspoon unsalted margarine
1 clove garlic, minced
8 scallions, chopped, including
  greens
½ tablespoon low-sodium
  mayonnaise
½ tablespoon sour cream
1½ teaspoons Chili Powder
  (page 210)

20 slices low-sodium butter pickles,
  chopped
¼ cup heavy cream
⅛ teaspoon garlic powder
1 tablespoon dried parsley
6 hard-cooked eggs, peeled and
  halved diagonally
1 teaspoon paprika

1. In skillet, heat margarine over low heat. Add garlic and sauté 3 minutes, or until garlic is lightly browned, stirring occasionally.
2. Stir in scallions and cook 1 minute more, stirring often. Transfer mixture to bowl.
3. Stir in all but last 2 ingredients, blending thoroughly.
4. Remove yolks from eggs. Mash into mayonnaise mixture.
5. Stuff egg halves with yolk mixture. Garnish with paprika and chill at least 1 hour.

Per serving: 79.2 calories; 34.5 mg. sodium; 3.6 gm. carbohydrates; 5.0 gm. fat.

Spiced Eggs, Peppers, and Cheese

SERVES 8

A Mexican omelet so pretty you will not want to eat it, so good you will not be able to stop.

1 tablespoon unsalted margarine
6 eggs, lightly beaten
1 teaspoon Chili Powder (page 210)
½ teaspoon dried oregano
Black pepper to taste
1 large green pepper, cut in ½-inch strips

2 ounces low-sodium Cheddar cheese, sliced thin
2 ounces low-sodium Gouda cheese, sliced thin
1 cup Sweet-and-Hot Chile Sauce (page 215)

1. Preheat oven to 350°.
2. In 5-inch soufflé dish, heat margarine over medium-low heat. Add eggs and cook 3 minutes, stirring occasionally.
3. Stir in chili powder, oregano, and black pepper. Cook 3 minutes more.
4. Add green pepper and both cheeses. Bake 5 minutes, or until eggs are set.
5. Pour chili sauce over all and bake 5 minutes more.

Per serving: 169.4 calories; 59.6 mg. sodium; 8.6 gm. carbohydrates; 10.7 gm. fat.

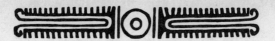

Desserts

Before the Spanish introduced flour, desserts in pre-Columbian Mexico consisted primarily of a selection of the succulent fresh fruits which flourished throughout the countryside. Fruit is still a favorite dessert today, its sweet refreshing taste a light and lovely way to end a hearty Mexican meal. Of course, fruit is prepared in more exotic ways than it once was and so is all the more delectable. Pineapple and Bananas in Sherry (page 253) and Broiled Oranges with Coconut (page 247) will have you licking your fingers.

Today, however, flour-based cakes and sweet breads are also very much part of the dessert menu. Many, like Kings' Ring (page 251), are associated with a feast day or religious holiday; but all of them need no reason other than your pleasure to be enjoyed.

Interestingly, flan—that most famous of all Mexican desserts—is not Mexican at all. This sugary-rich caramel custard is actually Spanish in origin, but one melting bite of Cinnamon-Pecan Flan (page 245), and you will not care where this confection was conceived.

In fact, that is how you will feel about all the delectable offerings in this chapter, for Mexican sweets are universal in their appeal. And don't overlook the special Dessert Empanadas (page 57).

Basic Flan
SERVES 12

Although Spanish in origin, flan is the most popular of Mexican desserts. It is wonderful in its simplest form, and becomes an exotic delight with the addition of a few ingredients. The basic recipe as well as some suggested variations are offered below.

⅓ cup water
1½ cups sugar, divided
5 cups low-fat milk

10 eggs, lightly beaten
1½ teaspoons vanilla extract

1. In saucepan, combine water and ¾ cup sugar. Turn heat to medium and cook until sugar melts, and mixture turns golden brown, stirring constantly.
2. Pour mixture into 12 small custard cups, tilting cups so that mixture covers bottoms and sides. When mixture stops running, turn cups upside down on a platter. Set aside.
3. In second saucepan, over medium-low heat, heat milk 5 minutes, or until film forms on top. Remove from heat.
4. In bowl, beat together remaining sugar and eggs. Then beat in milk and vanilla.
5. Preheat oven to 350°.
6. Pour milk mixture into caramelized cups.
7. Place cups in 9 x 13-inch ovenproof casserole. Fill casserole with hot water until it reaches halfway up the sides of the cups.
8. Bake 1 hour, or until knife inserted in center comes out clean.
9. Transfer cups to rack. Let stand ½ hour to cool. Then chill at least 2 hours.
10. To unmold, run a thin, sharp knife between the flan and the custard cups. Then place individual serving plates upside down on each cup and invert quickly.

Per serving: 209.3 calories; 95.7 mg. sodium; 33.6 gm. carbohydrates; 3.7 gm. fat.

Cinnamon-Pecan Flan
SERVES 12

⅓ cup water
1½ cups sugar, divided
5 cups low-fat milk
10 eggs, lightly beaten

½ teaspoon almond extract
½ teaspoon ground cinnamon
¼ cup unsalted, chopped pecans

1. Follow recipe for Basic Flan (page 244) through Step 3.
2. In Step 4, substitute almond extract and cinnamon for vanilla and beat in pecans.
3. Proceed with recipe for Basic Flan through Step 10.

Per serving: 229.7 calories; 95.7 mg. sodium; 34.0 gm. carbohydrates; 5.8 gm. fat.

Lemon-Coconut Flan
SERVES 12

⅓ cup water
1½ cups sugar, divided
5 cups low-fat milk
10 eggs, lightly beaten

½ teaspoon vanilla extract
1 teaspoon lemon peel powder
¼ cup shredded coconut

1. Follow the recipe for Basic Flan (page 244) through Step 3.
2. In Step 4, beat lemon peel powder and coconut into sugar and egg mixture.
3. Proceed with recipe for Basic Flan through Step 10.

Per serving: 235.8 calories; 95.7 mg. sodium; 36.2 gm. carbohydrates; 5.5 gm. fat.

Almond Pudding

SERVES 8

This elegant gelatin dish is like a pudding because of the creamy consistency the egg whites provide. It is usually accompanied by a custard sauce so rich that we have opted not to include it. However, we are sure you will enjoy the pudding for its own sake.

1 package unflavored gelatin	**½ teaspoon almond extract**
1 cup boiling water	**¼ teaspoon ground cinnamon**
6 egg whites	**2 ounces unsalted slivered almonds**
½ cup sugar	

1. In bowl, combine first 2 ingredients, stirring until gelatin is dissolved. Let stand 15 minutes.
2. In second bowl, beat egg whites until stiff peaks are formed.
3. Fold egg whites into gelatin mixture.
4. Beat in sugar, almond extract, and cinnamon. Chill at least 3 hours.
5. Garnish with almonds.

Per serving: 120.9 calories; 0.5 mg. sodium; 16.0 gm. carbohydrates; 4.1 gm. fat.

Anise Fritters

MAKES 12

Fritters are popular throughout Mexico. There are probably as many variations as there are cities, but the recipe which follows is an adaptation of the Spanish favorite.

1 cup dark brown sugar	**½ pound all-purpose flour**
¼ cup honey	**2 eggs, lightly beaten**
¼ teaspoon aniseed	**½ teaspoon low-sodium baking**
4 cups water, divided	**powder**
3 tablespoons shortening	**2 cups peanut oil**

1. In saucepan, combine first 3 ingredients plus 3 cups water. Turn heat to medium and cook 5 minutes, stirring constantly to dissolve sugar. Then let mixture come to a boil and continue boiling 10 minutes. Set aside.
2. In second saucepan, combine remaining water and shortening. Turn heat to medium and bring to a boil. Remove from heat.
3. Beat flour into shortening mixture. Let stand 10 minutes.

4. Beat eggs into flour mixture. Then beat in baking powder. Knead dough briefly.
5. In skillet, heat oil over medium heat until it crackles.
6. Break off small pieces of dough and roll into balls, 1 to 1½ inches around.
7. Flatten balls between fingers. Make holes in center of balls and drop into hot oil. Fry until balls are puffed and golden brown. Drain on paper towels.
8. Place fritters on warm platter and pour sugar mixture over all.

Per fritter: 256.9 calories; 15.8 mg. sodium; 36.6 gm. carbohydrates; 11.2 gm. fat.

Broiled Oranges with Coconut   SERVES 4

Simple and delightful and just as tasty if you substitute 4 peaches, halved and pitted, for the oranges.

2 oranges, halved	**4 tablespoons brandy**
2 tablespoons unsalted margarine	**4 tablespoons grated coconut**

1. Preheat oven to broil.
2. On baking sheet, place orange halves. Dot with margarine and broil 4 inches from heat 3 minutes.
3. Pour brandy over all and flame.
4. Garnish with coconut.

Per serving with oranges: 221.3 calories; 2.2 mg. sodium; 19.8 gm. carbohydrates; 11.6 gm. fat.
Per serving with peaches: 215.7 calories; 2.5 mg. sodium; 18.7 gm. carbohydrates; 11.5 gm. fat.

Coconut Soufflé   SERVES 12

This is one temptation you will not be able to resist. What's more, because it's so low in calories, you will not have to.

2 cups low-fat milk
½ cup sugar
⅛ teaspoon ground cinnamon

¼ cup shredded coconut
4 eggs, lightly beaten
2 tablespoons rum

1. In saucepan, combine first 3 ingredients. Turn heat to low and cook 10 minutes, or until sugar is dissolved, stirring often.
2. Stir in coconut and cook 10 minutes more, stirring often. Transfer mixture to 6-inch-square ovenproof casserole. Let stand 15 minutes.
3. Preheat oven to 350°.
4. Beat in eggs and rum.
5. In oven, place casserole in pan of water. Bake ½ hour, or until mixture is firm and knife inserted in center comes out clean.

Per serving: 96.1 calories; 38.2 mg. sodium; 10.9 gm. carbohydrates; 3.3 gm. fat.

Fried Bread
with Brandied Honey   MAKES 48

Crispy, crunchy, airy, light, and deliciously addictive.

2¼ cups all-purpose flour
3½ teaspoons low-sodium baking powder
1 tablespoon orange peel powder
1/16 teaspoon clove powder
2 tablespoons shortening

2¼ cups water, divided
2 cups vegetable oil
½ cup honey
1 tablespoon brandy
⅛ teaspoon ground nutmeg

1. In bowl, combine first 4 ingredients, blending thoroughly.
2. Cut in shortening. Then add 1¼ cups water to form dough.
3. Turn dough onto lightly floured board and knead until rubbery.
4. Place dough in greased bowl. Cover and let stand 1 hour.
5. Turn dough onto lightly floured board and roll to ¼-inch thickness. Cut into 3-inch squares.

6. In saucepan, heat oil over medium-high heat. When oil is crackling, with tongs, drop in bread squares, one at a time. Fry until squares puff. Drain on paper towels.
7. In second saucepan, combine remaining water, honey, brandy, and nutmeg. Turn heat to medium-low and cook 10 minutes, stirring occasionally. Serve as sauce for fried bread.

Per serving: 67.6 calories; 0.6 mg. sodium; 10.0 gm. carbohydrates; 2.5 gm. fat.

Fruit Puree

SERVES 12

The perfect refreshing ending to any meal.

1 pineapple, cored, peeled, and diced
2 bananas, peeled and diced
1 grapefruit, peeled and diced
2 oranges, diced, including rind
2 pears, cored and diced

½ teaspoon ground cinnamon
1 lime, diced, including rind
12 tablespoons sour cream

1. In blender, combine pineapple, bananas, and grapefruit. Puree a little at a time. Transfer to bowl.
2. In blender, combine remaining ingredients except sour cream. Puree. Combine with pineapple mixture, blending thoroughly.
3. Divide mixture among 12 dessert bowls. Garnish with sour cream.

Per serving: 140.2 calories; 6.6 mg. sodium; 23.7 gm. carbohydrates; 5.7 gm. fat.

Fruited Yam Pie

SERVES 12

A marvelous variation on fruit pie, with the yams adding a candy-like sweetness that recalls childhood holidays. Try this at Thanksgiving and start a memory book of your own.

2 pounds yams
½ cup hot water
¼ cup sugar
2 tablespoons honey
1 teaspoon vanilla extract
2 tablespoons rum
2 tablespoons banana liqueur
1 teaspoon orange peel powder

½ teaspoon ground cinnamon
¼ teaspoon ground nutmeg
⅓ cup unsalted chopped walnuts
¼ cup chopped dates
4 dried pears, chopped
12 dried apricots, chopped
¼ cup raisins*

1. Preheat oven to 350°.
2. Slit yams diagonally and bake 1 hour, or until fork-tender. Remove pulp and mash. Set aside.
3. In saucepan, combine water and sugar. Turn heat to low and cook 10 minutes, or until sugar is dissolved, stirring often.
4. Stir yams into sugar mixture, blending thoroughly.
5. Stir in remaining ingredients. Transfer to bowl. Cover and refrigerate at least 5 days.

Per serving: 188.7 calories; 3.5 mg. sodium; 37.5 gm. carbohydrates; 2.7 gm. fat.

* Preserved in non-sodium ingredient.

Kahlua Cream

SERVES 8

The most mouth-watering confection you will ever taste.

1 cup heavy cream
½ teaspoon orange peel powder
¾ teaspoon instant coffee
1/16 teaspoon ground cinnamon

¼ cup Kahlua
3 tablespoons sugar
2 egg whites
½ teaspoon ground nutmeg

1. In chilled bowl, beat together first 4 ingredients.
2. Beat in Kahlua and sugar.

3. In second bowl, beat egg whites until stiff. Fold into cream mixture. Cover and chill at least 2 hours. Then freeze for 10 minutes before serving.
4. Spoon mixture into 8 small bowls. Garnish with nutmeg.

Per serving: 146.2 calories; 9.2 mg. sodium; 6.3 gm. carbohydrates; 10.8 gm. fat.

Kings' Ring   SERVES 20

It is tradition to serve the Ring of Kings on Twelfth Night, marking the visit of the Three Kings to baby Jesus. Often a tiny doll, representing the infant king of kings, is baked in the cake and is a good luck charm for the recipient.

1 package active dry yeast	3 eggs
¼ cup warm water	¼ cup low-fat milk
2¾ cups all-purpose flour	1 cup mixed candied fruit, chopped
¼ cup sugar	4 tablespoons powdered sugar
1 tablespoon lemon peel powder	
1 teaspoon aniseed	
1 stick (¼ pound) unsalted margarine	

1. In bowl, combine first 2 ingredients. Set aside.
2. In second bowl, combine flour, sugar, lemon peel powder, and aniseed, blending thoroughly.
3. Cut in margarine.
4. Beat in eggs, milk, and fruit.
5. Stir in yeast mixture, blending to form a spongy dough.
6. Turn dough onto lightly floured board and knead until smooth.
7. Shape dough into a ring. Place on a greased and floured baking sheet. Cover and let stand in warm, dry place 2 hours, or until doubled in bulk.
8. Preheat oven to 350°.
9. Dust top of ring with powdered sugar and bake ½ hour, or until top is lightly browned.

Per serving: 222.9 calories; 11.8 mg. sodium; 37.4 gm. carbohydrates; 5.7 gm. fat.

Lemon-Prune Cake

SERVES 16

Instead of icing, top this lovely cake with fresh, chopped fruit or plain yogurt.

6 tablespoons unsalted margarine
⅓ cup sugar
2 cups all-purpose flour
4 teaspoons low-sodium baking
  powder

2 eggs
1½ teaspoons lemon peel powder
¼ cup low-fat milk
2 tablespoons lemon juice
12 prunes, pitted and chopped

1. Preheat oven to 350°.
2. In bowl, cream together margarine and sugar. Set aside.
3. In second bowl, combine flour and baking powder, stirring to blend.
4. Beat in eggs, lemon peel powder, milk, and lemon juice, blending thoroughly.
5. Beat in prunes.
6. Beat in sugar mixture, a little at a time.
7. Pour batter into greased and floured 9-inch-square baking pan. Bake 45 minutes, or until toothpick inserted in center comes out clean.

Per serving: 185.7 calories; 11.5 mg. sodium; 29.9 gm. carbohydrates; 5.3 gm. fat.

Mexican Sugar Cookies

MAKES 48

This is an unorthodox but tasty tribute to all the delicious variations of Mexican sugar cookies.

2 cups all-purpose flour
½ cup sugar
1½ teaspoons baking powder
¼ teaspoon clove powder
1 stick (¼ pound) unsalted margarine

2 eggs
⅓ cup unsalted slivered almonds
1 teaspoon mint extract
½ teaspoon vanilla extract

1. In bowl, combine first 4 ingredients, blending thoroughly.
2. Cream in margarine.
3. Beat in eggs. Then beat in remaining ingredients.
4. Preheat oven to 350°.

5. Break off one walnut-sized piece of dough at a time. Roll into ball. Place on greased and floured baking sheet. Flatten ball slightly.
6. Repeat Step 5 with remaining dough.
7. Bake 10 minutes, or until cookies are golden.

Per cookie: 67.3 calories; 3.1 mg. sodium; 9.1 gm. carbohydrates; 2.8 gm. fat.

Pineapple and Bananas in Sherry
SERVES 8

For a totally different taste-experience, substitute 4 large peaches, halved and pitted, for the bananas and 1 cup red raspberries for the pineapple.

2 tablespoons unsalted margarine
4 small firm bananas, halved
  diagonally
$\frac{1}{16}$ teaspoon ground nutmeg
2 tablespoons shredded coconut

1 can (8 ounces) crushed pineapple,
  including juice
2 tablespoons dry sherry

1. In skillet, heat margarine over low heat. Add bananas, cut side down, and cook 5 minutes.
2. Add nutmeg and coconut and cook 5 minutes more.
3. With spatula, turn bananas. Add pineapple, including juice, plus sherry. Raise heat to medium and cook 3 minutes more.

Per serving with pineapple and bananas: 89.9 calories; 1.3 mg. sodium; 12.9 gm. carbohydrates; 4.4 gm. fat.
Per serving with raspberries and peaches: 97.2 calories; 1.8 mg. sodium; 14.3 gm. carbohydrates; 4.5 gm. fat.

Rum Pears   SERVES 8

Apples instead of pears combined with pineapple juice instead of apple juice makes a lovely alternate to the recipe below.

4 pears, halved lengthwise and cored   **¼ cup light rum**
⅜ teaspoon ground nutmeg   **½ cup heavy cream**
4 teaspoons dark raisins*
1 cup apple juice

1. Preheat oven to 325°.
2. Sprinkle cut side of pears with nutmeg.
3. Spoon raisins into pear hollows. Then invert pears, cut side down, in 9-inch-square ovenproof casserole.
4. Pour juice and rum over all. Cover and bake 40 minutes, or until pears are fork-tender.
5. Divide pear halves among 8 plates. Spoon rum sauce over all.
6. Spoon cream over all.

Per serving with pears and apple juice: 150.4 calories; 7.6 mg. sodium; 20.8 gm. carbo-
    hydrates; 5.8 gm. fat.
Per serving with apples and pineapple juice: 148.7 calories; 6.5 mg. sodium; 20.7 carbo-
    hydrates; 6.0 gm. fat.

* Preserved in non-sodium ingredient.

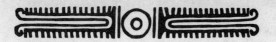

A Mexican Menu
for Entertaining

By its very nature, Mexican food *is* party food. Just think of the antojitos already so popular in this country: tacos, burritos, enchiladas, guacamole, brimming with spice and sparkle. They spell fiesta. The truth is Mexican food tingles with the gaiety, color, and exuberant abandon of its people. It is synonomous with celebration, which is why its appearance virtually guarantees the success of any party.

While good food is one important prerequisite to a good party, there is another your guests never see or taste: organization. With it, your party will roll merrily and triumphantly along. Without it, it will spin into chaos.

Organization is a frightening word to some people, who equate it with being complex, boring, unpleasant, and filled with minutiae. It may be so to them. But you should not think of it that way. To you, organization should simply mean the advance thought and preparation that will make your party flow effortlessly and leave you relaxed, confident, and in control before and during the festivities.

To realize this happy state of affairs, you need only remember a few tricks:

• *Balance your menu* for color and texture as well as for taste. Food is a sensual experience, best appreciated and heightened by contrast.

For example, the sweet, fibrous, creamy-green blend of Cabbage and Apples in Piquant Sour Cream Sauce (page 201) is a delightful companion for the more tangy and tender Chicken in Mustard Sauce (page 138) with its burnished yellow dressing.

• *Consider preparation time* and structure your menu to include dishes which can be made in advance and served cold, such as Green Bean and Sweet Pepper Salad (page 100), Fruit Soup (page 80), and Mixed Seafood in Lime Sauce (page 217); others which can simmer for hours, needing little of your attention, like Mexican Baked Beans (page 176) and Saucy Meat Balls (page 171).

You will find Mexican cuisine very cooperative in this regard because a majority of dishes are either marinated or cooked slowly in the relaxed, good-natured "mañana" tradition.

• *Rely on tried-and-true successes* which have proven themselves time after time. After all, entertaining is all about pleasure for your guests and for you, so sticking to dishes you already know will please them and reap the reward of their appreciation.

In this regard, Picadillo with Vegetables (page 169), Sour Cream-Chicken Enchiladas (page 60), Pickled Ceviche (page 43), and, of course, Beef Chile (page 150) are all sure to be among the permanent features on your party-planning agenda.

• *Make a checklist* of all the ingredients you will need at least one week ahead of time so you can properly stock up and avoid last-minute panic runs to the store.

Otherwise, relax. Mexican cooking requires no special equipment or instructions. The cuisine has no temperamental dishes which demand split-second precision. Just remember the four simple, commonsensical hints given here, and have fun at your own party.

And, oh, what a party when it is Mexican, as you are about to find out in this chapter. Brunches, lunches, formal dinners, cocktail parties, and buffets—40 menus for you to try, with preparation tips for each. Some menus are entirely Mexican; others are made memorable by the distinctive flair a Mexican dish or two can bring. All display the warmth and charm of our southern neighbors.

So take out your maracas, and let the mariachis play.

Brunch for 4

Eggs and Chorizo (page 232)
Green Bean and Sweet Pepper Salad (page 100)
Corn Tortillas (page 48)
Broiled Oranges with Coconut (page 247)

Preparation Tips:
1. Prepare Corn Tortillas up to 2 days before serving. Refrigerate 4 until ready to use. Freeze remainder.
2. Prepare Green Bean and Sweet Pepper Salad* 2 hours before serving. Cover and refrigerate until ready to use.
3. Prepare Eggs and Chorizo† 15 minutes before serving.
4. Prepare Broiled Oranges with Coconut 5 minutes before serving.

* The Oil and Vinegar Dressing (page 227) used in this recipe may be prepared and refrigerated any time before ready to use.

† The Chorizo (page 158) used in this recipe may be prepared and frozen up to 2 months before ready to use. The Basil-Tomato Sauce (page 212) called for may be prepared and refrigerated up to 2 weeks before ready to use.

>୧l■l■l©<

Brunch for 4

Eggs, Sweet Pepper, and Cheddar Cheese (page 235)
Shrimp Salad Mazatlan (page 106)
Golden Cinnamon Rolls (page 73)
Raspberries and Peaches in Sherry (page 253)

Preparation Tips:
1. Prepare Golden Cinnamon Rolls 2½ hours before serving. (Refrigerate or freeze additional rolls.)
2. Prepare Shrimp Salad Mazatlan,* through Step 2, 1½ hours before serving.
3. Finish preparation of Shrimp Salad Mazatlan ½ hour before serving. Cover and refrigerate until ready to serve.
4. Prepare Eggs, Sweet Pepper, and Cheddar Cheese 20 minutes before serving.
5. Prepare Raspberries and Peaches in Sherry† 15 minutes before serving.

* If you are not allowed shellfish, substitute 1 can (7¾ ounces) low-sodium salmon.
† Make ½ the recipe.

>୧l■l■l©<

Brunch for 4

Chicken Chilaquiles in Chile-Tomato Sauce (page 52)
Chile-Tuna Salad (page 107)
Cantaloupe and Red Grapes

Preparation Tips:
1. Prepare Chile-Tuna Salad 1½ hours before serving.
2. Prepare Chicken Chilaquiles* 20 minutes before serving.
3. Immediately before serving, slice 1 cantaloupe and surround with ¼ pound of red grapes.

* The Corn Tortillas (page 48) used in this recipe may be prepared and frozen up to 1 month before ready to use. Defrost 4 in the refrigerator up to 1 week before ready to use. The Chile-Tomato Sauce (page 213) called for may be prepared and refrigerated 2 weeks before ready to use.

>◦▮◼▮◼◦<

Brunch for 4

Scrambled Eggs with Asparagus (page 238)
Minced Meats with Fruit (page 170)
Paprika Potatoes

Preparation Tips:
1. Prepare Minced Meats with Fruit* through Step 1, 45 minutes before serving.
2. Boil 4 small new potatoes 40 minutes before serving. Drain.
3. Preheat oven to 325°.
4. Continue preparation of Minced Meats with Fruit through Step 5, 35 minutes before serving.
5. Place potatoes on roasting pan 30 minutes before serving. Sprinkle with paprika and roast until browned.
6. Finish preparation of Minced Meats with Fruit 25 minutes before serving.
7. Prepare Scrambled Eggs with Asparagus 20 minutes before serving.

* Make ½ the recipe. The Basic Salsa (page 210) used in this recipe may be prepared and refrigerated up to 3 weeks before ready to use.

>◦▮◼▮◼◦<

Brunch for 8

Fruit Salad Picante (page 102)
Scrambled Eggs Mexicana (page 238)
Picadillo with Vegetables (page 169)
Crescent Rolls (page 70)

Preparation Tips:
1. Prepare Crescent Rolls through Step 10, 3 hours before serving.
2. Prepare Picadillo with Vegetables 1½ hours before serving.
3. Prepare Fruit Salad Picante* through Step 2, 1 hour before serving.
4. Finish preparation of Crescent Rolls 20 minutes before serving. (Refrigerate or freeze additional rolls.)
5. Prepare Scrambled Eggs Mexicana† 15 minutes before serving.
6. Finish preparation of Fruit Salad Picante 5 minutes before serving.

* The Honey-Lime Dressing (page 229) option in this recipe may be prepared and refrigerated up to 1 month before ready to use; the Sweet Dressing (page 230) option may be prepared and refrigerated up to 2 weeks before ready to use.

† The Chile-Avocado Sauce (page 214) in this recipe may be prepared and refrigerated up to 2 hours before ready to use.

>◦■▮▯■◦<

Brunch for 8

Sour Cream-Chicken Enchiladas (page 60)
Christmas Eve Salad (page 103)
Broiled Tomatoes with Avocado (page 200)

Preparation Tips:
1. Prepare Christmas Eve Salad* through Step 1, 2 hours before serving.
2. Prepare Sour Cream-Chicken Enchiladas† through Step 7, 1 hour before serving.
3. Prepare Broiled Tomatoes with Avocado through Step 3, 40 minutes before serving.
4. Finish preparation of Sour Cream-Chicken Enchiladas 20 minutes before serving.
5. Finish preparation of Broiled Tomatoes with Avocado 10 minutes before serving.
6. Finish preparation of Christmas Eve Salad immediately before serving.

* The Sweet Dressing (page 230) used in this recipe may be prepared and refrigerated up to 2 weeks before ready to use.

† The Corn Tortillas (page 48) used in this recipe may be prepared and refrigerated up to 2 hours before ready to use. Freeze the remainder. Also, the Chile-Cheddar Dip (page 35) called for may be prepared and refrigerated up to 3 hours before ready to use.

>●▬▬▬●<

Brunch for 8

Chicken and Spiced Fruit (page 135)
Swordfish and Capers (page 122)
Avocado, Tomato, and Cheese Salad (page 98)
Boiled White Rice

Preparation Tips:
1. Prepare Chicken and Spiced Fruit* through Step 3, 2½ hours before serving.
2. Prepare Swordfish and Capers through Step 1, 1½ hours before serving.
3. Finish preparation of Chicken and Spiced Fruit 1 hour and 20 minutes before serving.
4. Prepare 2 cups of white rice ½ hour before serving.
5. Finish preparation of Swordfish and Capers 20 minutes before serving.
6. Prepare Avocado, Tomato, and Cheese Salad† 15 minutes before serving.

* The Chili Powder (page 210) used in this recipe should be a staple in your pantry.
† The Lemon Dressing (page 226) used in this recipe may be prepared and refrigerated any time before ready to use.

>⊜▮◢▮▩▮◖◄

Brunch for 8

Eggs Yucatan (page 236)
Burritos II (page 51)
Creamed Cauliflower and Sweet Peppers (page 204)
Fresh Strawberries

Preparation Tips:
1. Hull 1 pint of strawberries 2 hours before serving.
2. Prepare Burritos II* through Step 4, 1 hour before serving.
3. Prepare Creamed Cauliflower and Sweet Peppers 45 minutes before serving.
4. Finish preparation of Burritos II ½ hour before serving.
5. Prepare Eggs Yucatan† 20 minutes before serving.

* The Almond Sauce (page 218) used in this recipe may be prepared and refrigerated up to 1 week before ready to use. The White Flour Tortillas (page 49) called for may be prepared and 8 refrigerated up to 2 hours before ready to use. Freeze the remainder.
† The Tomato Sauce with Cayenne (page 212) used in this recipe may be prepared and refrigerated up to 3 weeks before ready to use.

>⊜▮◢▮▩▮◖◄

Brunch for 16

Grapefruit Sections
Chicken and Cheese Tamales (page 62)
Jicama and Chorizo Salad (page 105)

Preparation Tips:
1. Peel and section 8 grapefruit 2½ hours before serving. Place in bowl. Cover and refrigerate until ready to use.
2. Prepare Chicken and Cheese Tamales 2 hours before serving.
3. Prepare Jicama and Chorizo Salad* 25 minutes before serving.

* Double the recipe. The Chorizo (page 158) used in this recipe may be prepared and frozen up to 2 months before ready to use. The Oil and Vinegar Dressing (page 227) called for may be prepared and refrigerated any time before ready to use.

>●▬/▬●<

Brunch for 16

Low-Sodium Tomato Juice
Eggs in a Nest (page 234)
Broccoli and Mushrooms with Pork (page 200)
Mexican Sweet Bread (page 68)

Preparation Tips:
1. Chill 2 cans (64 ounces) low-sodium tomato juice 4 hours before serving.
2. Prepare Mexican Sweet Bread* 3½ hours before serving.
3. Prepare Broccoli and Mushrooms with Pork† 20 minutes before serving.
4. Prepare Eggs in a Nest† 15 minutes before serving.

* Refrigerate or freeze second loaf.
† Double the recipe.

>●▬/▬●<

Brunch for 16

Mixed Seafood in Lime Sauce (page 128)
Vegetable-Stuffed Chiles (page 195)
Corn Tortillas (page 48)
Pineapple and Bananas in Sherry (page 253)

Preparation Tips:
1. Prepare Corn Tortillas up to 2 days before serving. Refrigerate 16 until ready to use. Freeze remainder.
2. Prepare Mixed Seafood in Lime Sauce* through Step 1, 4 hours before serving.
3. Prepare Vegetable-Stuffed Chiles† 1½ hours before serving.
4. Finish preparation of Mixed Seafood in Lime Sauce 20 minutes before serving.
5. Prepare Pineapple and Bananas in Sherry‡ 15 minutes before serving.

* Double the recipe. The Lime Sauce (page 217) used in this recipe may be prepared and refrigerated up to 1 week before ready to use. If you are not allowed shellfish, substitute 1 pound of red snapper fillets, cut in 1-inch chunks, for the shrimp and oysters.
† The Chile-Avocado Sauce (page 214) used in this recipe may be prepared and refrigerated up to 2 hours before ready to use.
‡ Double the recipe.

Brunch for 16

Egg and Chicken Liver Casserole (page 232)
Salad of Colors (page 102)
Orange-Banana Wheat Rolls (page 69)
Almond Pudding (page 246)

Preparation Tips:
1. Prepare Almond Pudding through Step 4, 4 hours before ready to serve.
2. Prepare Orange-Banana Wheat Rolls 3 hours before serving. (Refrigerate or freeze additional rolls.)
3. Prepare Salad of Colors* through Step 3, 2½ hours before serving.
4. Prepare Egg and Chicken Liver Casserole† 1½ hours before serving.
5. Finish preparation of Salad of Colors ½ hour before serving.
6. Finish preparation of Almond Pudding immediately before serving.

* Double the recipe.

† Double the recipe. The Meat Stock (page 78) used in this recipe may be prepared and refrigerated up to 1 week before ready to use.

Lunch for 4

Creamy Carrot Soup (page 83)
Honey Fish (page 113)
Asparagus in Crumb Sauce (page 196)
Almond Pudding (page 246)

Preparation Tips:
1. Prepare Almond Pudding* through Step 4, 4 hours before serving.
2. Prepare Honey Fish through Step 4, 1 hour and 15 minutes before serving.
3. Prepare Creamy Carrot Soup† 45 minutes before serving.
4. Steam asparagus ½ hour before serving.
5. Finish preparation of Honey Fish 20 minutes before serving.
6. Finish preparation of Asparagus in Crumb Sauce 10 minutes before serving.
7. Finish preparation of Almond Pudding immediately before serving.

* Use ½ the recipe. Refrigerate or freeze remainder.

† The Chicken Stock (page 76) used in this recipe may be prepared and refrigerated up to 1 week before ready to use.

><8I■I■I8<

Lunch for 4

Parsley Chicken (page 144)
Rice with Mushrooms and Cheese (page 188)
Mixed Salad San Miguel (page 101)
Fruit Puree (page 249)

Preparation Tips:
1. Prepare Parsley Chicken 1 hour and 10 minutes before serving.
2. Prepare Fruit Puree* through Step 2, 1 hour before serving. Cover and refrigerate until ready to serve.
3. Prepare Rice with Mushrooms and Cheese ½ hour before serving.
4. Prepare Mixed Salad San Miguel† 20 minutes before serving.
5. Finish preparation of Fruit Puree immediately before serving.

* Use ⅓ the recipe. Refrigerate or freeze remainder.
† The Hot-and-Sweet Dressing (page 228) used in this recipe may be prepared and refrigerated any time before ready to use.

><8I■I■I8<

Lunch for 4

Fresh Fruit Cup
Flounder in Chile-Corn Sauce (page 110)
Watercress Salad with Lemon Juice
Mexican Sugar Cookies (page 252)

Preparation Tips:
1. Prepare Flounder in Chile-Corn Sauce through Step 1, at least 5 hours before serving.
2. Prepare fresh fruit cup with fruit of your choice 2½ hours before serving. Divide into 4 small bowls. Cover and refrigerate until ready to serve.
3. Prepare Mexican Sugar Cookies* 2 hours before serving.
4. Finish preparation of Flounder in Chile-Corn Sauce 45 minutes before serving.
5. Prepare watercress salad, using 4 bunches of watercress, 15 minutes before serving.

* Allow 2 cookies per serving. Store remainder in tightly closed container.

Lunch for 4

Puree of Spinach Soup (page 88)
Sherry Veal Chops (page 165)
Sliced Tomatoes and Cucumber
Parsley Potatoes

Preparation Tips:
1. Slice 2 tomatoes and 1 cucumber 1½ hours before serving. Refrigerate until ready to serve.
2. Prepare Sherry Veal Chops through Step 7, 1 hour before serving.
3. Boil 4 new potatoes 45 minutes before serving.
4. Prepare Puree of Spinach Soup ½ hour before serving.
5. Finish preparation of Sherry Veal Chops 20 minutes before serving.
6. Drain and peel potatoes 15 minutes before serving. Garnish with parsley.

Lunch for 8

Chicken in Mustard Sauce (page 138)
Cheesy Hot Noodles (page 182)
Cabbage and Apples in Piquant Sour Cream Sauce (page 201)
Mexican Sugar Cookies (page 252)

Preparation Tips:
1. Prepare Mexican Sugar Cookies 2½ hours before serving.
2. Prepare Chicken in Mustard Sauce through Step 1, 1½ hours before serving.
3. Prepare Cabbage and Apples in Piquant Sour Cream Sauce* through Step 1, 1 hour and 20 minutes before serving.
4. Finish preparation of Chicken in Mustard Sauce 1 hour and 15 minutes before serving.
5. Finish preparation of Cabbage and Apples in Piquant Sour Cream Sauce ½ hour before serving.
6. Prepare Cheesy Hot Noodles† 20 minutes before serving.

* The Piquant Sour Cream Sauce (page 224) used in this recipe should be prepared and refrigerated at least 2 hours before ready to use.

† The Tomato Sauce with Cayenne (page 212) used in this recipe may be prepared and refrigerated up to 3 weeks before ready to use.

>◦▮▰▮▰◦<

Lunch for 8

Mexican Vegetable Soup (page 87)
Flounder with Walnut-Orange Sauce (page 111)
Potatoes with Chiles (page 180)
Rum Apples (page 254)

Preparation Tips:
1. Prepare Flounder with Walnut-Orange Sauce through Step 1, 1½ hours before serving.
2. Prepare Mexican Vegetable Soup* 1 hour before serving.
3. Prepare Rum Apples 45 minutes before serving.
4. Finish preparation of Mexican Vegetable Soup 40 minutes before serving.
5. Continue preparation of Flounder with Walnut-Orange Sauce through Step 3, ½ hour before serving.
6. Prepare Potatoes with Chiles through Step 1, 25 minutes before serving.
7. Continue preparation of Flounder with Walnut-Orange Sauce through Step 7, 20 minutes before serving.
8. Finish preparation of Potatoes with Chiles 15 minutes before serving.
9. Finish preparation of Flounder with Walnut-Orange Sauce 5 minutes before serving.

* The Chicken Stock (page 76) used in this recipe may be prepared and refrigerated up to 1 week before ready to use.

>◦▮▰▮▰◦<

Lunch for 8

Low-Sodium Canned Tuna
Bean Salad (page 98)
Steamed Green Beans
Fresh Orange Sections

Preparation Tips:
1. Prepare Bean Salad* the day before serving.
2. Peel and section 8 oranges 1 hour before serving. Refrigerate until ready to serve.
3. Steam 1 pound of green beans ½ hour before serving.
4. Toss Bean Salad with 4 cans of drained low-sodium tuna immediately before serving.

* The Chili Powder (page 210) used in this recipe should be a staple in your pantry.

>⊙▮▮▮⊙<

Lunch for 8

Gazpacho (page 81)
Meat-Stuffed Chiles (page 194)
Boiled White Rice
Red and Green Grapes

Preparation Tips:
1. Prepare Gazpacho* 2 hours before serving.
2. Refrigerate 1 pound of grapes 1½ hours before serving.
3. Prepare Meat-Stuffed Chiles† 1 hour before serving.
4. Prepare 2 cups of white rice ½ hour before serving.

* The Chili Powder (page 210) used in this recipe should be a staple in your pantry.
† The Picadillo with Vegetables (page 169) used in this recipe may be prepared and set aside up to 3 hours before ready to use. The Basic Salsa (page 210) called for may be prepared and refrigerated up to 3 weeks before ready to use.

>⊙▮▮▮⊙<

Dinner for 4

Fruit Soup (page 80)
Baked Salmon in Mustard Sauce (page 116)
Mexican White Rice (page 186)
Asparagus and Mushrooms (page 196)

Preparation Tips:
1. Prepare Fruit Soup* 2 hours before serving. Keep refrigerated until ready to serve.
2. Prepare Baked Salmon in Mustard Sauce† through Step 6, ½ hour before serving.
3. Prepare Mexican White Rice* 25 minutes before serving.
4. Steam asparagus 20 minutes before serving.
5. Finish preparation of Baked Salmon in Mustard Sauce 15 minutes before serving.
6. Finish preparation of Asparagus and Mushrooms 10 minutes before serving.

* The Chicken Stock (page 76) used in this recipe may be prepared and refrigerated up to 1 week before ready to use.
† The Fish Stock (page 77) used in this recipe may be prepared and refrigerated up to 1 week before ready to use.

>◦▮▬▮◦<

Dinner for 4

Mint Lamb Chops with Peanuts (page 158)
Mexican Potato Salad (page 178)
Glazed Carrots with Minced Shrimp (page 202)
Mexican Sugar Cookies (page 252)

Preparation Tips:
1. Prepare Mexican Potato Salad the day before serving. Keep refrigerated until ready to serve.
2. Prepare Mexican Sugar Cookies* at least 2 hours before serving.
3. Prepare Mint Lamb Chops with Peanuts† through Step 3, 40 minutes before serving.
4. Prepare Glazed Carrots with Minced Shrimp‡ through Step 1, ½ hour before serving.
5. Finish preparation of Mint Lamb Chops with Peanuts 20 minutes before serving.
6. Finish preparation of Glazed Carrots with Minced Shrimp 10 minutes before serving.

* Allow 2 cookies per serving. Store remainder in tightly closed container.

† The Meat Stock (page 78) used in this recipe may be prepared and refrigerated up to 1 week before ready to use.

‡ Use ½ the recipe. Refrigerate or freeze remainder. If you are not allowed shellfish, substitute ¼ pound haddock, minced.

Dinner for 4

White Flour Tortillas (page 49)
Mixed Salad San Miguel (page 101)
Chicken with Figs and Lemons (page 141)
Saffron Noodles
Sponge Cake

Preparation Tips:
1. Prepare White Flour Tortillas up to 2 days before serving. Refrigerate 4 until ready to use. Freeze remainder.
2. Prepare sponge cake the day before serving. Keep refrigerated until ready to use.
3. Prepare Chicken with Figs and Lemons 1 hour and 20 minutes before serving.
4. Prepare 4 ounces of noodles with 1 strand of saffron added to the boiling water* 20 minutes before serving.
5. Prepare Mixed Salad San Miguel† 15 minutes before serving.

* Do not add salt to boiling water.
† The Hot-and-Sweet Dressing (page 228) used in this recipe may be prepared and refrigerated any time before ready to use.

Dinner for 4

Peppercorn Chicken Soup (page 94)
Broiled Sole with Lemon
Beans with Cheese (page 175)
Steamed Zucchini
Pineapple Gelatin

Preparation Tips:
1. Prepare pineapple gelatin the day before serving.
2. Prepare Peppercorn Chicken Soup 1 hour before serving.
3. Prepare Beans with Cheese* 25 minutes before serving.
4. Prepare broiled sole 20 minutes before serving. Garnish with lemon wedges.
5. Steam 2 zucchini, cut in 2-inch rounds, 10 minutes before serving.

* Use ½ the recipe. Refrigerate or freeze remainder. The Simple Beans (page 174) used in this recipe may be prepared and refrigerated the day before ready to use.

Dinner for 8

Puree of Squash Soup (page 89)
Sea Bass and Tomatoes (page 119)
Yellow Rice (page 190)
Rum Pears (page 254)

Preparation Tips:
1. Prepare Rum Pears through Step 3, 1¾ hours before serving.
2. Prepare Puree of Squash Soup through Step 1, 1 hour and 15 minutes before serving. Set aside.
3. Prepare Yellow Rice 1 hour before serving.
4. Continue preparation of Puree of Squash Soup through Step 2, 45 minutes before serving.
5. Finish preparation of Rum Pears 40 minutes before serving.
6. Prepare Sea Bass and Tomatoes ½ hour before serving.
7. Finish preparation of Puree of Squash Soup 15 minutes before serving.

Dinner for 8

Cucumber Salad La Jolla (page 100)
Mexican Pot Roast (page 153)
Spicy Potato Casserole (page 180)
Lima Beans and Tomatoes in Butter Sauce (page 199)
Pineapple and Bananas in Sherry (page 253)

Preparation Tips:
1. Prepare Mexican Pot Roast through Step 4, 2½ hours before serving.
2. Boil and mash potatoes 1 hour before serving. Set aside.
3. Finish preparation of Mexican Pot Roast 50 minutes before serving.
4. Finish preparation of Spicy Potato Casserole 40 minutes before serving.
5. Prepare Lima Beans and Tomatoes in Butter Sauce* ½ hour before serving.
6. Prepare Cucumber Salad La Jolla 15 minutes before serving.
7. Prepare Pineapple and Bananas in Sherry immediately before serving.

* The Chicken Stock (page 76) used in this recipe may be prepared and refrigerated up to 1 week before ready to use.

>◦▬◢▬◦<

Dinner for 8

Bread of the Dead (page 66)
Endive and Tomato Salad with Lemon Wedges
Chicken in Chile-Nut Sauce (page 139)
Vermicelli al dente
Steamed Green Beans with Unsalted Margarine
Kahlua Cream (page 250)

Preparation Tips:
1. Prepare Bread of the Dead* 4 hours before serving.
2. Prepare Kahlua Cream through Step 3, 2½ hours before serving.
3. Prepare Chicken in Chile-Nut Sauce through Step 2, 2 hours before serving.
4. Julienne endive and slice tomatoes 45 minutes before serving. Garnish with lemon wedges and refrigerate until ready to serve.
5. Finish preparation of Chicken in Chile-Nut Sauce ½ hour before serving.
6. Steam 1 pound of green beans 15 minutes before serving.
7. Boil 8 ounces of vermicelli† 10 minutes before serving.
8. Dab 1 tablespoon unsalted margarine over green beans immediately before serving.
9. Finish preparation of Kahlua Cream immediately before serving.

* Use ⅓ the recipe. Refrigerate or freeze remainder.
† Do not add salt to boiling water.

>◦▅▎▅◦<

Dinner for 8

Broccoli and Corn Soup (page 84)
Roast Pork Loin (page 162)
Baked Potatoes with Sour Cream
Salad of Colors (page 102)
Baked Apples

Preparation Tips:
1. Prepare Salad of Colors through Step 1, 3½ hours before serving.
2. Prepare Roast Pork Loin* through Step 6, 3 hours before serving.
3. Continue preparation of Salad of Colors through Step 3, 1½ hours before serving.
4. Prepare 8 small baked potatoes 1 hour before serving.
5. Prepare Broccoli and Corn Soup† 45 minutes before serving.
6. Prepare 8 baked apples ½ hour before serving.
7. Finish preparation of Roast Pork Loin 20 minutes before serving.
8. Finish preparation of Salad of Colors 5 minutes before serving.
9. Garnish each baked potato with 1 tablespoon of sour cream immediately before serving.

* The Meat Stock (page 78) used in this recipe may be prepared and refrigerated up to 1 week before ready to use.

† The Chicken Stock (page 76) used in this recipe may be prepared and refrigerated up to 1 week before ready to use. The Chili Powder (page 210) called for should be a staple in your pantry.

><|><|><|><|><

Buffet for 12

Mixed Salad San Miguel (page 101)
Oysters in Sherry-Tomato Sauce (page 129)
Cheese-Stuffed Chicken (page 132)
Mexican Baked Beans (page 176)
Fruit Puree (page 249)

Preparation Tips:
1. Prepare Mexican Baked Beans* 6 hours before serving.
2. Prepare Cheese-Stuffed Chicken† 1½ hours before serving.
3. Prepare Fruit Puree through Step 2, 1 hour before serving.
4. Prepare Oysters in Sherry-Tomato Sauce‡ through Step 3, 45 minutes before serving.
5. Finish preparations of Fruit Puree ½ hour before serving.
6. Prepare Mixed Salad San Miguel§ 15 minutes before serving.
7. Finish preparation of Oysters in Sherry-Tomato Sauce 5 minutes before serving.

* The Meat Stock (page 78) used in this recipe may be prepared and refrigerated up to 1 week before ready to use.

† Triple the recipe. The Chili Powder (page 210) used in this recipe should be a staple in your pantry.

‡ Double the recipe. The Chicken Stock (page 76) used in this recipe may be prepared and refrigerated up to 1 week before ready to use.

§ Triple the recipe. The Hot-and-Sweet Dressing (page 228) used in this recipe may be prepared and refrigerated any time before ready to use.

>◦▮▰▮▰▮◦<

Buffet for 12

Crudités
Cream Cheese Sauce (page 222)
Chicken and Shrimp Empanadas (page 54)
Beef Chile (page 150)
Sliced Peaches and Pears

Preparation Tips:

1. Prepare Cream Cheese Sauce* through Step 6, up to 2 weeks before serving. Keep refrigerated until ready to use.
2. Up to 2 days before serving, prepare crudités. Wrap in aluminum foil and keep refrigerated until ready to use.
3. Prepare Chicken and Shrimp Empanadas† through Step 7, 4½ hours before serving. Set aside.
4. Prepare Beef Chile 2½ hours before serving.
5. Finish preparation of Chicken and Shrimp Empanadas ½ hour before serving.
6. Finish preparation of Cream Cheese Sauce 5 minutes before serving.
7. Slice 6 peaches and core and slice 6 pears immediately before serving.

* Double the recipe.
† If you are not allowed shellfish, substitute ½ can (3¼ ounces) low-sodium tuna.

>◦▮▰▮▰▮◦<

Buffet for 16

Fish-Stuffed Eggplant (page 114)
Veal Loaf (page 167
Piquant Sour Cream Sauce (page 224)
Sweet Rice with Green Beans (page 189)
Raspberries and Peaches in Sherry (page 253)

Preparation Tips:

1. Prepare Piquant Sour Cream Sauce the day before serving. Cover and keep refrigerated until ready to use.
2. Prepare Fish-Stuffed Eggplant* 2 hours before serving.
3. Prepare Veal Loaf 1 hour and 15 minutes before serving.
4. Prepare Sweet Rice with Green Beans† ½ hour before serving.
5. Prepare Raspberries and Peaches in Sherry‡ 15 minutes before serving.

* Double the recipe. The Chili Powder (page 210) used in this recipe should be a staple in your pantry.
† Double the recipe. The Chicken Stock (page 76) used in this recipe may be prepared and refrigerated up to 1 week before ready to use.
‡ Double the recipe.

>◎▬▮▬◎<

Buffet for 16

Watercress and Mushroom Salad
Seafood Tamales (page 63)
Pineapple Chicken with Zucchini (page 145)
Boiled White Rice
Cabbage, Walnuts, and Pears (page 201)
Low-Sodium Cheddar Cheese

Preparation Tips:
1. Prepare Seafood Tamales* through Step 8, 3½ hours before serving. Set aside.
2. Chop and refrigerate 8 bunches of watercress and 16 mushrooms 1½ hours before serving.
3. Finish preparation of Seafood Tamales 1 hour and 20 minutes before serving.
4. Prepare Pineapple Chicken with Zucchini† through Step 1, 1 hour and 15 minutes before serving.
5. Prepare Cabbage, Walnuts, and Pears† 1 hour before serving.
6. Finish preparation of Pineapple Chicken with Zucchini 50 minutes before serving.
7. Prepare 4 cups of white rice ½ hour before serving.
8. Slice 1 pound of low-sodium Cheddar cheese immediately before serving.

* The Chile Powder (page 210) used in this recipe should be a staple in your pantry. If you are not allowed shellfish, replace the shrimp with 1 can (6½ ounces) low-sodium tuna.

† Double the recipe.

>◦▮▯▮◦<

Buffet for 24

Christmas Eve Salad (page 103)
Steak and Tomatoes (page 154)
Rice with Shrimp (page 187)
Creamed Cauliflower and Sweet Peppers (page 204)
Rum Apples (page 254)

Preparation Tips:
1. Prepare Christmas Eve Salad* 3 hours before serving. Keep refrigerated until ready to use.
2. Prepare Steak and Tomatoes† through Step 2, 2 hours before serving.
3. Prepare Rice with Shrimp‡ through Step 4, 1½ hours before serving.
4. Finish preparation of Steak and Tomatoes 1 hour before serving.
5. Prepare Rum Apples† 45 minutes before serving.
6. Prepare Creamed Cauliflower and Sweet Peppers† through Step 3, 40 minutes before serving.
7. Finish preparation of Rice with Shrimp 15 minutes before serving.
8. Finish preparation of Christmas Eve Salad 10 minutes before serving.
9. Finish preparation of Creamed Cauliflower and Sweet Peppers 5 minutes before serving.

* Triple the recipe. The Sweet Dressing (page 230) used in this recipe may be prepared and refrigerated up to 2 weeks before ready to use.
† Triple the recipe.
‡ Triple the recipe. The Chicken Stock (page 76) used in this recipe may be prepared and refrigerated up to 1 week before ready to serve. If you are not allowed shellfish, substitute 4 half chicken breasts, chopped into 2-inch pieces.

Buffet for 24

Mixed Green Salad with Grapefruit Sections
Festival Chicken in Wine (page 142)
Mexican Macaroni Salad (page 184)
Steamed Broccoli
Dessert Empanadas II (page 57)

Preparation Tips:
1. Prepare Mexican Macaroni Salad* the day before serving. Keep refrigerated until ready to use.
2. Prepare Dessert Empanadas II through Step 6, 3 hours before serving. Set aside.
3. Prepare Festival Chicken in Wine† 1½ hours before serving.
4. Prepare mixed greens with 3 grapefruits, peeled and sectioned, 45 minutes before serving. Keep refrigerated until ready to use.
5. Prepare 12 cups of broccoli flowerettes 20 minutes before serving.
6. Finish preparation of Dessert Empanadas II 15 minutes before serving.

* Double the recipe.
† Triple the recipe.

>◁▮▭▮▭▮◁<

Cocktails for 16

Corn Flour Tortillas (page 48)
Shrimp Salad Mazatlan (page 106)
Veal Balls in Sour Cream Sauce (page 166)
Vegetable-Stuffed Chiles (page 195)

Preparation Tips:
1. Prepare Corn Flour Tortillas up to 2 days before serving. Refrigerate 16 until ready to use. Freeze remainder.
2. Prepare Shrimp Salad Mazatlan* the day before serving. Keep refrigerated until ready to use.
3. Prepare Vegetable-Stuffed Chiles† through Step 8, 3 hours before serving. Set aside.
4. Prepare Veal Balls in Sour Cream Sauce‡ through Step 5, 2 hours before serving.
5. Finish preparation of Vegetable-Stuffed Chiles 45 minutes before serving.
6. Finish preparation of Veal Balls in Sour Cream Sauce 15 minutes before serving.

* Four times the recipe. If you are not allowed shellfish, substitute 4 cans (7¾ ounces each) low-sodium salmon.

† The Chile-Avocado Sause (page 214) used in this recipe may be prepared and refrigerated until ready to use.

‡ Double the recipe.

>⊙▉▮▯▉▮⊙<

Cocktails for 16

Crudités
Salmon and Caper Dip (page 36)
Guacamole (page 34)
Saucy Meat Balls (page 171)
Low-Sodium Swiss Cheese Cubes
Low-Sodium Crackers

Preparation Tips:

1. Prepare Guacamole* the day before serving. Keep refrigerated until ready to use.
2. Prepare Salmon and Caper Dip 4 hours before serving. Keep refrigerated until ready to use.
3. Prepare crudités of your choice 2½ hours before serving. Keep refrigerated until ready to use.
4. Prepare Saucy Meat Balls† 2 hours before serving.
5. Cut 1 pound of low-sodium Swiss cheese into 1-inch cubes 1 hour before serving. Let stand at room temperature until ready to use.

* Serve half the recipe. Refrigerate remainder up to 1 week. The Chile Powder (page 210) used in this recipe should be a staple in your pantry.

† Double the recipe. The Chicken Stock (page 76) used in this recipe may be prepared and refrigerated up to 1 week before ready to use.

>◦▬▮▬◦<

Cocktails for 24

Tacos (page 50)
Avocado, Cucumber, and Beet Dip (page 35)
Sour Cream Dip (page 37)
Chile-Tuna Salad (page 107)
Marinated Beef (page 44)
Mexican Deviled Eggs (page 240)

Preparation Tips:
1. Prepare Tacos, up to 2 days before serving, by dividing each corn tortilla ball into thirds and proceeding per directions. Keep refrigerated until ready to use.
2. Prepare Avocado, Cucumber, and Beet Dip,* Sour Cream Dip,* and Marinated Beef the day before serving.
3. Prepare Mexican Deviled Eggs† 3 hours before serving. Keep refrigerated until ready to use.
4. Prepare Chile-Tuna Salad‡ through Step 4, 2 hours before serving.
5. Finish preparation of Chile-Tuna Salad 5 minutes before serving.

* Double the recipe.
† Double the recipe. The Chili Powder (page 210) used in this recipe should be a staple in your pantry.
‡ Triple the recipe. The Chili Powder (page 210) used in this recipe should be a staple in your pantry.

>◠▮▬▮◠<

Cocktails for 24

Blanched Asparagus and Carrot Sticks
Low-Sodium Crackers
Chile-Cheddar Dip (page 35)
Sweet Hot Apple Relish (page 45)
Cold, Sliced London Broil
Low-Sodium Pickles
Tuna-Stuffed Mushrooms (page 39)

Preparation Tips:
1. Prepare Sweet Hot Apple Relish the day before serving. Refrigerate 4 cups until ready to use and freeze remainder.
2. Prepare London broil 2½ hours before serving. Slice thin and roll each slice around 1 low-sodium pickle slice. Cover and refrigerate until ready to use.
3. Blanch asparagus and carrot sticks 1½ hours before serving. Keep refrigerated until ready to use.
4. Prepare Chile-Cheddar Dip* through Step 1, 1 hour before serving.
5. Prepare Tuna-Stuffed Mushrooms† 45 minutes before serving.
6. Finish preparation of Chile-Cheddar Dip 20 minutes before serving.

* The Basic Salsa (page 210) used in this recipe may be prepared and refrigerated up to 3 weeks before ready to use.
† Double the recipe.

>●❮■❯/■❮●<

Cocktails for 32

Tacos (page 50)
Eggplant and Apple Dip (page 38)
Chicken Salad Cozumel (page 104)
Pickled Ceviche (page 43)
Beef and Cheese Tamales (page 62)

Preparation Tips:
1. Prepare Tacos up to 2 days before serving by dividing each corn tortilla ball into thirds and proceeding per directions. Keep refrigerated until ready to use.
2. Prepare Eggplant and Apple Dip* the day before serving. Keep refrigerated until ready to use.
3. Prepare Pickled Ceviche† 6 hours before serving. Keep refrigerated until ready to use.
4. Prepare Chicken Salad Cozumel‡ through Step 1 only, 5 hours before serving. Keep refrigerated until ready to use.
5. Prepare Beef and Cheese Tamales§ 4 hours before serving.

* Serve 4 cups. Refrigerate remainder up to 1 week. The Chili Powder (page 210) used in this recipe should be a staple in your pantry.

† Four times the recipe.

‡ Four times the recipe. The Sweet Dressing (page 230) used in this recipe may be prepared and refrigerated up to 3 weeks before ready to use.

§ Double the recipe and cut each tamale in half.

>⊲▮▬▮▰▮◖<

Cocktails for 32

Low-Sodium Crackers
Low-Sodium Cottage Cheese and Scallion Dip
Picadillo with Vegetables (page 169)
Avocado and Caper Canapés (page 40)
Cucumber and Chorizo Canapés (page 41)
Fruit Juice Chicken Wings (page 44)

Preparation Tips:
1. Prepare Avocado and Caper Canapés* through Step 2, 3 hours before serving. Keep refrigerated until ready to use.
2. Prepare low-sodium cottage cheese and scallion dip, 2½ hours before serving, by mixing 4 pints of low-sodium cottage cheese with 1 tablespoon of dried dill and 6 scallions, chopped, including greens. Cover and keep refrigerated until ready to use.
3. Prepare Picadillo with Vegetables through Step 3, 1½ hours before serving.
4. Prepare Cucumber and Chorizo Canapés† through Step 2, 45 minutes before serving. Set aside.
5. Finish preparation of Picadillo with Vegetables ½ hour before serving.
6. Prepare Fruit Juice Chicken Wings‡ 20 minutes before serving.
7. Finish preparation of Cucumber and Chorizo Canapés 10 minutes before serving.

* Double the recipe.
† Four times the recipe.
‡ Double the recipe. The Fruit Juice Dressing (page 226) used in this recipe may be prepared and refrigerated up to 3 weeks before ready to use.

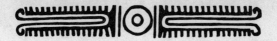

A Mexican Diet

On the surface, dieting and Mexican food are antithetical: one signaling restriction, deprivation, and lackluster meals; the other, sumptuous, rich, and, yes, fattening fare. Yet, break down the elements of Mexican cuisine, and you will discover the fundamentals of good nutrition to underscore what can be a thoroughly soul-satisfying dietary way of life.

Since the days of the Mexican Indian, corn and beans have been the mainstays of the people's diet. These complex carbohydrates fuel the brain and body with energy and help metabolize fat.

Recent studies at the University of Kentucky indicate that navy and pinto beans may contribute to the body's well-being in other ways as well. On the one hand, they may slow production of cholesterol in the liver; on the other, they can speed up removal of excess cholesterol in the blood. This same research also suggests that beans help keep blood sugar under control.

In addition to beans and corn, complex carbohydrates are found in rice, potatoes, grains and wheat, fruit, and vegetables. In Mexico's temperate climate, these essential foods flourish in the fertile lowlands along the enormous stretches of the country's coastline. Accordingly, based on production alone, the Mexican diet is more than able to meet the nutrition and medical standards which recommend that complex carbohydrates comprise one half to two thirds of our daily food consumption.

If the body does not get the proper amount of carbohydrates, it starts to feed off its own protein, resulting in weakened muscles, flabbiness, and malnutrition. Athletes have long known this, which is why their main meal, especially before a competition, contains a generous amount of these necessary and, yes, slenderizing nutrients.

So forget the myth. Potatoes, pasta, beans and rice are not loaded with fattening calories. The truth is that they provide more mileage per calorie than any other food, and make up the one group your body cannot live without.

The Pacific Ocean and the warm waters of the Gulf of Mexico spawn a rich selection of seafood which provides much of the country's protein. In fact, fish is a perfect food for dieters because it is high in protein but low in calories, fat, and sodium. Fish is also a valuable source of bone-building calcium. What is more, certain oily species, like salmon and mackerel, contain fatty acids which help lower cholesterol in the bloodstream.

Shellfish, though delicious, are not as good for everyone. Their relatively high sodium content makes them taboo for many low-sodium dieters. In addition, some people suffer severe allergic reactions to the concentrated levels of iodine that shellfish contain.

However, on balance, the seas which buttress Mexico on three sides yield one of nature's healthiest harvests.

Cattle which graze on the vast coastal and central plains, pigs which thrive in the mountain regions, and chickens which roost everywhere, also contribute the protein so necessary for developing muscle and toning the body. The truth is, Mexicans have such an array of fish, meat, and poultry from which to choose that they tend to consume somewhat more protein than is good for them.

Too much protein forces fluids—and, accordingly, important nutrients like potassium and calcium—from the body by putting extreme pressure on the kidneys. As a result, the body becomes dehydrated and vulnerable to toxicity, and the kidneys may sustain irreparable damage. Moreover, this sequence can set off a chain reaction which exerts severe stress on other vital organs, ultimately destroying them.

That is why we should always be wary of the high-protein and/or car-bohydrate-deficient fad diets which trick the body into rapid weight loss (generally water only, not fat). Such diets always fail in the end, but not before they can render permanent injury.

For all these reasons, in this book, we have adjusted the amount of protein in every dish and in this diet to correspond with the 20 to 25 percent daily protein allotment most experts prescribe.

Even the most rigid of diets requires some fat, both to grease the way for easier ingestion of other nutrients and to supply concentrated energy. Indeed, fat should account for 25 to 30 percent of our daily intake.

However, the type of fat is important. Vegetable fats, including corn and olive oils, margarine and mayonnaise, are much preferred to animal fats, like lard and butter. Very simply, the former either lower or have no effect on the level of cholesterol in the blood. The latter definitely increase it.

Thus, while the jury is still out on cholesterol's link to heart disease, it pays to be safe rather than sorry. Consequently, when adapting an authentic Mexican recipe which calls for animal (saturated) fats, we have taken the liberty of switching to one of the healthier (polyunsaturated or monounsaturated) cooking oils noted above.

If nutritional balance is important, so are eating habits which, in Mexico, are impeccable. To wit, Mexicans have always known that a hearty, robust breakfast, packed with nutritional value and energy, is the best way to start one's day. Their menu—eggs for protein, tortillas and/or beans for carbohydrates, fruit and vegetables for fiber, a little fat to grease the way—is sure to convince you that a Mexican breakfast is also the tastiest way to greet the sun.

Moreover, *comida*, the day's main meal, is served in the afternoon between 2:00 and 4:00. This custom is rooted, in part, in the superstition that eating late at night in the country's high altitudes will make one ill. That may or may not be the case. However, the practice is a good one because digestion and efficient burning of calories are easier and healthier during the day than in the evening when we in the United States eat our heaviest meal. So it is that Mexicans also end the day wisely with their lightest meal. Called the *cena*, it generally consists of a light snack accompanied by a beverage.

Mexican food is such a wonderful experience, it deserves to be relished bite by delectable bite. In this regard, we can take our lead from the Mexicans themselves, who really know how to enjoy their food.

In their homes, mealtime is a leisurely affair, each dish savored slowly in the midst of rollicking socializing with family and friends. This tradition is not only pleasant, but healthy as well and sets an excellent example for those of us who wolf down our food, scarcely knowing or tasting what we are eating.

What we eat and how are the keys to a healthy diet. However, those of us with special diet needs have a few additional considerations.

To explain, those of us with hypertension, cardiovascular disease, arteriosclerosis, kidney dysfunction, or edema must limit not only our salt intake but fat and calories as well. Those with hypoglycemia or diabetes must monitor and control sugar and/or complex carbohydrate consumption, and must also be prudent about fat, salt, and calories.

The common denominator for us all is to avoid weight gain and, for some of us, to shed health-threatening pounds. The reason is simple. Extra pounds quite literally weigh us down, and our bodies have to exert extra effort to carry the load. Think how much easier it is to lift an empty suitcase than it is to struggle up a flight of stairs with one crammed full, and you will begin to understand the burden a mere five pounds can put on that delicate machine we call the body.

Such strain can create physical anxiety and stress, which in turn, can cause blood pressure to soar, blood sugar to shoot up, and the vital organs —like the heart, lungs and kidneys—to work unnaturally hard to rid the body of waste and impurities.

If this sounds a little frightening, calm yourself. The body is as resilient as it is delicate and will respond to care and respect. The simplest and wisest way to address our individual and, in some instances, mutual requirements is to follow a balanced and healthy eating program.

You are probably thinking, easier said than done. Indeed, which one of us has not experienced the physical and emotional rigors of dieting. Bland, tasteless food, predictable, inflexible routines, and chronic hunger pains eventually lead to cheating or total abandonment. In short, most diets are a perfect Catch-22, wickedly designed to trap us into failure.

However, history does not have to repeat itself because, with a few minor adjustments, Mexican food is excellent for dieters, whatever their concerns may be. As we explained, the nutritional basics are there, and, happily, the variety of taste experiences in Mexican cuisine will take the onus off dieting—so much so, it will not seem like dieting at all. With a minor change here and there, a Mexican diet will help you to easily make the transition to a healthier, happier, and thinner way of life.

As for the particulars, using the recipes in this book, we have prepared a diet based on the following:

1. *Two weeks' duration* because it takes at least this long for your palate to adjust to the absence of salt and to appreciate new flavors. After the initial two-week period, you can repeat the basic plan with different dishes.
2. *Under 1200 calories* to show you how much food and satisfaction you can have and still lose weight.

   To determine the proper calorie level for yourself, keep the following points in mind:

   • If you want to maintain your weight, multiply your ideal weight by 13.5 to determine your daily calorie level.
   • If you want to lose weight—or gain it for that matter—just remember that slowly and steadily is the safest, healthiest way to reach and hold on to your goal. That translates to a one-and-a-half-pound gain or loss over a two-week period.

     Add to that the knowledge that 3,500 calories equal one pound. So if you cut out 250 calories per day, you will lose that pound in 14 days; add the same 250 calories, you will gain that pound in the pre-scribed time.

3. *Under 500 milligrams sodium* to prove how easy it is to live and dine happily and deliciously on a so-called restricted diet.

   If your sodium limits—self-imposed or otherwise—are more liberal, consult a sodium guide (some of which are listed in this book's bibliography) to see what additional options are available to you.

   For example, if you love calf's liver or shrimp, enjoy them. Just remember to stay within your limits and not to exceed 1,500 milligrams per day, more than enough sodium for anyone.

   If, like me, you must get by with less than 500 milligrams sodium per day, just replace all shellfish on the menu with meat, poultry, or another fish. Or delete some dairy products. It is just that simple.

At the end of these two weeks, we hope you will realize that a diet is neither a curse nor a punishment. It is not one of life's aberrations but rather the way of life which is healthiest and best for you.

With Mexican food, it can also be fun and more tasty than you would have thought possible.

Note: The menus on the following pages were specifically designed for the salt-free dieter. Thus, if you do use sugar substitutes, please be sure they are not only sugar-free but low-sodium (calcium saccharin or Nutra-sweet) as well.

In addition, much consideration was given to the needs of those with diabetes, which accounts for the carbohydrate snacks throughout the day. (By the way, deliciously healthy, energy-releasing snacking is good for all of us and helps cut down the urge to splurge.) But if you are a diabetic, pass on sugary desserts and, in fact, check this program with your own doctor or nutritionist to see if adjustments are necessary.

One final word. Read the entire diet before you begin. It contains a lot of tips, such as using leftovers and switching meals, designed to save you time and work, and make it both easy and pleasant for you to stick to your goal.

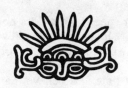

TIPS FOR DAY ONE

Take a deep breath and smile, for the diet you are about to begin will hardly seem like a diet at all, being so chock full of tasty, even so-called fattening foods like potatoes, beans, rice, and cheese.

Just remember a few tips:

1. Do not skip meals or snacks. Diet does not mean starvation. Rather, the body needs proper nourishment now and always.

2. Enjoy yourself. You will see that bland, boring foods are *not* the price you have to pay for a slim, healthy body.

3. Take it one day at a time and believe that at the end of two weeks, you will feel and look better than ever. You will also know the secret and have the control for staying that way.

4. Now—go for it.

	Calories	Sodium (mg.)	Carbo-hydrates (gm.)	Fat (gm.)
BREAKFAST				
½ grapefruit	62.9	1.4	16.4	0.14
1 boiled egg	78.0	55.0	0.4	4.3
1 Corn Tortilla*	86.1	1.2	17.3	0.2
Coffee or tea	—	—	—	—
1 teaspoon sugar substitute	2.0	0	1.4	0
1 tablespoon low-fat milk	6.3	7.1	0.75	0.1
Total	235.3	64.7	36.3	4.7

* See index for recipe page number.

	Calories	Sodium (mg.)	Carbo-hydrates (gm.)	Fat (gm.)
LUNCH				
Chile-Tuna Salad*	183.2	61.8	11.5	6.5
1 cup steamed broccoli	36.6	0.3	6.7	17.1
Coffee or tea	—	—	—	—
1 teaspoon sugar substitute	2.0	0	1.4	0
1 tablespoon low-fat milk	6.3	7.1	0.75	0.1
Total	228.1	69.2	20.4	23.7
SNACK				
½ ounce low-sodium Swiss cheese	50.7	4.0	0.3	3.9
2 low-sodium crackers	22.0	1.7	2.9	1.0
Iced tea with lemon	—	—	—	—
Total	72.7	5.7	3.2	4.9
DINNER				
½ cup chopped watercress	9.5	26.0	0.3	0.2
½ cup shredded lettuce	9.0	4.5	1.8	0.2
2 tablespoons Hot-and-Sweet Dressing*	64.0	0.8	0.6	6.2
Sherry Veal Chops* (use apricots)	240.8	58.7	16.7	14.0
Spicy Potato Casserole*	107.8	12.4	23.2	0.4
Lime Eggplant with Tomatoes*	68.0	13.8	14.4	1.0
Mexican Sugar Cookies* (1)	67.3	3.1	9.1	2.8
Coffee or tea	—	—	—	—
1 teaspoon sugar substitute	2.0	0	1.4	0
1 tablespoon low-fat milk	6.3	7.1	0.75	0.1
Total	574.7	126.4	68.3	24.9
SNACK				
1 pear	62.0	2.0	15.3	0.4
Grand Total	1,172.8	268.0	143.5	58.6

* See index for recipe page number.

TIPS FOR DAY TWO

The first day was not so hard, was it? You should be feeling your first rush of confidence. Well done.

If you have leftover Chile-Tuna Salad, you may store it in a plastic container and refrigerate up to three days. You can also enjoy it today for lunch in place of Cabbage Soup Veracruz or on Day Four for lunch instead of Snapper Yucatan.

Day Two awaits your pleasure.

	Calories	Sodium (mg.)	Carbo-hydrates (gm.)	Fat (gm.)
BREAKFAST				
3½ ounces low-sodium tomato juice	19.0	3.0	4.3	0.1
¼ cup low-sodium cottage cheese	45.0	31.0	4.0	1.0
1 Crescent Roll*	126.9	7.3	22.8	1.6
Coffee or tea	—	—	—	—
1 teaspoon sugar substitute	2.0	0	1.4	0
1 tablespoon low-fat milk	6.3	7.1	0.75	0.1
Total	199.2	48.4	33.3	2.8

* See index for recipe page number.

	Calories	Sodium (mg.)	Carbo-hydrates (gm.)	Fat (gm.)
LUNCH				
Cabbage Soup Veracruz*	171.5	55.6	16.5	7.9
Cauliflower Salad*	137.8	26.9	12.5	9.0
Coffee or tea	—	—	—	—
1 teaspoon sugar substitute	2.0	0	1.4	0
1 tablespoon low-fat milk	6.3	7.1	0.75	0.1
Total	317.6	89.6	31.2	17.0
SNACK				
½ cup pineapple	26.0	0.5	6.9	0.1
DINNER				
1 cup chopped lettuce	18.0	9.0	3.5	0.3
1 tablespoon lemon juice	1.7	0.1	0.7	0.1
1 tablespoon Sour Cream Dressing*	26.5	3.0	2.4	2.2
Chicken in Orange-Mint Sauce*	236.4	57.2	35.0	3.2
Cheesy Hot Noodles*	149.1	14.3	24.5	2.3
Asparagus in Crumb Sauce*	114.0	10.0	11.9	6.4
Coffee or tea	—	—	—	—
1 teaspoon sugar substitute	2.0	0	1.4	0
1 tablespoon low-fat milk	6.3	7.1	0.75	0.1
Total	554.0	100.7	80.2	14.6
SNACK				
Raspberries and Peaches in Sherry*	97.2	1.8	14.3	4.5
Grand Total	1,194.0	241.0	165.9	39.0

* See index for recipe page number.

TIPS FOR DAY THREE

With two days behind you and a day full of sumptuous meals ahead, you might be wondering if you will really lose weight on a diet so pleasant. Well, do not worry. You will. Think back to what we said on Day One: dieting is not punishment.

Now for Day Three:

If you have leftover Cabbage Soup Veracruz, you may store it in a plastic container and refrigerate up to one week, or serve it for lunch on Day Seven in place of Swordfish and Capers.

If you have leftover Cauliflower Salad and Cheesy Hot Noodles, these, too, can be refrigerated in plastic containers up to one week. Or enjoy both for lunch today in place of the Poached Chicken in Chile-Cream Sauce and the green beans. You might also reheat the Cheesy Hot Noodles for dinner on Day Seven instead of the Simple Beans.

In other words, as long as the nutritional values are about the same and you maintain a balanced diet, you can always exchange dishes at will.

As for the Raspberries and Peaches in Sherry, this dish is so delicious you might want to have it every day. If not, it too will keep up to one week if refrigerated in a plastic container.

One thing more, if you need to limit your daily sodium intake to 250 milligrams, substitute ¾ cup white rice and ½ cup Basic Salsa* for the Beans with Chorizo and Salsa listed on the dinner menu.

	Calories	Sodium (mg.)	Carbo-hydrates (gm.)	Fat (gm.)
BREAKFAST				
½ cup strawberries	20.8	0.7	5.5	0.3
½ cup oatmeal	62.9	2.0	11.1	1.1
¼ cup low-fat milk	25.0	28.6	3.0	0.5
Coffee or tea	—	—	—	—
1 teaspoon sugar substitute	2.0	0	1.4	0
1 tablespoon low-fat milk	6.3	7.1	0.75	0.1
Total	117.0	38.4	21.8	2.0

* See index for recipe page number.

	Calories	Sodium (mg.)	Carbo-hydrates (gm.)	Fat (gm.)
LUNCH				
1 cup chopped lettuce	18.0	9.0	3.5	0.3
Poached Chicken in Chile-Cream Sauce*	223.7	66.8	10.5	8.1
1 cup steamed green beans	32.0	7.0	0.2	7.1
Coffee or tea	—	—	—	—
1 teaspoon sugar substitute	2.0	0	1.4	0
1 tablespoon low-fat milk	6.3	7.1	0.75	0.1
Total	282.0	89.9	16.4	15.6
SNACK				
½ ounce low-sodium mozzarella cheese	42.5	4.3	0.3	3.5
1 Corn Tortilla*	86.1	1.2	17.3	0.2
Iced tea with lemon	—	—	—	—
Total	128.6	5.5	17.6	3.7
DINNER				
1 cup chopped lettuce	18.0	9.0	3.5	0.3
¼ green pepper, sliced	11.0	6.5	2.4	0.1
2 tablespoons red wine vinegar	2.0	2.0	1.6	0
Snapper Yucatan*	198.4	94.4	14.8	5.4
Beans with Chorizo and Salsa*	256.6	45.9	32.2	8.2
Coffee or tea	—	—	—	—
1 teaspoon sugar substitute	2.0	0	1.4	0
1 tablespoon low-fat milk	6.3	7.1	0.75	0.1
Total	494.3	164.9	56.7	14.1
SNACK				
Almond Pudding*	120.9	0.5	16.0	4.1
Grand Total	1,142.8	299.2	128.5	39.5

* See index for recipe page number.

TIPS FOR DAY FOUR

By now, although you might not see a weight loss on the scale, you should feel thinner and less weighed down. And when you feel good, you generate that feeling to everyone, and they return it to you.

So keep up the good work. The first pound or two will be slipping off soon.

If you still have any Poached Chicken in Chile-Cream Sauce, you may store it up to two days in the refrigerator, tightly wrapped in aluminum foil. Or you may want to have it for dinner tonight or tomorrow in place of the main dishes suggested.

Leftover Beans with Chorizo and Salsa will keep up to two days in the refrigerator, or may be frozen up to one month in plastic containers.

As for the Almond Pudding, it will not stay fresh much more than a day. But there is very little chance of any waste. It is so good, you will no doubt have plenty of hungry helpers.

If you need to reduce your sodium, substitute the Chile-Tuna Salad leftover from Day One for the Snapper Yucatan at lunch; and replace the cucumber at dinner with two radishes.

Have a good day.

	Calories	Sodium (mg.)	Carbo-hydrates (gm.)	Fat (gm.)
BREAKFAST				
3½ ounces cranberry juice	65.0	1.0	16.5	0.1
Huevos Rancheros*	241.6	64.8	24.7	10.3
Coffee or tea	—	—	—	—
1 teaspoon sugar substitute	2.0	0	1.4	0
1 tablespoon low-fat milk	6.3	7.1	0.75	0.1
Total	314.9	72.9	43.4	10.5

* See index for recipe page number.

	Calories	Sodium (mg.)	Carbo-hydrates (gm.)	Fat (gm.)
LUNCH				
1 cup shredded lettuce	18.0	9.0	3.5	0.3
½ tomato, chopped	15.7	2.1	3.4	0.1
1 scallion, chopped, including greens	10.3	1.4	0.6	2.3
2 tablespoons lemon juice	3.3	0.1	1.3	0.1
Snapper Yucatan*	198.4	94.4	14.8	5.4
Coffee or tea	—	—	—	—
1 teaspoon sugar substitute	2.0	0	1.4	0
1 tablespoon low-fat milk	6.3	7.1	0.75	0.1
Total	254.0	114.1	25.8	8.3
SNACK				
1 banana	86.0	1.0	22.0	0.2
DINNER				
1 cup shredded lettuce	18.0	9.0	3.5	0.3
¼ cucumber, sliced	41.0	17.7	2.9	0.1
¼ green pepper, sliced	11.0	6.5	2.4	0.1
2 tablespoons Onion Sauce*	24.2	4.6	3.2	1.4
Festival Chicken in Wine*	218.8	64.5	23.4	3.6
Potatoes with Chiles*	119.0	12.2	36.6	11.8
Coffee or tea	—	—	—	—
1 teaspoon sugar substitute	2.0	0	1.4	0
1 tablespoon low-fat milk	6.3	7.1	0.75	0.1
Total	440.3	121.6	74.2	17.4
SNACK				
1 orange	98.0	2.0	24.4	0.4
Grand Total	1,193.2	311.6	189.8	36.8

* See index for recipe page number.

TIPS FOR DAY FIVE

Almost through the first week, and you are probably noticing some changes other than what your scale and mirror tell you. For one thing, I would bet you attack your meals with gusto and are really enjoying your food for the first time in years. Tasting it, too, for without salt, which masks it, the true, good flavor of food comes through.

What is more, I am also sure this is the first diet you have been on without experiencing hunger pains.

Feeling pretty good about yourself? Well, you have every right.

Any leftover Potatoes with Chiles can be reheated for dinner tonight in place of Rice with Tomatoes.

	Calories	Sodium (mg.)	Carbo-hydrates (gm.)	Fat (gm.)
BREAKFAST				
½ cup blueberries	62.0	1.0	15.3	0.5
¼ cup plain yogurt	70.9	53.7	5.6	3.9
1 slice Comb Bread*	110.5	3.2	19.9	1.4
Coffee or tea	—	—	—	—
1 teaspoon sugar substitute	2.0	0	1.4	0
1 tablespoon low-fat milk	6.3	7.1	0.75	0.1
Total	251.7	65.0	43.0	5.9

* See index for recipe page number.

	Calories	Sodium (mg.)	Carbo-hydrates (gm.)	Fat (gm.)
LUNCH				
1 cup shredded lettuce	18.0	9.0	3.5	0.3
½ tomato, sliced	15.7	2.1	3.4	0.1
2 tablespoons lemon juice	3.3	0.1	1.3	0.1
Festival Chicken in Wine*	218.8	64.5	23.4	3.6
Coffee or tea	—	—	—	—
1 teaspoon sugar substitute	2.0	0	1.4	0
1 tablespoon low-fat milk	6.3	7.1	0.75	0.1
Total	264.1	82.8	33.8	4.2
SNACK				
½ grapefruit	62.9	1.4	16.4	0.14
DINNER				
Steak with Chile Strips*	253.9	58.1	4.6	12.8
Rice with Tomatoes*	226.4	20.3	44.7	3.2
Cabbage, Walnuts, and Pears*	82.0	14.7	13.5	3.2
Coffee or tea	—	—	—	—
1 teaspoon sugar substitute	2.0	0	1.4	0
1 tablespoon low-fat milk	6.3	7.1	0.75	0.1
Total	570.6	100.2	65.0	19.3
SNACK				
1 serving low-sodium lime gelatin	9.0	11.0	0	0
Grand Total	1,158.3	260.4	158.2	29.5

* See index for recipe page number.

TIPS FOR DAY SIX

Now is the time to think about a treat for yourself as you close in on Week One. Maybe a sweater you have had your eye on, or tickets to a play. Reward is a wonderful incentive, and you deserve it.

	Calories	Sodium (mg.)	Carbo-hydrates (gm.)	Fat (gm.)
BREAKFAST				
½ cup grapes	39.4	1.7	9.0	0.6
¼ cup low-sodium cottage cheese	45.0	31.0	4.0	1.0
1 Crescent Roll*	126.9	7.3	22.8	1.6
Coffee or tea	—	—	—	—
1 teaspoon sugar substitute	2.0	0	1.4	0
1 tablespoon low-fat milk	6.3	7.1	0.75	0.1
Total	219.6	47.1	38.0	3.3
LUNCH				
½ cup chopped watercress	9.5	26.0	0.3	0.2
Chicken Salad Cozumel*	253.3	45.8	22.5	12.7
Coffee or tea	—	—	—	—
1 teaspoon sugar substitute	2.0	0	1.4	0
1 tablespoon low-fat milk	6.3	7.1	0.75	0.1
Total	271.1	78.9	25.0	13.0

* See index for recipe page number.

	Calories	Sodium (mg.)	Carbo-hydrates (gm.)	Fat (gm.)
SNACK				
½ ounce low-sodium Swiss cheese	50.7	4.0	0.3	3.9
2 low-sodium crackers	22.0	1.7	2.9	1.0
Iced tea with lemon	—	—	—	—
Total	72.7	5.7	3.2	4.9
DINNER				
Green Bean and Sweet Pepper Salad*	75.5	12.7	8.8	4.6
Swordfish and Capers*	171.7	11.8	7.4	5.3
Baked Stuffed Potatoes*	183.0	21.9	19.3	9.2
Lima Beans and Tomatoes in Butter Sauce*	85.5	7.9	12.1	3.4
Coffee or tea	—	—	—	—
1 teaspoon sugar substitute	2.0	0	1.4	0
1 tablespoon low-fat milk	6.3	7.1	0.75	0.1
Total	524.0	61.4	49.8	22.6
SNACK				
1 peach	43.4	1.1	11.1	0.1
Grand Total	1,130.8	194.2	127.1	43.9

* See index for recipe page number.

TIPS FOR DAY SEVEN

One week down and one to go. And to celebrate, delectable dining throughout the day.

If you have leftover Baked Stuffed Potatoes, wrap tightly in aluminum foil and refrigerate up to four days. Reheat and serve for dinner in place of beans or rice on Days Seven, Eight, or Eleven, if you desire.

As for the Lima Beans and Tomatoes in Butter Sauce, they will keep up to three days if refrigerated in plastic containers. You might want to substitute them for the Peas and Almonds at dinner on Day Ten.

Clear sailing from here. So hoist your sails and anchors aweigh.

	Calories	Sodium (mg.)	Carbo- hydrates (gm.)	Fat (gm.)
BRUNCH				
½ grapefruit	62.9	1.4	16.4	0.14
Pork and Cheese Tamales*	218.5	16.0	25.4	8.5
Coffee or tea	—	—	—	—
1 teaspoon sugar substitute	2.0	0	1.4	0
1 tablespoon low-fat milk	6.3	7.1	0.75	0.1
Total	289.7	24.5	44.0	8.7

* See index for recipe page number.

	Calories	Sodium (mg.)	Carbo-hydrates (gm.)	Fat (gm.)
LUNCH				
1 cup shredded lettuce	18.0	9.0	3.5	0.3
¼ green pepper, chopped	11.0	6.5	2.4	0.1
2 tablespoons cider vinegar	2.0	2.0	1.6	0
Swordfish and Capers*	171.7	11.8	7.4	5.3
Creamed Cauliflower and Sweet Peppers*	66.5	22.5	5.8	4.5
Coffee or tea	—	—	—	—
1 teaspoon sugar substitute	2.0	0	1.4	0
1 tablespoon low-fat milk	6.3	7.1	0.75	0.1
Total	277.5	58.9	22.9	10.3
SNACK				
Melon Soup*	93.4	43.3	10.4	3.8
DINNER				
Cucumber Salad La Jolla*	98.3	22.6	6.0	4.3
Pineapple Chicken with Zucchini*	190.6	62.5	14.2	3.4
Simple Beans*	143.8	12.1	24.6	2.6
Coffee or tea	—	—	—	—
1 teaspoon sugar substitute	2.0	0	1.4	0
1 tablespoon low-fat milk	6.3	7.1	0.75	0.1
Total	441.0	104.3	47.0	10.4
SNACK				
¼ cup low-sodium cottage cheese	45.0	31.0	4.0	1.0
2 low-sodium crackers	22.0	1.7	2.9	1.0
Total	67.0	32.7	6.9	2.0
Grand Total	1,168.6	263.7	131.2	35.2

* See index for recipe page number.

TIPS FOR DAY EIGHT

As you start your second week, you should be on a mental and physical high—actually feeling stronger and confident you can reach your goal.

Those feelings will continue to build. So hang in there.

If you have leftover Cucumber Salad La Jolla, you may have it for dinner tonight instead of the suggested mixed salad. Leftover Simple Beans may be stored in a plastic container and refrigerated up to one week, or frozen up to one month. You may choose to serve them for dinner on Days Eleven or Twelve instead of the respective rice and bean dishes recommended. If so, reheat with one cup of Chicken Stock for a new and fresh flavor.

For today, if the sodium count exceeds your limit, simply eliminate the egg at breakfast and replace it with ½ ounce low-sodium Cheddar cheese plus one pat unsalted margarine.

	Calories	Sodium (mg.)	Carbo-hydrates (gm.)	Fat (gm.)
BREAKFAST				
½ cup strawberries	20.8	0.7	5.5	0.3
1 boiled egg	78.0	55.0	0.4	4.3
1 slice Mexican Sweet Bread*	133.1	6.3	24.0	1.8
Coffee or tea	—	—	—	—
1 teaspoon sugar substitute	2.0	0	1.4	0
1 tablespoon low-fat milk	6.3	7.1	0.75	0.1
Total	240.2	69.1	32.1	6.5

* See index for recipe page number.

	Calories	Sodium (mg.)	Carbo-hydrates (gm.)	Fat (gm.)
LUNCH				
1 cup shredded lettuce	18.0	9.0	3.5	0.3
Pineapple Chicken with Zucchini*	190.6	62.5	14.2	3.5
Coffee or tea	—	—	—	—
1 teaspoon sugar substitute	2.0	0	1.4	0
1 tablespoon low-fat milk	6.3	7.1	0.75	0.1
Total	216.9	78.6	19.9	3.9
SNACK				
½ ounce low-sodium Gouda cheese	56.9	6.0	0.3	4.6
2 low-sodium crackers	22.0	1.7	2.9	1.0
Iced tea with lemon	—	—	—	—
Total	78.9	7.7	3.2	5.6
DINNER				
1 cup shredded lettuce	18.0	9.0	3.5	0.3
½ tomato, chopped	15.7	2.1	3.4	0.1
2 radishes, sliced	4.9	5.1	0.03	1.0
2 tablespoons cider vinegar	2.0	2.0	1.6	0
Haddock in Walnut Sauce*	194.5	87.7	12.4	5.9
Rice with Eggplant*	225.7	25.0	44.6	3.2
Coffee or tea	—	—	—	—
1 teaspoon sugar substitute	2.0	0	1.4	0
1 tablespoon low-fat milk	6.3	7.1	0.75	0.1
Total	469.1	138.0	67.7	10.6
SNACK				
½ cup grapes	39.4	1.7	9.0	0.6
Grand Total	1,044.5	295.1	131.9	27.2

* See index for recipe page number.

TIPS FOR DAY NINE

There is a special treat in store for dessert tonight just to prove how much food you can enjoy with your newfound life-style. And since by now you have surely seen a weight loss and know the diet works, you can relish this goody without guilt or fear.

If you need to reduce your sodium intake today, replace the yogurt and crackers on the breakfast menu with one slice of low-sodium bread and one pat unsalted margarine. In addition, substitute ½ cup shredded lettuce for the watercress at lunch.

By the way, leftover Rice with Eggplant can be refrigerated up to three days if stored in a plastic container. You might want to enjoy it again on Day Eleven instead of Yellow Rice. If so, try baking it for 45 minutes at 325° with ½ cup Chicken Stock to keep it moist.

You are in the swing of things now. Keep it up.

	Calories	Sodium (mg.)	Carbo- hydrates (gm.)	Fat (gm.)
BREAKFAST				
½ cup pineapple	26.0	0.5	6.9	0.1
¼ cup plain yogurt	70.9	53.7	5.6	3.9
2 low-sodium crackers	22.0	1.7	2.9	1.0
Coffee or tea	—	—	—	—
1 teaspoon sugar substitute	2.0	0	1.4	0
1 tablespoon low-fat milk	6.3	7.1	0.75	0.1
Total	127.2	63.0	17.6	5.1

* See index for recipe page number.

	Calories	Sodium (mg.)	Carbo-hydrates (gm.)	Fat (gm.)
LUNCH				
½ cup chopped watercress	9.5	26.0	0.3	0.2
¼ cucumber, sliced	41.0	17.7	2.9	0.1
2 tablespoons lime juice	3.3	0.1	1.3	0.01
Haddock in Walnut Sauce*	194.5	87.7	12.4	5.9
Green Beans and Corn*	86.5	12.1	20.0	1.8
Coffee or tea	—	—	—	—
1 teaspoon sugar substitute	2.0	0	1.4	0
1 tablespoon low-fat milk	6.3	7.1	0.75	0.1
Total	343.1	150.7	39.1	8.1
SNACK				
1 plum	66.0	2.0	0.2	11.9
Iced tea with lemon	—	—	—	—
Total	66.0	2.0	0.2	11.9
DINNER				
1 cup shredded lettuce	18.0	9.0	3.5	0.3
1 Corn Tortilla*	86.1	1.2	17.3	0.2
Picadillo with Vegetables*	286.6	65.0	31.0	10.9
Kahlua Cream*	146.2	9.2	6.3	10.8
Coffee or tea	—	—	—	—
1 teaspoon sugar substitute	2.0	0	1.4	0
1 tablespoon low-fat milk	6.3	7.1	0.75	0.1
Total	545.2	91.5	60.3	22.3
SNACK				
½ ounce low-sodium Cheddar cheese	56.9	6.0	0.3	4.6
½ apple, sliced	58.0	1.0	14.5	0.6
Total	114.9	7.0	14.8	5.2
Grand Total	1,196.4	314.2	132.0	52.6

* See index for recipe page number.

TIPS FOR DAY TEN

If you have any Green Beans and Corn left over, it will keep up to one week refrigerated in plastic containers. Leftover Kahlua Cream can be frozen up to one month in plastic containers.

You can see the finish line from here. So just relax. Start believing that your new body, your new energy are here to stay.

	Calories	Sodium (mg.)	Carbo-hydrates (gm.)	Fat (gm.)
BREAKFAST				
½ cup blueberries	62.0	1.0	15.3	0.5
¼ cup low-sodium cottage cheese	45.0	31.0	4.0	0.1
2 low-sodium crackers	22.0	1.7	2.9	1.0
Coffee or tea	—	—	—	—
1 teaspoon sugar substitute	2.0	0	1.4	0
1 tablespoon low-fat milk	6.3	7.1	0.75	0.1
Total	137.3	40.8	24.4	1.7
LUNCH				
1 cup shredded lettuce	18.0	9.0	3.5	0.3
1 Corn Tortilla*	86.1	1.2	17.3	0.2
Picadillo with Vegetables*	286.6	65.0	31.0	10.9
Coffee or tea	—	—	—	—
1 teaspoon sugar substitute	2.0	0	1.4	0
1 tablespoon low-fat milk	6.3	7.1	0.75	0.1
Total	399.0	82.3	54.0	11.5

* See index for recipe page number.

	Calories	Sodium (mg.)	Carbo-hydrates (gm.)	Fat (gm.)
SNACK				
3½ ounces low-sodium tomato juice	19.0	3.0	4.3	0.1
DINNER				
Mixed Salad San Miguel*	157.8	44.8	19.4	8.6
Chicken Ancho*	199.9	75.9	18.4	4.2
1 boiled potato	76.0	3.0	17.1	0.1
Peas and Almonds*	97.6	1.6	9.7	4.9
Coffee or tea	—	—	—	—
1 teaspoon sugar substitute	2.0	0	1.4	0
1 tablespoon low-fat milk	6.3	7.1	0.75	0.1
Total	539.6	132.4	66.8	17.9
SNACK				
Pineapple and Bananas in Sherry*	89.9	1.3	12.9	4.4
Grand Total	1,184.8	259.8	162.4	35.6

* See index for recipe page number.

TIPS FOR DAY ELEVEN

It is not too soon to plan for the gift from you to you that will mark the successful completion of these two weeks and a wonderful beginning for the rest of your life. What shall it be: an hour-long massage? A long weekend in the sun to show off the new you? Whatever it is, focus on it and smile.

Leftover Peas and Almonds can be refrigerated in a plastic container up to three days. Or you might choose to have it for dinner on Day Fourteen in place of Broiled Tomato with Avocado. If there is anything left of Pineapple and Bananas in Sherry, store in a plastic container up to three days. Or substitute for the late-night snacks on either Days Thirteen or Fourteen.

To reduce today's sodium total, change your breakfast egg to the simple soft-boiled variety, and replace the lunch soup and salad with one cup shredded lettuce and Chicken with Figs and Lemons.

No problem. Right?

	Calories	Sodium (mg.)	Carbo-hydrates (gm.)	Fat (gm.)
BREAKFAST				
3½ ounces apple juice	47.0	1.0	11.9	0.1
Egg and Chicken Liver Casserole*	128.6	73.4	6.3	6.5
1 slice Comb Bread*	110.5	3.2	19.9	1.4
Coffee or tea	—	—	—	—
1 teaspoon sugar substitute	2.0	0	1.4	0
1 tablespoon low-fat milk	6.3	7.1	0.75	0.1
Total	294.4	84.7	40.3	8.1

* See index for recipe page number.

	Calories	Sodium (mg.)	Carbo-hydrates (gm.)	Fat (gm.)
LUNCH				
Peppercorn Chicken Soup*	94.5	27.4	10.7	4.1
Jicama and Chorizo Salad*	192.1	55.6	21.9	7.7
Coffee or tea	—	—	—	—
1 teaspoon sugar substitute	2.0	0	1.4	0
1 tablespoon low-fat milk	6.3	7.1	0.75	0.1
Total	294.9	90.1	34.8	11.9
SNACK				
½ ounce low-sodium mozzarella cheese	42.5	4.3	0.3	3.5
2 low-sodium crackers	22.0	1.7	2.9	1.0
Iced tea with lemon	—	—	—	—
Total	64.5	6.0	3.2	4.5
DINNER				
½ cup shredded lettuce	9.0	4.5	1.8	0.2
Green Bean and Sweet Pepper Salad*	75.5	12.7	8.8	4.6
Sea Bass in Red Wine Sauce*	216.2	69.2	20.1	6.0
Yellow Rice*	187.8	11.0	36.2	4.4
Coffee or tea	—	—	—	—
1 teaspoon sugar substitute	2.0	0	1.4	0
1 tablespoon low-fat milk	6.3	7.1	0.75	0.1
Total	496.8	104.5	69.1	15.3
SNACK				
¼ cantaloupe	42.9	17.1	10.7	0.1
Grand Total	1,193.5	302.4	158.1	39.9

* See index for recipe page number.

TIPS FOR DAY TWELVE

Almost there. You should be dancing around, light as a feather.

It is time to start trusting your own instincts and imagination. That is, if today's sodium total is more than you should have, change the menu to suit your needs. For example, your dinner menu could just as easily consist of Avocado, Tomato, and Cheese Salad,* Chicken and Bananas,* the Refried Beans, and one cup of steamed broccoli. The sodium will be slightly less than 250 milligrams, and the calories will drop by about 100. Fat and carbohydrates will be about the same.

Just take charge. It is easier and more fun for you if you do.

By the way, if you have leftover Yellow Rice or Jicama and Chorizo Salad, both will keep up to five days if refrigerated in plastic containers.

	Calories	Sodium (mg.)	Carbo-hydrates (gm.)	Fat (gm.)
BREAKFAST				
1 peach	43.4	1.1	11.1	0.1
½ cup oatmeal	62.9	2.0	11.1	1.1
¼ cup low-fat milk	25.0	28.6	3.0	0.5
Coffee or tea	—	—	—	—
1 teaspoon sugar substitute	2.0	0	1.4	0
1 tablespoon low-fat milk	6.3	7.1	0.75	0.1
Total	139.6	38.8	27.4	1.8

* See index for recipe page number.

	Calories	Sodium (mg.)	Carbo-hydrates (gm.)	Fat (gm.)
LUNCH				
1 cup shredded lettuce	18.0	9.0	3.5	0.3
½ tomato, sliced	15.7	2.1	3.4	0.1
2 tablespoons lemon juice	3.3	0.1	1.3	0.01
Sea Bass in Red Wine Sauce*	216.2	69.2	20.1	6.0
Coffee or tea	—	—	—	—
1 teaspoon sugar substitute	2.0	0	1.4	0
1 tablespoon low-fat milk	6.3	7.1	0.75	0.1
Total	261.5	87.5	30.5	6.5
SNACK				
½ ounce low-sodium Cheddar cheese	56.9	6.0	0.3	4.6
2 low-sodium crackers	22.0	1.7	2.9	1.0
Iced tea with lemon	—	—	—	—
Total	78.9	7.7	3.2	5.6
DINNER				
Christmas Eve Salad*	233.8	28.1	33.2	11.6
Parsley Chicken*	211.8	87.3	21.7	5.8
Refried Beans*	167.2	21.0	26.1	4.6
Sherried Carrots in Rum Cream*	73.6	36.2	8.9	3.1
Coffee or tea	—	—	—	—
1 teaspoon sugar substitute	2.0	0	1.4	0
1 tablespoon low-fat milk	6.3	7.1	0.75	0.1
Total	694.7	179.7	92.1	25.2
SNACK				
1 cup low-sodium chicken bouillon	18.0	5.0	2.0	1.0
Grand Total	1,192.7	318.7	155.2	40.1

* See index for recipe page number.

TIPS FOR DAY THIRTEEN

Have you decided on your present yet? Get ready because there are only two more days to go.

If you need to cut back on today's sodium total, substitute ½ ounce of Cheddar cheese for the yogurt at breakfast.

As for leftovers, both the Christmas Eve Salad and Sherried Carrots in Rum Cream will stay fresh about two days if refrigerated in plastic containers. The Refried Beans can be refrigerated up to one week, or frozen up to one month.

What a wonderful day this is: the next to last day of a major personal victory.

	Calories	Sodium (mg.)	Carbo-hydrates (gm.)	Fat (gm.)
BREAKFAST				
1 plum	66.0	2.0	0.2	11.9
¼ cup plain yogurt	70.9	53.7	5.6	3.9
1 Corn Tortilla*	86.1	1.2	17.3	0.2
Coffee or tea	—	—	—	—
1 teaspoon sugar substitute	2.0	0	1.4	0
1 tablespoon low-fat milk	6.3	7.1	0.75	0.1
Total	231.3	64.0	25.3	16.1

* See index for recipe page number.

	Calories	Sodium (mg.)	Carbo- hydrates (gm.)	Fat (gm.)
LUNCH				
1 cup shredded lettuce	18.0	9.0	3.5	0.3
¼ green pepper, sliced	11.0	6.5	2.4	0.1
2 tablespoons cider vinegar	2.0	2.0	1.6	0
Fish Soup*	167.3	61.3	15.3	5.5
Coffee or tea	—	—	—	
1 teaspoon sugar substitute	2.0	0	1.4	0
1 tablespoon low-fat milk	6.3	7.1	0.75	0.1
Total	206.6	85.9	25.0	6.0
SNACK				
½ ounce low-sodium Gouda cheese	56.9	6.0	0.3	4.6
2 low-sodium crackers	22.0	1.7	2.9	1.0
Iced tea with lemon	—	—	—	—
Total	78.9	7.7	3.2	5.6
DINNER				
1 cup shredded lettuce	18.0	9.0	3.5	0.3
Cucumber Salad La Jolla*	98.3	22.6	6.0	4.3
Roast Pork Loin*	307.2	80.5	17.3	14.6
1 small boiled potato	76.0	3.0	17.1	0.1
½ small zucchini, steamed	17.0	1.0	3.6	0.1
Coffee or tea	—	—	—	—
1 teaspoon sugar substitute	2.0	0	1.4	0
1 tablespoon low-fat milk	6.3	7.1	0.75	0.1
Total	524.8	123.2	49.7	19.5
SNACK				
Rum Apples*	148.7	6.5	20.7	6.0
Grand Total	1,190.3	287.3	123.9	53.2

* See index for recipe page number.

TIPS FOR DAY FOURTEEN

Hats off to you. You have come to the end of this road, fortified to make your own way from now on.

I am sure you are thinner than when you started this journey. But equally important, you are feeling and thinking thinner. It is this attitude which assures you continued success.

So do not despair if you have not yet lost a lot of weight. You will. Concentrate on how good you feel and remember it usually takes three weeks for your body to fully adjust to a new diet. You might not see a major drop in weight (two pounds) until then.

But you can be sure that on a good, well-balanced diet like this one, the pounds you lose slowly and steadily will stay off. No more bouncing up and down the scales. No more double wardrobes. In these two weeks, you have embarked on a new way of life.

To get back to today, if you need to lower your sodium intake, substitute ½ ounce of low-sodium Swiss cheese for your morning egg, and enjoy the added benefit of a few less calories. If refrigerated in plastic containers, the Fruit Salad Picante will stay fresh about one week, the Rice with Mushrooms and Cheese about three days; but the Broiled Tomato with Avocado should be eaten the next day (perhaps chopped and tossed with some lettuce). If there is anything left of the Coconut Soufflé, serve it again tomorrow night. No one will mind.

Whatever you do, the decisions and power are now in your very capable hands. You can start your own meal planning by following the guidelines in this chapter. Or you can repeat or adapt the first two weeks of this diet until you are ready to experiment.

You can do it. One look in the mirror will tell you so.

	Calories	Sodium (mg.)	Carbo-hydrates (gm.)	Fat (gm.)
BRUNCH				
¼ cantaloupe	42.9	17.1	10.7	0.1
Eggs with Lemon-Pepper Chicken*	137.6	69.4	1.2	8.1
1 slice Mexican Sweet Bread*	133.1	6.3	24.0	1.8
Coffee or tea	—	—	—	—
1 teaspoon sugar substitute	2.0	0	1.4	0
1 tablespoon low-fat milk	6.3	7.1	0.75	0.1
Total	321.9	99.9	38.1	10.1
LUNCH				
Fruit Salad Picante*	198.0	12.8	45.8	28.0
Coffee or tea	—	—	—	—
1 teaspoon sugar substitute	2.0	0	1.4	0
1 tablespoon low-fat milk	6.3	7.1	0.75	0.1
Total	206.3	19.9	48.0	28.1
SNACK				
1 cup low-sodium chicken bouillon	18.0	5.0	2.0	1.0
DINNER				
1 cup shredded lettuce	18.0	9.0	3.5	0.3
2 tablespoons lemon juice	3.3	0.1	1.3	0.01
Flounder in Green Garlic Sauce*	183.6	95.0	6.1	8.4
Rice with Mushrooms and Cheese*	245.7	32.4	41.0	5.8
Broiled Tomatoes with Avocado*	98.0	5.6	8.4	7.2
Coffee or tea	—	—	—	—
1 teaspoon sugar substitute	2.0	0	1.4	0
1 tablespoon low-fat milk	6.3	7.1	0.75	0.1
Total	556.9	149.2	62.5	21.8
SNACK				
Coconut Soufflé*	96.1	38.2	10.9	3.3
Grand Total	1,199.2	312.2	161.5	64.3

* See index for recipe page number.

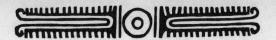

Tables of
Nutritional Values

The tables on the following pages provide an easy reference for nutritional values of all foods used (or suggested) in this book. Specifically included are the calorie, sodium, carbohydrate, and fat content per 100 grams (approximately 3½ ounces).

We ask that you note the following:

1. Nutritional values are based on raw ingredients unless otherwise noted.
2. Zero connotes no presence.
3. A dash connotes trace amounts.

	Calories	Sodium (mg.)	Carbo- hydrates (gm.)	Fat (gm.)
ALCOHOLIC BEVERAGES				
Banana Liqueur	295.0	1.0	—	0
Brandy	295.0	1.0	—	0
Kahlua	295.0	1.0	—	0
Rum	249.0	1.0	—	0
Tequila	249.0	1.0	—	0
Vermouth	85.0	5.0	4.2	0
Wine (dry sherry, red and white)	85.0	5.0	4.2	0

	Calories	Sodium (mg.)	Carbo- hydrates (gm.)	Fat (gm.)
CONDIMENTS				
Capers[1]	10.0	10.0	2.0	0.2
Chili Powder[2]	427.0	497.0	79.8	12.6
Honey	304.0	5.0	82.3	0
Hot cherry peppers, low-sodium	19.6	24.5	4.9	0
Jam and preserves	272.0	12.0	70.0	0.1
Jelly	273.0	17.0	70.6	0.1
Ketchup				
Chili, low-sodium	56.0	30.0	1.0	0
Regular, low-sodium	42.0	20.0	1.0	0
Marmalade	257.0	14.0	70.1	0.1
Mayonnaise, low-sodium	100.0	3.0	0	11.0
Molasses	232.0	37.0	60.0	0
Mustard, low-sodium	91.0	7.0	5.3	6.3
Pickles, butter, low-sodium	73.0	5.0	2.2	0.2
Sugar				
Regular	385.0	1.0	99.5	0
Substitute[3]	42.0	0	9.8	0
Sweet pepper slices, low-sodium	35.0	24.5	8.8	0
Tomato paste, low-sodium	91.0	10.0	18.6	0.4
Tomato puree, low-sodium	39.0	6.0	8.9	0.2
Tomato sauce, low-sodium	39.0	6.0	8.9	0.2

[1] Preserved in vinegar only.
[2] Without salt.
[3] Low-sodium as well as sugar-free.

	Calories	Sodium (mg.)	Carbo-hydrates (gm.)	Fat (gm.)
CONDIMENTS (*continued*)				
Vinegar				
Cider and red	14.0	1.0	5.9	0
White	12.0	1.0	5.0	0
Worcestershire sauce, low-sodium	304.0	5.0	82.3	0

	Calories	Sodium (mg.)	Carbo-hydrates (gm.)	Fat (gm.)
DAIRY				
Cheese				
Cheddar, low-sodium	398.0	18.0	2.1	32.2
Cottage, low-sodium	106.0	18.0	2.9	4.2
Cream, low-sodium	374.0	12.0	2.1	37.7
Gouda, low-sodium	345.0	35.0	1.7	28.0
Mozzarella, low-sodium	106.0	12.0	2.9	4.2
Muenster, low-sodium	345.0	12.0	2.2	28.0
Swiss, low-sodium	355.0	30.0	1.7	28.0
Cream	352.0	32.0	3.1	37.6
Egg[4]	163.0	122.0	0.9	11.5
Margarine, unsalted	720.0	15.0	0.4	81.0
Milk, low-fat	48.0	145.0	5.5	1.0
Sour cream	352.0	32.0	3.1	37.6
Yogurt, plain, low-fat	50.0	143.0	5.2	1.7

[4] One medium egg is approximately 2 ounces.

	Calories	Sodium (mg.)	Carbo-hydrates (gm.)	Fat (gm.)
FISH AND SEAFOOD				
Bass				
Sea	93.0	68.0	0	1.2
Striped	105.0	—	0	2.7
White	98.0	68.0	0	2.3

	Calories	Sodium (mg.)	Carbo-hydrates (gm.)	Fat (gm.)
FISH (*continued*)				
Cod	78.0	70.0	0	0.3
Flounder	79.0	78.0	0	0.8
Haddock	79.0	61.0	0	0.1
Halibut	100.0	54.0	0	1.2
Mackerel, canned, low-sodium	180.0	120.0	0	10.0
Oysters, shucked	66.0	73.0	3.4	1.8
Red snapper	93.0	67.0	0	0.9
Salmon				
Raw	217.0	64.0	0	13.4
Canned, low-sodium	145.0	70.0	0	5.9
Sardines, canned, low-sodium	203.0	120.2	—	11.1
Scrod	78.0	70.0	0	0.3
Shrimp	91.0	140.0	1.5	0.8
Sole	79.0	78.0	0	0.8
Squid	84.0	—	1.5	0.9
Swordfish	118.0	—	0	4.0
Tuna				
Raw	145.0	37.0	0	4.1
Canned, low-sodium	108.0	51.0	0	0.8

	Calories	Sodium (mg.)	Carbo-hydrates (gm.)	Fat (gm.)
FRUIT				
Apple	58.0	1.0	14.5	0.6
Apricots				
Canned, in juice	54.0	1.0	13.6	0.2
Dried[5]	260.0	26.0	66.5	0.5
Banana	85.0	1.0	22.0	0.2
Cantaloupe	30.0	12.0	7.5	0.1
Coconut, dried	548.0	—	53.2	39.1
Dates[6]	275.0	1.0	72.9	0.5
Figs, raw[7]	80.0	2.0	20.3	0.3

[5] 1 cup equals 3 ounces; 5 dried equal 1 ounce.
[6] 1 cup equals 6½ ounces.
[7] 1 fig equals 3½ ounces.

	Calories	Sodium (mg.)	Carbo-hydrates (gm.)	Fat (gm.)
FRUIT (*continued*)				
Grapefruit				
Canned, in water	30.0	4.0	7.6	0.1
Raw	44.0	1.0	11.5	0.1
Lemon	27.0	5.0	8.2	0.3
Lime	28.0	2.0	9.5	0.2
Orange	49.0	1.0	12.2	0.2
Peach				
Canned, dietetic	31.0	2.0	8.1	0.1
Raw	38.0	1.0	9.7	0.1
Pear				
Canned, dietetic	32.0	1.0	8.3	0.2
Raw	62.0	2.0	15.3	0.4
Pineapple				
Canned, in water	39.0	1.0	10.2	0.1
Raw	52.0	1.0	13.7	0.2
Plum				
Canned, in water	46.0	2.0	11.9	0.2
Raw	66.0	2.0	17.8	—
Pomegranate	63.0	3.0	16.4	0.3
Prunes[8]	255.0	8.0	67.4	0.6
Raisins[9]	289.0	27.0	77.4	0.2
Raspberries				
Frozen, in syrup	445.0	5.0	111.6	0.9
Raw[10]	251.0	4.0	59.8	2.2

[8] 3 prunes equal 1 ounce.
[9] 1 cup equals 6 ounces.
[10] 1 cup equals 3 ounces.

	Calories	Sodium (mg.)	Carbo-hydrates (gm.)	Fat (gm.)
JUICE				
Apple	47.0	1.0	11.9	—
Grapefruit	42.0	1.0	10.2	0.1
Lemon	23.0	1.0	7.6	0.1
Lime	26.0	1.0	9.0	0.1
Orange	48.0	1.0	11.2	0.2

	Calories	Sodium (mg.)	Carbo-hydrates (gm.)	Fat (gm.)
JUICE (*continued*)				
Pineapple	55.0	1.0	13.5	0.1
Tomato	19.0	3.0	4.3	0.1

	Calories	Sodium (mg.)	Carbo-hydrates (gm.)	Fat (gm.)
MEAT				
Beef				
Bottom round	197.0	65.0	0	12.3
Chuck (ground beef)	286.0	47.0	0	20.3
Flank (London broil)	191.0	65.0	0	6.6
Short ribs	193.0	65.0	0	11.6
Sirloin	353.0	65.0	0	27.5
Lamb				
Leg	192.0	75.0	0	7.7
Loin	197.0	75.0	0	8.6
Rib	224.0	75.0	0	12.1
Shoulder	215.0	75.0	0	11.2
Liver, chicken	129.0	70.0	2.9	3.7
Pork				
Loin	254.0	70.0	0	14.2
Shoulder	244.0	70.0	0	14.3
Spareribs	440.0	70.0	0	38.9
Veal				
Rib	207.0	90.0	0	14.0
Shoulder (ground veal)	240.0	90.0	0	18.0

	Calories	Sodium (mg.)	Carbo-hydrates (gm.)	Fat (gm.)
NUTS[11]				
Almonds	598.0	4.0[12]	19.5	54.2
Cashews	561.0	15.0[12]	29.3	45.7
Peanuts	582.0	5.0[12]	20.6	48.7

[11] ¼ cup equals approximately 2 ounces.
[12] Unsalted only.

	Calories	Sodium (mg.)	Carbo-hydrates (gm.)	Fat (gm.)
NUTS (continued)				
Pecans	687.0	—[12]	14.6	71.2
Pine Nuts	552.0	0[12]	11.6	47.4
Sesame Seeds	582.0	—[12]	17.6	53.4
Walnuts				
Black	628.0	3.0[12]	14.8	59.3
English	651.0	2.0[12]	15.8	64.0

[12] Unsalted only.

	Calories	Sodium (mg.)	Carbo-hydrates (gm.)	Fat (gm.)
POULTRY				
Chicken[13]				
Fryers				
Flesh and skin (whole)	126.0	58.0	0	5.1
Flesh only (whole)	107.0	78.0	0	2.7
Breast	110.0	50.0	0	2.4
Drumstick	115.0	67.0	0	3.9
Thigh	128.0	67.0	0	5.6
Wing	146.0	50.0	0	7.4
Roasters				
Flesh and skin (whole)	197.0	58.0	0	12.6
Flesh only (whole)	131.0	58.0	0	4.5
Dark meat, without skin	132.0	67.0	0	4.7
Light meat, without skin	128.0	50.0	0	3.2
Turkey[14]				
Total edible	218.0	66.0	0	14.7
Dark meat, without skin	128.0	81.0	0	4.3
Light meat, without skin	116.0	51.0	0	1.2

[13] Approximately 60 percent of a whole chicken is actually meat.
[14] Approximately 50 percent of a whole turkey is actually meat.

	Calories	Sodium (mg.)	Carbo-hydrates (gm.)	Fat (gm.)
VEGETABLES				
Asparagus	26.0	2.0	5.0	0.2
Avocados	167.0	4.0	6.3	16.4
Beans				
Black[15]	339.0	25.0	61.2	1.5
Kidney[15]	343.0	10.0	61.9	1.5
Pink[15]	343.0	10.0	61.9	1.5
Pinto[15]	349.0	10.0	63.7	1.2
White[15]	340.0	19.0	61.3	1.6
Beets, canned, low-sodium	32.0	46.0	7.8	—
Broccoli[16]	32.0	15.0	5.9	0.3
Cabbage[17]	24.0	20.0	5.4	0.2
Carrots	42.0	43.0	9.7	0.2
Cauliflower[18]	27.0	13.0	5.2	0.2
Chiles				
Dried	321.0	373.0	59.8	9.1
Raw, green	37.0	25.0	9.1	0.2
Raw, red	65.0	25.0	15.8	0.4
Corn, canned, low-sodium	57.0	2.0	13.6	0.5
Cucumbers	48.0	20.6	3.4	0.1
Eggplant	25.0	2.0	5.6	0.2
Garlic	137.0	19.0	30.8	0.2
Green beans	32.0	7.0	7.1	0.2
Jicama	44.0	—	16.7	0.1
Leeks	52.0	5.0	11.2	0.3
Lentils[15]	340.0	30.0	60.1	1.1
Lettuce[19]	18.0	9.0	3.5	0.3
Lima beans[15]	123.0	2.0	22.1	0.5
Mushrooms[20]	28.0	15.0	4.4	0.3
Okra	36.0	3.0	7.6	0.3
Onions	38.0	10.0	17.4	0.2
Parsley (cilantro)	44.0	45.0	8.5	0.6
Pasta				
Cooked	148.0	2.0	30.1	0.5
Raw	362.0	2.0	75.2	1.2
Peas	84.0	2.0	14.4	0.4

[15] 1 cup equals 6 ounces.
[16] 1 spear equals 5 ounces; 1 head equals 20 ounces.
[17] 1 cup equals 4 ounces.
[18] 1 cup equals 4 ounces; 1 head equals 24 ounces.
[19] 1 cup equals 3½ ounces; 1 head equals 1 pound.
[20] 2 mushrooms equal 1 ounce.

	Calories	Sodium (mg.)	Carbo-hydrates (gm.)	Fat (gm.)
VEGETABLES (*continued*)				
Peppers				
Bell, green	22.0	13.0	4.8	0.2
Bell, red	31.0	25.0	7.1	0.3
Potatoes				
Baked	93.0	4.0	21.7	1.0
Boiled	76.0	3.0	17.1	1.0
Radishes	17.0	18.0	3.6	0.1
Rice				
Cooked[21]	109.0	5.0	24.2	0.1
Raw[15]	363.0	5.0	80.4	0.4
Scallions	36.0	5.0	8.2	0.2
Spinach	26.0	71.0	4.3	0.3
Squash				
Butternut	54.0	1.0	14.0	0.1
Yellow	20.0	1.0	4.3	0.2
Zucchini	17.0	1.0	3.6	0.1
Tomatoes	22.0	3.0	4.7	0.2
Yams	101.0	—	23.2	0.2

[21] 1 cup equals 8 ounces.

	Calories	Sodium (mg.)	Carbo-hydrates (gm.)	Fat (gm.)
WHEAT AND GRAIN				
Bread, low-sodium[22]	241.0	3.5	49.3	2.6
Bread crumbs, low-sodium[23]	364.0	35.0	77.0	7.0
Crackers, low-sodium[24]	195.0	4.3	25.5	9.0
Oatmeal, cooked	55.0	4.0	9.7	1.0
Rice, puffed, salt-free	399.0	2.0	89.5	0.4
Wheat, puffed, salt-free	363.0	4.0	78.5	1.5

[22] 1 slice equals 1 ounce.
[23] 1 cup equals 4 ounces.
[24] Eleven equal 1 ounce.

	Calories	Sodium (mg.)	Carbo-hydrates (gm.)	Fat (gm.)
MISCELLANY				
Baking powder, low-sodium	83.0	40.0	20.1	—
Bouillon				
Beef, low-sodium[25]	378.0	210.0	42.0	21.0
Chicken, low-sodium[26]	378.0	105.0	42.0	21.0
Candied fruit	314.0	290.0	80.2	0.3
Chocolate, bittersweet, low-sodium	490.0	140.0	56.0	28.0
Flour				
All-purpose	365.0	2.0	74.5	1.2
Corn (masa harina)	368.0	1.0	76.8	2.6
Wheat	333.0	3.0	71.0	2.0
Gelatin, unflavored[27]	335.0	2.0	0	0.1
Oil	884.0	0	0	100.0
Shortening	902.0	—	0	100.0
Yeast	282.0	52.0	38.9	1.6

[25] Content per tablespoon equals 54 calories, 30 milligrams sodium, 3 grams carbohydrates, 3 grams fat.
[26] Content per tablespoon equals 54 calories, 15 milligrams sodium, 3 grams carbohydrates, 3 grams fat.
[27] One package equals 2 tablespoons equals 1 ounce.

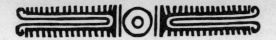

Bibliography

American Diabetes Association, Inc., and The American Dietetic Association. *A Guide for Professionals: The Effective Application of "Exchange Lists for Meal Planning,"* 1977.

American Diabetes Association, Inc., and The American Dietetic Association. *Exchange Lists for Meal Planning*, 1976.

American Heart Association. *Cooking Without Your Salt Shaker.* Dallas, Texas: American Heart Association's Communication Division, 1978.

American Heart Association Booklets: *Your 500 Milligrams Sodium Diet, Your 1000 Milligrams Sodium Diet, Your Mild Sodium-Restricted Diet.* Dallas, Texas: American Heart Association, 1957.

American Spice Trade Association Booklets: *A Glossary of Spices. A Guide to Spices. A History of Spices. The Art of Seasoning Low-Sodium Diets*, reprinted from Hospital Management Magazine. *Calorie Watcher's Spice Chart*, reprinted from Restaurant Hospitality. 580 Sylvan Avenue, Englewood Cliffs, New Jersey 07632.

Ashley, Richard, and Duggal, Heidi. *Dictionary of Nutrition.* New York: Pocket Books, 1975.

Bayrd, Edwin. *The Thin Game.* New York: Avon Books, 1978.

Bieler, Henry G., M.D. *Food Is Your Best Medicine.* New York: Vintage Books, 1975.

Bowen, Angela, M.D. *The Diabetic Gourmet.* New York: Harper & Row, Publishers, 1970, 1980.

Brody, Jane. *Jane Brody's Nutrition Book.* New York: W. W. Norton & Company, Inc., 1981.

Brunswick, J. Peter; Love, Dorothy; and Weinberg, Assa, M.D. *How to Live 365 Days a Year the Salt-Free Way.* New York: Bantam Books, Inc., 1977.

Calderon de la Barca, Frances. *Life in Mexico.* Edited by Howard T. Fisher and Marion Hall Fisher. New York: Doubleday, 1966.

Eisner, Will. *What's in What You Eat.* New York: Bantam Books, Inc., 1983.

Fodor's Travel Guides. *Fodor's Mexico 1985.* New York: Fodor's Travel Guides, 1984.

Foster, Lynne V., and Foster, Lawrence. *Fielding's Mexico 1985*. New York: Fielding Travel Books c/o William Morrow & Company, Inc., 1985.

Heiss, Kay Beauchamp, and Heiss, C. Gordon. *Eat to Your Heart's Content. The Low-Cholesterol Gourmet Cookbook*. New York: New American Library, 1972.

James, Janet, and Goulder, Lois. *The Dell Color-Coded Low-Salt-Living Guide*. New York: Dell Publishing, Inc., 1980.

Joslin Clinic. *Diabetic Diet Guide*. Boston, Mass.

Kennedy, Diana. *The Cuisines of Mexico*. New York: Harper & Row Publishers, Inc., 1972.

Kraus, Barbara. *Calories and Carbohydrates*. Fifth Revised Edition. New York: New American Library, 1983.

Kraus, Barbara. *Sodium Guide to Brand Names and Basic Foods*. Expanded Edition. New York: New American Library, 1983.

Kritchersky, David. *Dietary Fiber: What It Is and What It Does*. Volume 300, pages 283–289. New York: *Annals of the New York Academy of Sciences*, 1977.

Middleton, Katharine, and Hess, Mary Abbott. *The Art of Cooking for the Diabetic*. New York: New American Library, 1978.

Ornish, Dean, M.D. *Stress, Diet and Your Heart*. New York: New American Library, 1982.

Rechtschaffen, Joseph S., M.D. and Carola, Robert. *Dr. Rechtschaffen's Diet for Lifetime Weight Control and Better Health*. New York: Random House, Inc., 1980.

Revell, Dorothy. *Cholesterol Control*. Denver, Colorado: Royal Publications, Inc., 1961.

Roth, Harriet. *Deliciously Low. The Gourmet Guide to Low-Sodium, Low-Fat, Low-Cholesterol, Low-Sugar Cooking*. New York: New American Library, 1983.

Roth, June. *Salt-Free Cooking with Herbs and Spices*. Chicago: Contemporary Books, Inc., 1975.

Schell, Merle. *Tasting Good. The International Salt-Free Diet Cookbook*. New York: New American Library, 1981.

———. *The Chinese Salt-Free Diet Cookbook*. New York: New American Library, 1985.

Simon, Kate. *Mexico Places and Pleasures*. Third Edition. New York: Harper Colophon Books, 1979.

Sullivan, Margaret. *The New Carbohydrate Gram Counter*. New York: Dell Publishing, Inc., 1980.

United States Department of Agriculture. *Handbook No. 8*. U.S. Government Printing Office. Washington, D.C. 20402, 1963.

U.S. Department of Health and Human Services. *Cookbooks for People with Diabetes*. Selected Annotations. NIH Publications. No. 81-2177. Bethesda, Maryland 20205: National Diabetes Information Clearinghouse, 1981.

U.S. Department of Health and Human Services. *Diet and Nutrition for People with Diabetes.* Selected Annotations. NIH Publication No. 80–1872. Washington, D.C.: National Diabetes Information Clearinghouse, 1979.

U.S. Department of Health, Education and Welfare. *Medicine for the Layman. Heart Attacks.* Bethesda, Maryland: National Institute of Health, 1979.

Vaillant, George Clapp. *Aztecs of Mexico.* Middlesex, England: Penguin Books, Ltd., 1962.

Veterans' Administration. *Regional Diet Handbook.* Medical District 1—Region 1, 1981.

Whitney, Eleanor Noss, and Hamilton, Eva May Nunnelley. *Understanding Nutrition.* St. Paul: West Publishing Company, 1977.

Williams, Roger J. *Nutrition in a Nutshell.* New York: Dolphin Books, 1962.

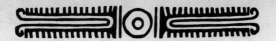

INDEX

A

Achiote, about, 10
Adapting your favorite Mexican
    recipes, 25–26
Alcoholic beverages
    about, 10, 15, 17–18
    about nutritional value, 319
Allspice, about, 10
Almond
    pudding, 246
    sauce, 218
    -sherry chicken, 132
Ancho chicken, 133
Anise fritters, 246–47
Aniseed (fennel seed), about, 10
Appetizers and Snacks (antojitos),
        69–95. See also Canapés, Dips
    apple relish, sweet hot, 45
    fruit juice chicken wings, 44
    guacamole, 34
    marinated beef, 44
    meat balls, saucy, 171
    pickled ceviche, 43
    tuna-stuffed (or chicken-stuffed)
        mushrooms, 39
Apple(s)
    and cabbage in piquant sour cream
        sauce, 201
    relish, sweet hot, 45
    rum, 254
    and veal (or beef) in green sauce,
        166
Apricots, tuna and, 124
Asparagus
    in crumb sauce, 196–97
    and mushrooms, 196
    scrambled eggs with, 238–39
Avocado
    about, 10
    broiled tomatoes with, 200
    and caper canapés, 40
    and cheese enchiladas, 59
    -chile sauce, 214–15
    cucumber and beet dip, 35
    and green peppers, 198
    guacamole dip (sauce), 34
    and pork soup, 95
    and prunes, snapper with, 120
    soup, puree of, 88
    stuffed, salad, 104
    tomato and cheese salad, 98

B

Baked beans, Mexican, 176–77
Baked green peppers with raisins, 197
Baked lamb in drunken sauce, 156–57
Baked rice with Chicken and
        Chorizo, 185
Baked salmon in mustard sauce, 116
Baked stuffed potatoes, 179
Banana(s)
    about, 11
    and chicken, 134
    orange wheat rolls, 69
    and pineapple in sherry, 253
Basic flan, 244
Basic salsa, 210
Basil-tomato sauce, 212
Bass. See Sea bass

Bay leaf, about, 11
Bean(s). *See also* Lentils
    about, 11; nutritional value of, 324
    black, soup, 79
    with cheese, 175
    with chorizo and salsa, 175
    green. *See* Green beans
    lamb and tomato soup, 91
    lima, and tomatoes in butter sauce,
        199
    Mexican baked (with pork),
        176–77
    with pork (or chicken) in lime
        sauce, 176
    refried, 177
    salad, 98
    simple, 174
    -stuffed chiles (or peppers), 192
Beef
    about nutritional value, 323
    and apples in green sauce, 166
    balls in sour cream sauce, 166
    boiled, 151
    and cheese tamales, 62
    chile (con carne), 150
    marinated (ground), 44
    minced, canapés, 42–43
    and pecans, 160
    pot roast, Mexican, 153
    steak with chile strips, 156
    steak, citrus, 152
    steak guacamole with dates, 155
    steak and tomatoes, 154
Beets, low-sodium, 19
Beverages. *See* Alcoholic beverages
Black bean soup, 79
Boiled beef, 151
Bouillon, unsalted beef and chicken,
    19–20
Breads and Rolls, 65–69. *See also*
    Tamales, Tortillas
    about nutritional value, 326
    bread of the dead, 66
    bread fried with brandied honey
        (dessert), 248–49
    cinnamon rolls, golden, 73
    comb bread (peineta), 67
    crescent rolls, 70; sugar-glazed, 71
    fruit logs, 72
    Mexican sweet bread, 68
    orange-banana wheat rolls, 69

Broccoli
    and corn soup, 84
    in cream cheese sauce, 206
    creamed corn and chicken, 205
    and mushrooms with pork, 200
Broiled oranges with coconut, 247
Broiled tomatoes with avocado, 200
Brunch menus, 256–62
Buffet menus, 273–77
Burritos I, 50; burritos II, 51

C

Cabbage
    and apples in piquant sour cream
        sauce, 201
    soup Veracruz, 84–85
    walnuts and pears, 201
Cake, bread of the dead, 66
Cake, lemon-prune, 252
Camarones. *See* Shrimp
Canapés
    avocado and caper, 40
    chile-chicken, 40
    cucumber (or zucchini, red pepper)
        and chorizo, 41
    fruit juice chicken wings, 44
    marinated beef, 44
    minced veal (or beef), 42
    sweet pepper and mackerel, 42
    tuna-stuffed (or chicken-stuffed)
        mushrooms, 39
Carrot(s)
    glazed with minced shrimp, 202
    in rum cream, sherried, 203
    soup, creamy, 83
Cayenne pepper, about, 11
Cauliflower
    creamed, and sweet peppers, 204
    salad, 99
    and tomatoes in butter sauce, 199
Celery seed, about, 20
Ceviche, pickled, 43
Cheddar cheese soup, 85
Cheddar-chile dip, 35
Cheese
    about, 11, 20
    and avocado enchiladas, 59
    beans with, 175

Cheddar-chile dip, 35
Cheddar, soup, 85
cream, and nut sauce, chiles with, 193
cream, sauce, 222
with red and green chicken, 147
-stuffed chicken, 132–33
tamales, chicken (or beef, pork, veal) and, 62
Cheesy hot noodles, 182
Chicken
about nutritional value, 324
almond-sherry, 132
ancho, 133
and bananas, 134
with beans in lime sauce, 176
burritos II, 51
cheese-stuffed, 132–33
and cheese tamales, 62
chilaquiles in chile-tomato sauce, 52
-chile, canapés, 40
in chile-nut sauce, 139
and chorizo, 134
and chorizo, baked rice with, 185
Colombian, 137
creamed corn, eggplant (or broccoli) and, 205
festival, in wine, 142
with figs and lemons, 141
lemon-pepper, eggs with, 236
liver and egg casserole, 232
mint, 143
molé, 140
in mustard sauce, 138
in orange-mint sauce, 138–39
parsley, 144
pineapple with zucchini, 145
poached in chile cream sauce, 144
pueblo, 146
red and green, with cheese, 147
rice with, 187
salad Cozumel, 104
and shrimp empanadas, 54
soup, peppercorn, 94
-sour cream enchiladas, 60
and spiced fruit, 135
and squash, 136
stock, 76
-stuffed mushrooms, 39
and vegetable stew, spiced, 148
-walnut soup, 94
wings, fruit juice canapés, 44
Chilaquiles, chicken (or pork) in chile-tomato sauce, 52
Chile(s)
about (varieties), 12; dried, 15
about nutritional value, 324
-avocado sauce, 214–15
bean-stuffed, 192
beef (con carne), 150
-Cheddar dip, 35
-chicken canapés, 40
-cinnamon pork (or lamb) chops, 159
corn, creamed, 204
with cream cheese and nut sauce, 193
meat-stuffed, 194
potatoes with, 180
rice with shrimp and cheese, 184
sauce, sweet-and-hot, 215
strips, steak with, 156
-tomato sauce, 213
-tuna salad, 107
-vegetable sauce, 214
vegetable-stuffed, 195
Chili powder, 210
about, 12–13
Chimichangas, 50
Chocolate, about, 13
Chorizo (sausage), 158–59
about, 13
with beans and salsa, 175
and chicken, 134
and chicken, baked rice with, 185
and cucumber (or zucchini, red pepper) canapés, 41
and eggs, 232–33
and jicama salad, 105
spaghetti and, 181
Christmas Eve salad, 103
Chutney. See Relish
Cilantro (coriander), 13, 14
Cinnamon
about, 13
-chile pork (or lamb) chops, 159
-pecan flan, 245
rolls, golden, 73
Citrus beef steak (or pork, veal), 152
Cloves, about, 13
Cocktail party menus, 278–83

Coconut soufflé, 248
Colombian chicken, 137
Comb bread (peineta), 67
Condata leg of lamb, 157
Condiments. *See* Herbs and Spices
  about nutritional value, 320
Cookies, sugar, Mexican, 252–53
Cooking equipment, Mexican, 23
Coriander, about, 14
Corn
  about, 14, 20
  and broccoli soup, 84
  creamed chile, 204
  creamed, eggplant (or broccoli) and
    chicken, 205
  flour (masa harina), about, 16
  and green beans, 202
  husks, 14
  soup, 82–83
  tortillas, 48. *See also* Enchiladas
  zucchini and tomatoes casserole,
    208
Cozumel chicken salad, 104
Cream cheese sauce, 222
Cream, Mexican, about, 14
Creamed cauliflower and sweet
    peppers, 204
Creamed chile corn, 204
Creamed corn, eggplant, and chicken,
    205
Creamy carrot soup, 83
Creamy wine sauce, 221
Crescent rolls, 70; sugar-glazed, 71
Cucumber
  and chorizo canapés, 41
  salad, La Jolla, 100
  soup, 86–87
Cumin seed, about, 14–15

coconut soufflé, 248
empanadas I, 57; empanadas II, 57
flan, basic, 244
fried bread with brandied honey,
    248
fruit puree, 249
fruited yam pie, 250
Kahlua cream, 250–51
kings' ring (for Christmas), 251
lemon-coconut flan, 245
lemon-prune cake, 252
oranges (or peaches) broiled with
    coconut, 247
pineapple and bananas in sherry,
    253
raspberries and peaches in sherry,
    253
rum pears (or apples), 254
sugar cookies, Mexican, 252–53
Diet foods, 19–22, 27–30
Diet menus (2-week), 290–317
Diet, Mexican, 285–88
  calories to consume on, 288
  length of, 288
  menus for day one to day fourteen,
    290–317
  sodium limits on, 288
Dinner menus, 267–72
Dips
  avocado, cucumber, and beet, 35
  chile-Cheddar, 35
  eggplant and apple, 38
  guacamole, 34
  salmon (or sardine) and caper, 36
  sour cream, 37
  sweet hot apple relish, 45
Dressings. *See* Sauces
Dried chiles, about, 15
Drunken sauce, 220

D

Dairy products, about nutritional
    value, 320–21
Dates, steak with, 155
Desserts, 243–54
  almond pudding, 246
  anise fritters, 246–47
  cinnamon-pecan flan, 245

E

Eating out, 30
Eggplant
  and apple dip, 38
  baked with raisins, 197
  creamed corn and chicken, 205
  fish-stuffed, 114

lime, with tomatoes, 198
rice with, 188–89
Eggs, 231–41
and chicken liver casserole, 232
and chorizo, 232–33
huevos rancheros, 237
with lemon-pepper chicken, 236
Mexican deviled, 240
in a nest, 234
peppers and cheese, spiced, 241
potatoes and onion, 234–35
scrambled with asparagus, 238–39
scrambled with green sauce, 239
scrambled Mexicana, 238
and shrimp with yogurt sauce, 233
sweet pepper and Cheddar cheese,
235
Yucatan, 236–37
Empanada(s)
about, 53
chicken and shrimp, 54
dessert I, 57; dessert II, 57
dough, 53
meat and cheese, 55
vegetable, 56
Enchiladas
avocado and cheese, 59
meat in pungent chile sauce, 58
sour cream-chicken (or fish), 60
Entertaining, 255–63
brunches, 256–63
for 4, 256–58
for 8, 258–61
for 16, 261–63
buffets, 273–77
for 12, 273–74
for 16, 274–75
for 24, 276–77
cocktails, 278–83
for 16, 278–79
for 24, 280–81
for 32, 282–83
dinners, 267–72
for 4, 267–69
for 8, 270–72
general tips for
lunches, 263–67
for 4, 263–65
for 8, 265–67
Epazote, about, 15

F

Fennel seed, about, 10
Festival chicken, in wine, 142
Festival soup, three-color, 86
Figs and lemons, chicken with, 141
Fish and Shellfish, 109–29. *See also*
name of fish
about nutritional value, 321
ceviche, pickled, 43
honey, 113
seafood mixed in lime sauce, 128
seafood tamales, 63
soup, 93
stock, 77
-stuffed eggplant, 114
topping, sour cream dip, 37
Flan
basic, 244
cinnamon-pecan, 245
lemon-coconut, 245
Flounder
in chile-corn sauce, 110
in green garlic sauce, 110–11
honey fish, 113
pickled ceviche, 43
-sour cream enchiladas, 60
with walnut-orange sauce, 111
Flour, white, tortillas, 49. *See also*
Burritos
Fried bread with brandied honey,
248–49
Fritters, anise, 246–47
Fritters, potato, 178
Fruit. *See also* name of fruit
about nutritional value, 321–22
juice chicken wings canapés, 44
juice dressing, 226
logs, 72
minced meats with, 170
puree, 249
salad picante, 102
soup, 80
spiced, chicken and, 135
-vegetable salad, Christmas Eve,
103
-vegetable salad of colors, 102
Fruited yam pie, 250

G

Garlic, about, 15
Garlic dressing, 228
Garlic soup, 82
Gazpacho, 81
Glazed carrots with minced shrimp, 202
Golden cinnamon rolls, 73
Grapefruit, swordfish with, 123
Green beans
   and corn, 202
   in cream cheese sauce, 206
   mushrooms and sweet peppers, 203
   and sweet pepper salad, 100
   sweet rice with, 189
Green peppers. *See* Peppers, green
Green rice, 186
Green sauce I, 216; green sauce II, 217
Green tomatoes (tomatillos), about, 15
Guacamole dip (sauce), 34
Guacamole, steak, with dates, 155

H

Haddock
   pickled ceviche, 43
   tomato-fried, 112-13
   in walnut sauce, 112
Halibut, fish-stuffed eggplant, 114
Herbs and spices, about, 10, 11, 13–17, 25,
   nutritional value of condiments, 320
Honey fish, 113
Honey-lime dressing, 229
Hors d'oeuvres, *see* Appetizers, Canapés, Dips
Hot-and-sweet dressing, 228
Hot cherry peppers, about, 12
Huevos rancheros, 237

I

Ingredients and where
   to find them, 9–22

a low-sodium pantry, 19–22
a Mexican pantry, 10–19

J

Jicama, about, 15
Jicama and chorizo salad, 105

K

Kahlua, about, 15
Kahlua cream, 250–51
Ketchup, about, 20
Kings' ring (Christmas dessert), 251

L

Lamb
   about nutritional value, 323
   baked in drunken sauce, 156–57
   chops, cinnamon-chile, 159
   chops, mint with peanuts, 158
   leg of, condata, 157
   tomato and bean sauce, 91
Lasagna, Mexican, 183
Leg of lamb condata, 157
Lemon(s)
   -coconut flan, 245
   dressing, 226
   and figs, chicken with, 141
   -prune cake, 252
Lemon peel powder, about, 21
Lentil soup with okra, 90
Lima beans and tomatoes in butter sauce, 199
Lime eggplant with tomatoes, 198
Lime sauce, 217
Lime-honey dressing, 229
Low-sodium pantry, about stocking, 19–22, 27–29
Lunch menus, 263–67

M

Macaroni salad, Mexican, 184
Mackerel and sweet pepper canapés, 42

Marinade, garlic dressing, 228
Marinated beef canapés (steak tartare), 44
Masa harina, about, 16
Mayonnaise, about, 21
Mazatlan shrimp salad, 106
Meat(s). *See also* name of meat
  about nutritional value, 323
  balls, saucy, 171
  and cheese empanadas, 55
  enchiladas in pungent chile sauce, 58
  loaf, south-of-the-border, 172
  minced with fruit, 170
  minced, noodles with, 182
  picadillo with vegetables, 169
  stock, 78
  -stuffed chiles, 194
  topping, sour cream dip, 37
Melon soup, 80
Menus, *see* Diet, Mexican, Entertaining
Mexican
  baked beans, 176–77
  brunch menus, 256–62
  buffet menus, 273–77
  cocktail menus, 278–83
  cuisine, about, 1, 6–7
  deviled eggs, 240
  diet, about, 285–88
  diet menus (2-week), 290–317
  dinner menus, 267–72
  history and culture, 1–5
  kitchen utensils, 23
  lasagna, 183
  lunch menus, 263–67
  macaroni salad, 184
  menus, about entertaining, 255–56
  pantry, about stocking, 10–22; low-sodium, 19–22
  pot roast, 153
  potato salad, 178
  recipes, how to adapt, 25–26
  stock pot, 91
  sugar cookies, 252–53
  sweet bread, 68
  vegetable soup, 87
  white rice, 186
Minced veal (or beef) canapés, 42–43
Mint
  about, 16

chicken, 143
  lamb chops with peanuts, 158
Mixed salad San Miguel, 101
Mixed seafood in lime sauce, 128
Mole, about, 16
Mole chicken (or turkey), 140
Mushrooms
  and asparagus, 196
  and broccoli with pork, 200
  and cheese, rice with, 188
  green beans and sweet peppers, 203
  tuna-stuffed (or chicken-stuffed), 39
Mustard, about, 21

N

Noodles, cheesy hot, 182
Noodles with minced meats, 182
Nutmeg, about, 16
Nutritional value of foods, 319–26
Nuts, about, 16; nutritional value, 323. *See also* name of nut

O

Oil and vinegar dressing, 227
Omelet. *See* Eggs
Onions, about, 17
Onion sauce, 219
Orange(s)
  -banana wheat rolls, 69
  broiled with coconut, 247
  Seville, about, 17–18
Orange peel powder, about, 21
Oregano, about, 17
Oysters
  with rice, 187
  in sherry-tomato sauce, 129
  in wine sauce, 128–29

P

Paprika, about, 17
Parsley chicken, 144
Pasta. *See also* Macaroni, Noodles, Spaghetti
  about nutritional value, 325

Peaches broiled with coconut, 247
Peaches and raspberries in sherry, 253
Pears, cabbage, and walnuts, 201
Pears, rum, 254
Peas
    and almonds, 206
    in cream cheese sauce, 206
    and tomatoes in butter sauce, 199
Pecan-cinnamon flan, 245
Pecans, pork (or beef) and, 160
Peineta (comb bread), 67
Pepper(s), green
    and avocado, 198
    baked with raisins, 197
    bean-stuffed, 192
    with cream cheese and nut sauce, 193
    squid salad with, 106–07
    vegetable-stuffed, 195
Pepper(s), hot cherry, 20
Pepper(s), sweet
    creamed cauliflower and, 204
    eggs and Cheddar cheese, 235
    and green bean salad, 100
    green beans and mushrooms, 203
    halves, about, 21
    and mackerel canapés, 42
    and peanuts, shrimp with, 127
    red, and chorizo canapés, 41
    red, squid salad with, 106–07
Peppercorn chicken soup, 94
Peppercorns, about, 17
Picadillo with vegetables, 169
Pickled ceviche, 43
Pie, fruited yam, 250
Pineapple and bananas in sherry, 253
Pineapple chicken with zucchini, 145
Piquant sour cream sauce, 224
Pork
    about nutritional value, 323
    and avocado soup, 95
    balls in sour cream sauce, 166–77
    beans with, in lime sauce, 176
    broccoli and mushrooms with, 200
    burritos I, 50
    and cheese tamales, 62
    chilaquiles in chile-tomato sauce, 52
    chile, 150
    chops, cinnamon-chile, 159
    chorizo, 158–59
    citrus, steak, 152

    loin, roast, 162
    Mexican baked beans, 176–77
    and pecans, 160
    with rice, 187
    shredded, 163
    stew, 161
    stew, sweetly hot, 164
Pot roast. *See* Beef
Potato(es)
    baked stuffed, 179
    casserole, spicy, 180–81
    with chiles, 180
    fritters, 178–79
    onion and eggs, 234–35
    salad, Mexican, 178
    sauce, 223
    topping, sour cream dip, 37
    -tuna casserole, 125
Poultry, *see* Chicken, Turkey
Preparation and assembly of
    ingredients, 24
Prune-lemon cake, 252
Prunes and avocado, snapper with, 120
Pudding, almond, 246
Pueblo chicken, 146
Puree of avocado soup, 88
Puree of spinach soup, 88–89
Puree of squash soup, 89

R

Raspberries and peaches in sherry, 253
Recipes, about using, 31–32
Recipes, Mexican, how to adapt, 25
Red pepper and chorizo canapés, 41
Red snapper
    honey fish, 113
    with prunes and avocado, 120
    Yucatan, 121
Refried beans, 177
Relish, sweet hot apple, 45
Rice
    about, 17; nutritional value, 325
    baked with chicken and chorizo, 185
    with chicken (or oysters, pork, shrimp), 187

chile, with shrimp and cheese,
    184–85
  green, 186
  with green beans, sweet, 189
  Mexican white, 186
  with mushrooms and cheese, 188
  with tomatoes (or eggplant),
    188–89
  yellow, 190
Roast pork loin, 162
Rolls. *See* Bread and Rolls
Rum, about, 17
Rum pears (or apples), 254

S

Salad, 97–107
  avocado, stuffed, 104
  avocado, tomato, and cheese, 98
  bean, 98–99
  cauliflower, 99
  chicken Cozumel, 104
  chile-tuna, 107
  Christmas Eve, 103
  of colors, 102
  cucumber, La Jolla, 100
  dressing, oil and vinegar, 227
  fruit, picante, 102–03
  green bean and sweet pepper, 100
  jicama and chorizo, 105
  macaroni, Mexican, 184
  mixed, San Miguel, 101
  potato, Mexican, 178
  shrimp Mazatlan, 106
  squid with peppers, 106–07
Salmon
  baked in mustard sauce, 116
  and caper dip, 36
  fillets, honey fish, 113
  with vegetables Veracruz, 117
Salsa. *See* Sauces
The Salt-Free Diet Cookbook, 24, 28,
    29
Salt-reduced (low-sodium) pantry,
    19–22, 27–29
Salt replacement tips, 25
Sardine and caper dip, 36

Sauces, 209–30
  about, 209
  almond, 218
  basic salsa, 210
  basil-tomato, 212
  chile-avocado, 214–15
  chile, sweet-and-hot, 215
  chile-tomato, 213
  chile-vegetable, 214
  cream cheese, 222
  creamy wine, 221
  drunken, 220
  fruit juice dressing, 226–27
  garlic dressing, 228
  green I, 216; green II, 217
  guacamole, 34
  honey-lime dressing, 229
  hot-and-sweet dressing, 228
  lemon dressing, 226
  lime, 217
  oil and vinegar dressing, 227
  onion, 219
  piquant sour cream, 224
  potato, 223
  sour cream dressing, 225
  sour cream topping, 37
  sweet dressing, 230
  tomato with cayenne, 212
  tomato, sweet, 211
Saucy meat balls, 171
Sausage, 158. *See also* Chorizo
Scrambled eggs. *See* Eggs
Scrod
  fish-stuffed eggplant, 114
  in pecan sauce, 118
  and potatoes in spicy cheese sauce,
    115
Sea bass
  in red wine sauce, 118–19
  and tomatoes, 119
Seafood
  about nutritional value, 321
  mixed, in lime sauce, 128
  tamales, 63
  See Fish and Shellfish, individual
    names, e.g., Flounder; Haddock
Seville oranges, about, 17–18
Shellfish. *See* Fish and Shellfish, name
    of shellfish, e.g., Oysters; Shrimp
Sherried carrots in rum cream, 203

Sherry
about, 18
-almond chicken, 132
pineapple and bananas (or peaches
and raspberries) in, 253
veal chops, 165
Shredded pork, 163
Shrimp
and cheese, chile rice with, 184
and chicken empanadas, 54
in creamy wine sauce, 126
and eggs with yogurt sauce, 237
minced, glazed carrots with, 202
with peppers and peanuts, 127
with rice, 187
salad Mazatlan, 106
soup, 92
in spice sauce, 126
Simple beans, 174
Snacks. See Appetizers and Snacks
Snapper. See Red snapper
Sodium (low). See Salt-reduced
Sole, pickled ceviche, 43. See also
Flounder
Soufflé, coconut, 248
Soup, 75–95
avocado, puree of, 88
black bean, 79
broccoli and corn, 84
cabbage Veracruz, 84–85
carrot, creamy, 83
Cheddar cheese, 85
chicken, peppercorn, 94–95
chicken-walnut, 94
corn, 82–83
cucumber, 86–87
festival, three-color, 86
fish, 93
fruit, 80
garlic, 82
gazpacho, 81
lamb, tomato, and bean, 91
lentil with okra, 90
melon, 80
pork and avocado, 95
shrimp, 92
spinach, puree of, 88–89
squash, puree of, 89
stock, chicken, 76; fish, 77; meat,
78
vegetable, Mexican, 87

Sour cream
-chicken (or fish) enchiladas, 60
dip, 37
dressing, 225
sauce, piquant, 224
South-of-the-border meat loaf, 172
Spaghetti and chorizo, 181
Spice, chili powder, 210
Spiced
chicken and vegetable stew, 148
eggs, peppers, and cheese, 241
fruit, chicken and, 135
Spices. See Herbs and Spices
Spicy potato casserole, 180
Spinach in almond-cream sauce, 207
Spinach soup, puree of, 88–89
Squash
baked with raisins, 197
butternut, chicken and, 136
soup, puree of, 89
Squid salad with peppers, 106–07
Steak
with chile strips, 156
citrus, 152
guacamole with dates (or just
dates), 155
and tomatoes, 154
Stew. See Chicken, Pork, Veal, etc.
Stock
chicken, 76
fish, 77
meat, 78
pot, Mexican, 91
Stuffed avocado salad, 104
Stuffed potatoes, baked, 179
Sugar
cookies, Mexican, 252–53
-glazed crescent rolls, 71
substitutes, 21
Sweet
bread, rolls. See Bread and Rolls
dressing, 230
hot apple relish, 45
-and-hot chile sauce, 215
peppers. See Peppers, sweet
rice with green beans, 189
-and-spicy veal stew, 168
tomato sauce, 211
pepper and mackerel canapés, 42
Sweetly hot pork stew, 164

Swordfish
and capers, 122
with grapefruit, 123

T

Tacos and Tostadas, about, 50
Tamales, 18, 61. *See also* Tortillas
about, 18–19
chicken (or pork, beef, veal) and
cheese, 62
dough, 61
seafood, 63
Tequila, about, 18
Three-color festival soup, 86
Tomatillos (green tomatoes), about,
15
Tomato(es)
about, 18
with avocado, broiled, 200
-basil sauce, 212
-chile sauce, 213
fried haddock, 112–13
green (tomatillos), about, 15
lamb and bean soup, 91
paste, about, 21–22
and lima beans (or cauliflower,
peas) in butter sauce, 199
lime eggplant with, 198
puree, about, 22
rice with, 188
sauce, about, 22
sauce with cayenne, 212–13
sauce, sweet, 211
sea bass and, 119
zucchini and corn casserole, 208
Tortillas. *See also* Burritos,
Chilaquiles, Tamales
about, 18
corn, 48
white flour, 49
Tostadas and Tacos, about, 50
Travel, about, 29–30
Tuna
and apricots, 124
casserole, 125
-chili salad, 107
-stuffed mushrooms, 39

Turkey, about nutritional value, 324
Turkey mole, 140–41
Turnovers. *See* Empanadas

U

Utensils for Mexican cooking, 23–24

V

Vanilla, about, 19
Veal
about nutritional value, 323
and apples in green sauce, 166
and cheese tamales, 62
balls in sour cream sauce, 166
chops, sherry, 165
citrus steak, 152
loaf, 167
minced, canapés, 42–43
stew, 161
stew, sweet-and-spicy, 168
Vegetable(s)
about nutritional value, 324–25
and chicken stew, spiced, 148
-chile sauce, 214
empanadas, 56
-fruit salad, Christmas Eve, 103
-fruit salad of colors, 102
picadillo with, 169
salad, mixed, San Miguel, 101
salmon with, Veracruz, 117
soup, Mexican, 87
soup, three-color festival, 86
-stuffed chiles (or peppers), 195
Vinegar, about, 19
Vinegar and oil dressing, 227

W

Walnuts, pears, and cabbage, 201
Wheat rolls, orange-banana, 69
White flour tortillas, 49
Wine sauce, creamy, 221

Y

Yam pie, fruited, 250
Yellow rice, 190
Yucatan
    citrus steak, 152
    eggs, 236
    snapper, 121

Z

Zucchini
    in cheese sauce, 207
    and chorizo canapés, 41
    pineapple chicken with, 145
    tomatoes and corn casserole, 208